Midlife

This book is a rare and intriguing account of the midlife experience from a multidisciplinary perspective. It represents an insightful construal of midlife from the disciplines of philosophy, psychology, neuroscience, literature, sociology and the fine arts.

This volume provides an in-depth understanding of the middle phase of human lives which is the transitional phase at which a crucial transformation happens in the perspective towards life, society and the world at large. It encompasses multiple methodological perspectives including empirical studies, descriptive and interpretative narratives, text analyses and revisiting existing literature. Since it addresses the issues of midlife from a multidisciplinary perspective, it would enable a wide variety of readers to connect with it.

This book would be useful to students, researchers and teachers of psychology, philosophy, neuroscience, literature, sociology, social work, film studies and the fine arts. It would also be an invaluable companion to professionals working in the fields of Counselling Gerontology, Health and Social care, and NGOs.

Sanjukta Das is Professor at University of Calcutta, India. She is an eminent professor known for her vital contribution to the field of psychology. She has more than 25 years' research and teaching experience of in the areas of clinical psychology, adult personal growth, midlife crisis, disturbed childhood, mental health crises and psychosocial intervention. Gradually her research focus has matured into multidisciplinary intervention approaches with an emphasis on community service. Her work has been published at national and international levels.

Nabamita Chakraborty is Assistant Professor at Gokhale Memorial Girls' College, India. Her doctoral research focused on psycho-socio-emotional growth and developmental outcomes of midlifers. Her research interests focus on lifespan development and its multiple facets along with community mental health, wellbeing and positive psychology. As a researcher her work has been published at national and international levels.

Midlife

Multidisciplinary Theories, Thoughts and Issues

Edited by Sanjukta Das and Nabamita Chakraborty

Routledge
Taylor & Francis Group
LONDON AND NEW YORK

First published 2025
by Routledge
4 Park Square, Milton Park, Abingdon, Oxon OX14 4RN

and by Routledge
605 Third Avenue, New York, NY 10158

Routledge is an imprint of the Taylor & Francis Group, an informa business

British Library Cataloguing-in-Publication Data
A catalogue record for this book is available from the British Library

ISBN: 978-1-032-85247-8 (hbk)
ISBN: 978-1-032-93958-2 (pbk)
ISBN: 978-1-003-56836-0 (ebk)

DOI: 10.4324/9781003568360

Typeset in Sabon
by Deanta Global Publishing Services, Chennai, India

Contents

List of Figures *vii*
List of Table *viii*
List of Contributors *ix*
Preface *xiii*
Foreword *xv*

PART I
Fundamental Issues of Midlife 1

1 **Midlife and the Lifespan: An Overview** 3
SANJUKTA DAS AND NABAMITA CHAKRABORTY

2 **An Overview of the Theoretical Perspectives in Middle Adulthood** 9
SARANYA BANERJEE AND NABAMITA CHAKRABORTY

3 **Midlife from a Philosophical Perspective** 20
ANUP DHAR

4 **Midlife through a Sociological Lens** 31
MALLARIKA SARKAR (DAS) AND SRITAMA CHAUDHURI

5 **Brain, Ageing and Maturity in Middle Adulthood** 44
MASROOR JAHAN AND ASHISH SILSWAL

PART II
The Experience of the Intra- and Interpersonal Spaces: Some Crucial Insights 67

6 **Attachment, Intimacy and Close Relationships in Midlife** 69
POULOMI BHAR, SWETA SAH AND SUBRATA DASGUPTA

7 **Attachment in Workspace and Midlife** 83
DEEPSHIKHA RAY

8 Midlife and Parenthood 97
RUDRANI CHATTERJEE AND ZAINAB AHMED

9 Spirituality and Midlife Transition 110
DEEPSHIKHA RAY AND SANJUKTA DAS

PART III
Challenges, Community and Midlife 119

10 Crises and Challenges in Midlife 121
PAPRI DAS AND SANJUKTA DAS

11 COVID-19 and Midlife 142
MASROOR JAHAN, AMOOL R. SINGH AND RAHUL SHARMA

12 Conversations on Marginalization: Dovetailing Lived Experiences of Marginal Urban Groups of India 167
RITWIK SAHA, JAYEETA NASKAR DAS AND ANINDITA CHAUDHURI

13 Community Intervention, Support and Wellbeing in Midlife 180
RUDRANI CHATTERJEE AND RUDRA P. GOSWAMI

PART IV
The Creative Portrayal of Midlife 197

14 Midlife Transitions in Men and their Representations in Literature across Centuries 199
SUKANYA SAHA

15 Midlife, Stereotypes and Agencies in *English Vinglish* (2012), *The Lunch Box* (2013) and *Three of Us* (2022) 214
SUBHAM DUTTA AND NABAMITA CHAKRABORTY

16 The Socio-political Canvas of Middle Adulthood: An Analysis through Tagore's Literary Lens 229
TANAYA ROY CHOWDHURY AND RUDRANI CHATTERJEE

17 Cinematherapy: A Sustainable Way to Overcome Midlife Woes in Women 238
SUKANYA SAHA

Index *251*

Figures

11.1 Impact of COVID-19 147
13.1 PRISMA flow diagram 186

Table

13.1 Systematic review of community-based participatory research on middle-aged adults: feasibility and outcome studies 187

Contributors

Zainab Ahmed is a clinical psychologist with nearly two decades of experience and works in the West Bengal government health sector with children and adults. She has researched extensively on women's experiences of childlessness, aiming to support those affected.

Saranya Banerjee is currently working as an Assistant Professor in the Clinical Psychology Centre of University of Calcutta, India. She is also an RCI Registered Clinical Psychologist currently engaged in clinical practice and deals with emotional distress and behavioural issues of midlifers and other populations.

Poulomi Bhar is an Assistant Professor in Psychology, Vivekananda College for Women, India and has a 15 years' experience in the fields of undergraduate and postgraduate teaching. She has published several works in her research interest area, the field of social and community psychology.

Rudrani Chatterjee is a Clinical Psychologist with a focus on dynamic psychology and a multi-faceted view of reality. She is actively engaged in clinical care and interested in translation of clinical care into community participation and intervention. Currently she is working as an Assistant Professor, Institute of Human Behavior & Allied Sciences, India.

Anindita Chaudhuri is currently working as an Associate Professor at the University of Calcutta, India. Her principal areas of interest include research on identity, marginalisation, happiness and wellbeing. Her work has appeared in many research publications, she has delivered lectures in many eminent institutes, and she has had active research collaborations with national and international scholars of various institutions.

Sritama Chaudhuri is a PhD scholar, Department of Sociology, University of Calcutta, India. Researching the influence of online food delivery apps on the food consumption pattern of a city. Her research interests include food studies, technology–culture intersection, ethnography and sustainability. Her writings have already been published in various reputed journals. She also teaches sociology and social entrepreneurship.

Papri Das is an Assistant Professor of Psychology at a prestigious private university in Kolkata, India. In addition to three years of experience in academia, she is an RCI Licensed Clinical Psychologist, pursuing her doctoral studies in psychology. She is also a certified Mindfulness-Based Cognitive Therapy practitioner, certified by the National Institution for Transforming India, and a dedicated compassion cultivator.

Subrata Dasgupta is a Professor in Applied Psychology with 25 years' experience in postgraduate teaching and research, and has published numerous works in the fields of applied social psychology, community psychology, cross-cultural psychology, school psychology, creativity, and art and music.

Anup Dhar has training in medicine and is a former Professor of Philosophy and Psychology. He is a Fellow of the Hans Kilian and Lotte Köhler Center for Cultural Psychology and Historical Anthropology, Ruhr-Universität Bochum, Germany. He is also Distinguished Visiting Professor of Philosophy at BML Munjal University, India. He has published 13 books and more than 80 papers. He is completing a book on Girindrasekhar Bose titled *Aboriginal Psychoanalysis*.

Subham Dutta teaches English Literature at Gokhale Memorial Girls' College affiliated to University of Calcutta, India. His research interests include South Asian literature, film studies and gender studies. His work has appeared in national and international publications.

Rudra P. Goswami is a medical doctor specialising in rheumatology who also works in methodology and biomedical statistics and is interested in psychosocial aspects of health. He is an Associate Professor, All India Institute of Medical Sciences, New Delhi, India.

Masroor Jahan has been a teaching faculty member of repute in the field of mental health (clinical psychology) for more than 25 years. She has been an office bearer and member of related international and national associations. She is an Additional Professor, Ranchi Institute of Neuropsychiatric & Allied Sciences, India. Her main areas of interest include clinical neuropsychology, psychological assessment, and psychological management of psychiatric disorders and psychological problems.

Jayeeta Naskar Das is a Research Scholar at Calcutta University, India and a former Fellow of the Indian University Grants Commission. She is pursuing a PhD research project, "The Lived Experiences and Emotions of Becoming Young: An Ethnography in Kolkata Metropolis". Her research interests are diverse, including emotions, social experiences, identities and cultural heritage.

Deepshikha Ray is currently an Associate Professor at the University of Calcutta, India. She is the co-investigator in two Indian Council of

Medical Research-funded projects: one exploring social information processing deficits in schizophrenia and their first-degree relatives, and the search for a novel endophenotype, and the other exploring developmental disorders in amygdala-prefrontal connectivity in impulse control disorders – adolescent screening for intervention. She has supervised several doctoral research projects.

Tanaya Roychowdhury is currently pursuing a PhD from the Department of Psychology, University of Calcutta, India, and also has a post at the District Mental Health Programme, North 24 Paraganas in West Bengal, India. She has a deep interest in music, literature, theatre and the nuanced observation of human behaviour.

Sweta Sah is an Assistant Professor in Psychology at Sister Nivedita University, India, and Rehabilitation Council of India-registered rehabilitation psychologist with six years' teaching experience and 11 years' experience in industry. She teaches therapeutic clinical and rehabilitation psychology and her work has appeared in a number of research publications.

Ritwik Saha has been working as an Assistant Professor at the Dr. A.P.J. Abdul Kalam Government College in New Town, India since December 2018 and is currently pursuing a PhD at the University of Calcutta, India. His work has appeared in two international publications, and his research interests include social realities of marginalised groups, wellbeing, and social and community psychology.

Sukanya Saha is an experienced faculty member of English and a mentor, Amity University, Kolkata, India. She is actively involved in guiding PhD, undergraduate and postgraduate students in critical thinking, writing and literary analysis, empowering them to find their voice and purpose. She is passionate about teaching English literature and composition, helping students grow as readers, writers and thinkers.

Mallarika Sarkar (Das) is an Assistant Professor of Sociology, University of Calcutta, India. Her areas of interest are the sociology of ageing, urban sociology, social exclusion and social research methods. She has participated in national and international seminars and conferences and delivered lectures as invited speaker in renowned institutions. She has published several articles in reputable journals and contributed chapters in books.

Rahul Sharma is a Rehabilitation Council of India-licensed clinical psychologist. He is a research scholar, and his interests lie in public health (mental health) and psychological assessment (tool construction). He has been closely working with patients suffering from various mental illnesses and their caregivers.

Ashish Silswal is a Rehabilitation Council of India-licensed clinical psychologist and a research scholar. His major areas of interest are neuropsychology, and psychotherapy and counselling of psychiatric patients as well as the general population. He is a member of the Somatic Inkblot Society.

Amool R. Singh is an eminent professor who has worked in the field of mental health (clinical psychology) for more than 30 years. His main areas of work include psychological assessment and psychological management of various psychiatric and psychological problems. He has been office bearer and member of various international and national associations.

Preface

The book is about the life-phase of middle adulthood. The purpose of the book is to address the life trajectory of midlifers through a multidisciplinary perspective. It contains a construal of midlife from the disciplines of philosophy, psychology, neuroscience, literature, sociology, and cinema.

Midlife has been conceptualized as a transitional phase at which a crucial transformation happens in the perspective towards life, society, and the world at large. It is at this point that the lifegoals become more focused on the future of society, culture, and the world as a whole. The changes introduced in the psyche of the midlifer should have a significant impact on the overall productivity of the community at large. The in-depth understanding of this phase, therefore, will be insightful for the growth, well-being, and evolution of the human species.

This volume has been divided into four parts. Part I, 'The Fundamental Issues of Midlife', focus on creating a basic understanding of the phase of middle adulthood. It includes a multifaceted understanding of midlife from the psychological, sociological, philosophical, and neuroscientific perspectives.

Part II, 'The Experience of the Intra and Interpersonal Spaces: Some Crucial Insights', involves an elaboration of the intra- and interpersonal spaces' midlife. Psychosocial constructs like attachment (personal and professional), intimate and close relationships, and parenthood. The last chapter in this part is on human spirituality and how human connectedness evolves beyond the immediate social life-context during midlife.

Part III of the volume titled, 'Challenges, Community and Midlife', includes a vivid discussion on how the midlifers from the different sections of society deal with the crises and challenges peculiar to those sections, how the rapidly changing contemporary life-contexts poses as a challenge during this life-phase. Chapter 13, Community Interventions, Support and Well-being', includes an enriching outline on the community support systems.

Part IV, 'The Creative Portrayal of Midlife', probes into national and international cinematic and literary representations of the intriguing phase of midlife – how the protagonists, of the past and present, grapple and come to terms with the challenges inherent in midlife.

The book encompasses multiple methodological perspectives. Revisiting existing literature, descriptive and interpretative narratives, text analyses, descriptive and phenomenological analyses, and so on are embedded in the chapters from the different disciplines. The contributors share their thoughts, insights, and empirical understanding on the pertinent issues salient to the midlife journey.

Sanjukta Das
Nabamita Chakraborty

Foreword

Dr Oliver C. Robinson

President of the European Society for Research in Adult Development

Midlife is a truly fascinating period of life. What makes it so interesting is that it is characterised by paradoxes, tensions and conflicts, which all bring the potential for developmental growth. This interdisciplinary book expertly conveys the dynamics and juxtapositions of midlife in the context of contemporary India. It covers some of the established topics that relate to midlife, such as parenthood, midlife crisis and career, and some less-covered domains such as spirituality, cinematherapy and marginalised groups.

I resonate with many of the topics covered in this book in a personal sense. I am 47 years old and can observe the paradoxes of midlife in myself. For example, I am continuing to develop in important ways, particularly in terms of becoming aware of my own biases and psychological frailties that were repressed when I was younger. I am also still improving in my leadership abilities and my capacity to remain calm and reflective in difficult leadership situations at work. However, while continuing to develop, I am ageing too. I can observe the visible effects of ageing in my skin, voice and hair loss, and am aware of having less energy than when I was younger. I also have less motivation to undertake certain long-term projects that require a lot of creative tension, because I am more inclined to enjoy the present moment rather than push for a future achievement at the expense of my current wellbeing.

I am lucky to be thoroughly enjoying midlife, but between 40 and 44 I was going through a transitional period that resembles many of the features described by James Hollis in *The Middle Passage* (1993). This brilliant book looks at the complex inner dynamics of midlife. My own experiences reflect what Hollis says in terms of midlife being a time to deal with issues that were, as a younger adult, relegated to the unconscious, but can no longer be buried, so must be faced consciously.

One of the most problematic characteristics of midlife in the UK where I live, and in many other Western countries too, is that midlife is the peak of life in terms of suicide rates, with men showing this peak even more than women (Samaritans, 2022). The pattern is similar in India too (Yadav et al., 2023). Tragically, I personally know of two people who committed suicide. Both were men in their forties, fitting this pattern exactly. Midlife male suicide represents how managing midlife has serious consequences. In many ways, midlife is a challenge to change. A person can continue with the coping strategies that worked when they were younger (in UK men, this is often the use of alcohol, workaholism, and an avoidance of talking about distress or difficulties), or they can seek to grow into a more mature and conscious version of themselves via a challenging process of letting go of old habits and facing the unknown. Where individuals end up with midlife depression, anxiety or even suicide, this can sometimes represent a situation where this opportunity for midlife change was not taken.

For this and many other reasons, developing an understanding of the inner and outer dynamics of midlife remains a vital concern for researchers worldwide, and I am certain that this book is going to be an essential contribution to the literature and will be read by many researchers and practitioners across the world for years to come.

References

Hollis, J. (1993). *The middle passage: From misery to meaning in mid-life*. Inner City Books.

Yadav, S., et al. (2023). Changing pattern of suicide deaths in India. *The Lancet Regional Health Southeast Asia*, August 17. https://doi.org/10.1016/j.lansea.2023.100265

Samaritans. (2022). Suicide in England. https://media.samaritans.org/documents/Suicide_Stats_England_2022_FINAL.pdf

PART I

Fundamental Issues of Midlife

1 Midlife and the Lifespan

An Overview

Sanjukta Das and Nabamita Chakraborty

The Relevance of Midlife?

Midlife as a life phase remains dynamic and vague, as its understanding is contingent on the chronological age boundaries of youth and later adulthood. The dictionary defines midlife as a period between youth and old age (Lachman, 2015). Being a relatively new concept in the developmental research literature (Cohen, 2012), the phase is sensitive to social transitions. Crucial social variables such as family living, career milestones, nature and skill demands of jobs, and diversified context-dependent demands and responsibilities make this life phase particularly challenging along with deficiencies in addressing of them by scientific research. Moreover, there are temporal variations in the onset of the active phase of the stable challenges of adulthood across societies, cultures and geographies. Therefore, robust representations through voices from across all corners of the globe would create a more inclusive and advanced knowledge base about this life phase, highlighting the precedence of novel perspectives, models and theories, and thereby informing upcoming policies.

Adulthood and Midlife

Adulthood is a considerably vast phase of life, rich in opportunities for tremendous life changes, growth and decline. This phase has been broken down into briefer sub-phases, such as emerging adulthood (Arnett, 2000), early/young adulthood, middle adulthood and later adulthood, based on the unique characteristic features of such phases. This volume on middle adulthood aims to challenge the existing, traditional frameworks of reference to midlife and initiate a re-evaluation of these. Scholarly work on the life course has devoted more attention to the two ends of this life phase than the middle. The different life phases within the larger phase of adulthood, have undergone revisions over time with a new phase of adulthood emerging in the 2020s called "established adulthood" (aged 30–45 years) (Mehta, 2020). Research, primarily done on exclusively developed geographies and socio-economies, has attested to the idea that the pinnacle of stable maturity and responsibility is attained in these years (Mehta et al., 2020).

DOI: 10.4324/9781003568360-2

Though the scientific work focusing on middle adulthood has its roots embedded in the recent few decades, historically, the phrase has been recognised since the beginning of the 20th century. Individual development is shaped not only by biological and idiosyncratic influences but also by history-graded influences affecting all members of a certain birth cohort in similar ways (Baltes et al., 1980, 1988) or dissimilar ways. The formidable change caused by historical factors has been reported by numerous studies (e.g., Baltes, 1968; Caspi, 1987; Elder, 1998; Riegel, 1972; Schaie, 1965). So a comprehensive, holistic approach combining historical, biological, psychological, social, genetic, cultural and environmental factors can enrich the understanding of middle adulthood.

Age-related Norms at Midlife

Neugarten's theory suggests that neither the quality nor the frequency of events decide the course of midlife. Importance has been given to appropriate timing for psychosocial adjustment. According to Neugarten, there exists a "prescriptive timetable for the ordering of major life events" embedded throughout the cultural fabric of adult life (Neugarten et al., 1965). Social clocks are of particular relevance in midlife as those at both of ends of the chronological continuum comprising of younger and older adults are granted a degree of lenience either to try themselves out or due to health-related frailty. Thus, societal expectations tend to be much more codified and structured in middle age (Diehl et al., 2001).

There is some reason to believe, that midlife across historical times is a period of the lifespan that is most closely associated with the carrying out and maintaining of social structures. In this vein, both Neugarten and Havighurst have argued for the relevance and validity of social norms in midlife. The latter argues that midlifers, through social experience, become not only more skilled at but also more compliant with social conventions. In sum, Neugarten (1968) and Havighurst (1973) both suggested that adherence to social norms is of crucial importance during midlife, and non-adherence might entail serious consequences for a person's wellbeing and challenge psychosocial adjustment and personal growth.

Recent Literature and Its Focus: Change in the Contemporary Social Context

Contemporary society has undergone dramatic and significant changes over time. Such changes have instilled crucial debates about ageing and its psychosocial correlates. Under this transitory cultural backdrop, the self is also scrutinised and reconstrued. A complex, interconnected set of factors is responsible for promoting growth or decline across the middle adulthood phase. Such factors create an intricate, multilayered matrix that can manipulate the overall developmental trajectory. Cross-generational cohort effects can be relevant to this discourse. Members of the Greatest Generation (born

1901–1924), Silent Generation (1925–1945), Baby Boomers (1946–1964), Generation X (1965–1980), Millennials (1981–1996), Generation Z (1997–2012) and Generation Alpha (2013–2025) will all have experienced distinctive socio-historical and cultural contexts of living that have affected their wellbeing, life satisfaction and their experiential journey through life.

The rising awareness about gender equality and flexible gender roles has created a platform for more fairness and uniformity in the representation of all social strata in the workforce. This has led to a higher demand for work–home balance in the growing workforce. Such a massive social transition has bolstered the need to think beyond all existing age and gender stereotypes, and also challenged family and cultural prototypes. This social scenario has considerably diversified pre-existing notions about caregiving in the family system. Caregiving, restricted initially only to the mother, could be passed on to multiple other sources of support found in the still active grandparents, the father or outsourced agents such as nurses or governesses and organisations dedicated to caregiving. Members of the family who are aged, or suffering from ill-health can be cared for not only by family members but also by the widely accepted outsourced alternatives. The socio-economic context has undergone revisions due to this and altered the power equations within the family scenario. Society readjusts its pince-nez to usher in the values of economic independence and individual identity, thereby triggering Individualism and its concomitants.

Romantic spaces of attachment are inclined more towards the goals of intimacy and self-realization rather than those of security and reliability (Lachman, 2020). Marriages lean more emphatically towards psychological compatibility and emotional connectedness with the partner, marital alliances have become diverse socio-demographically, and the hierarchical relationship structure is replaced by a more egalitarian and androgynous role in the family. Marriage is redefined from the perspective of gender fluidity, with a reduced demand for the homogeneity of backgrounds of the partners. Childbearing ceases to be the ultimate culmination of the marital bond, and the success of marriage and womanhood no longer depend on it. The marital alliance loses most of its evolutionary relevance, in terms of species survival and propagation as newer forms of parenthood get introduced. The emergent concept of reproductive identity (Athan, 2020), allows for a wider range of options concerning reproduction and parenthood. This was wisely expressed by Lachman (2020) as "whether, when and in what interpersonal contexts to have children". Parenting is not a life-defining task any longer.

Generativity

Generativity refers primarily to "the concern in establishing and guiding the next generation" (Erikson, 1950). Moreover, generativity is said to include the more popular synonyms of productivity and creativity, which, however, cannot replace generativity. From a psychoanalytic perspective, Erikson argued that "the ability to lose oneself in the meeting of bodies and minds leads to a gradual expansion of ego interests and to a libidinal investment in that which is being generated" (Erikson, 1950). The virtue of this period is *care*. D.P. McAdams also focused on generativity, concern and commitment for future generations and developed a new model, that draws on Erikson's theory. Yet he also makes some significant departures from it. Rather than supposing a specific stage of generativity in middle adulthood, McAdams suggests that generativity becomes an important issue at that time because of increased cultural demand for it. Beginning with individual and shared desires to guide one to find occasions to care for others and cultural demands for assuming responsibility for the next generation as one gets older, generativity leads to conscious concern for the next generation.

Generativity is the concern for and commitment to promoting future generations through parenting, teaching, mentoring, and generating products and outcomes that aim to benefit youth and foster the wellbeing and development of individual and social systems that will outlive the self (McAdams & de St. Aubin, 1998). From a psychological standpoint, generativity may be experienced both as an inner desire or proclivity on the one hand and an age-appropriate expectation or demand on the other. From the standpoint of society and culture, generativity is a critical resource that may undergird social institutions, encourage citizens' contribution and commitments to the public good, motivate efforts to sustain continuity from one generation to the next and initiate social change. Consequently, generativity is a psychosocial concept in two related senses. First, adults can be generative only in social arenas that sustain their generative efforts. Second, social contexts and institutions themselves may be more or less generative. Likewise, there are people, groups, situations, and even societies that are more or less lacking or deficient in generativity (Kotre, 1999; Moran, 1998).

Positive Plasticity

The age-old conceptions of middle adulthood are burdened with the typical baggage of the "empty nest", "sandwich generation" and others that come together to conjure a bleak and crisis-laden view of the phase. Recent research updates, however, open up novel channels of thought about midlife. Firstly, average life expectancy has increased with the advancing vigour of medical science, gradual improvement in health, hygiene and the environment, and heightened levels of overall awareness. The literature indicates that by 2040, average life expectancy will reach 84–87 years (Foreman et al., 2018; World Bank, 2019; CDC, 2019; Staudinger, 2020). Such an expansion in the expected years of healthy functioning provides new opportunities for changing or co-creating bio-social developmental premises that mobilize new adaptive resources. Positive plasticity, initially introduced by Lasker (1969) has been re-emphasised in the recent research literature (Staudinger, 2020; Hogg & Vaughan, 1995; Li, 2003; Staudinger et al., 1995). This concept of positive plasticity evolved from the biosocial perspective that has been around for several decades. Bio-scientists have been interested in the attribute of human evolutionary adaptability which is common to all primates. Such research has implicated "an evolutionary tendency to shift human adaptability from genetic selection to ontogenetic plasticity to reversible adaptability" (Lasker, 1969). Interactions between organism, context and person determine developmental outcomes, simultaneously limited and promoted by biological and contextual precursors. The following model, adapted from Staudinger (2020), explains the dynamic interplay of the multiple layers of interactions determining the level of positive plasticity. In this model, three different tiers – *organism* (including organs, organ systems, cells, tissues and molecules), *person* (including behaviour, habits, attitudes, cognition, emotion, motivation and decisions) and *context* (including institutions, laws and values) – define the pathway of positive plasticity.

The existing literature also suggests direction and degree of plasticity are functions of vulnerabilities and resources embedded in the person's internal and external developmental contexts (Baltes et al., 1980; Lerner, 1984; Staudinger et al., 1995). Plasticity can vary from one individual to another, and thus the notion of "personalised plasticity" (Staudinger, 2020) has come into existence. Inter-cultural and longitudinal cohort research would enrich the existing understanding of the phase of midlife, along with leveraging positive plasticity in them. This would help them to combat the emergent issues of the extended lifespan successfully and help the genesis of balance between individuals' generative selves and their wellbeing.

References

Arnett, J. J. (2000). Emerging adulthood: A theory of development from the late teens through the twenties. *American Psychologist*, *55*(5), 469.

Athan, A. M. (2020). Reproductive identity: An emerging concept. *American Psychologist*, *75*(4), 445.

Baltes, P. B. (1968). Longitudinal and cross-sectional sequences in the study of age and generation effects. *Human Development*, *11*(3), 145–171.

Baltes, P. B., Reese, H. W., & Lipsitt, L. P. (1980). Life-span developmental psychology. *Annual Review of Psychology*, *31*(1), 65–110.

Centre for Disease Control and Prevention (2019). Life Expectancy at birth by race and Hispanic origin. Retrieved from CDC website.

Cohen, P. (2012). *In our prime: The invention of middle age*. Simon and Schuster.

Diehl, M., Hastings, C. T., & Stanton, J. M. (2001). Self-concept differentiation across the adult life span. *Psychology and Aging*, *16*(4), 643.

Erikson, E. H. (1950). *Childhood and society* (Vol. 2). Norton.

Foreman, K. J., Marquez, N., Dolgert, A., Fukutaki, K., Fullman, N., McGaughey, M., & Murray, C. J. (2018). Forecasting life expectancy, years of life lost, and all-cause and cause-specific mortality for 250 causes of death: reference and alternative scenarios for 2016–40 for 195 countries and territories. *The Lancet*, *392*(10159), 2052–2090.

Havighurst, R. J. (1973). History of developmental psychology: Socialization and personality development through the life span. In P. B. Baltes & O. G. Brim (Eds.), *Life-span developmental psychology* (pp. 3–24). Academic Press.

Hogg, M. A., & Vaughan, G. M. (1995). *Social psychology: An introduction*. Harvester Wheatsheaf.
Infurna, F. J., Gerstorf, D., & Lachman, M. E. (2020). Midlife in the 2020s: Opportunities and challenges. *American Psychologist*, *75*(4), 470.
Kotre, J. (1999). Generativity and the gift of meaning. *Generations: Journal of the American Society on Aging*, *23*(4), 65–70.
Lachman, M. E. (2015). Mind the gap in the middle: A call to study midlife. *Research in Human Development*, *12*(3–4), 327–334.
Lasker, G. W. (1969). Human biological adaptability: The ecological approach in physical anthropology. *Science*, *166*(3912), 1480–1486.
Lerner, R. M. (1984). *On the nature of human plasticity*. Cambridge University Press.
Li, S. C. (2003). Biocultural orchestration of developmental plasticity across levels: The interplay of biology and culture in shaping the mind and behavior across the life span. *Psychological Bulletin*, *129*(2), 171–194. https://doi.org/10.1037/0033-2909.129.2.171
McAdams, D. P., & de St Aubin, E. D. (1998). *Generativity and adult development*. American Psychological Association.
Mehta, C. M., Arnett, J. J., Palmer, C. G., & Nelson, L. J. (2020). Established adulthood: A new conception of ages 30 to 45. *American Psychologist*, *75*(4), 431.
Moran, G. F. (1998). Cares for the rising generation: Generativity in American history, 1607–1900. In D. P. McAdams & E. de St. Aubin (Eds.), Generativity and adult development: How and why we care for the next generation (pp. 311–333). American Psychological Association.
Neugarten, B. L. (Ed.). (1968). *Middle age and aging* (Vol. 10). University of Chicago Press.
Neugarten, B. L., Moore, J. W., & Lowe, J. C. (1965). Age norms, age constraints, and adult socialization. *American Journal of Sociology*, *70*(6), 710–717.
Riegel, K. F., & Riegel, R. M. (1972). Development, drop, and death. *Developmental Psychology*, *6*(2), 306.
Schaie, K. W. (1965). A general model for the study of developmental problems. *Psychological Bulletin*, *64*(2), 92.
Staudinger, U. M. (2020). The positive plasticity of adult development: Potential for the 21st century. *American Psychologist*, *75*(4), 540.
Staudinger, U. M., Marsiske, M., & Baltes, P. B. (1995). Resilience and reserve capacity in later adulthood: Potentials and limits of development across the life span. *Developmental Psychopathology*, 2, 801–847.
World Bank (2019). Life Expectancy a birth, total (years). Retrieved from World Bank website.

2 An Overview of the Theoretical Perspectives in Middle Adulthood

Saranya Banerjee and Nabamita Chakraborty

Middle adulthood or midlife, one of the most under-researched areas in the field of developmental psychology, is devoid of even basic theoretical concepts like a proper demarcation about age range. Multiple research projects have come up with multiple perspectives over the years. As early as 1965, in a study by Neugarten, Moore and Lowe on the subjective conceptions of when midlife begins and when midlife ends, it was observed that while respondents had a clear cognisance of what constitutes 'young age' and 'old age', there were great disparities in their understanding of midlife. Shanan and Keder in 1980 reported that participants in their study considered 50–60 years as middle adulthood, whereas Cameron (1969) and Drevenstedt (1976) through their studies shared their observations that middle adulthood constitutes the age range 40–55 years. Even current studies on midlife over the last few years do not not mention any proper age categorisation.

However, this does not undervalue the significance of this stage but rather shows our naivety and lack of exploration in this area. One of the erroneous notions about midlife is that it is one of the peaceful phases of life, since in the previous phases, much of the stability in terms of career, finances and relationships have been attained. In this phase, there are also fewer biological changes and more social and environmental factors impacting life situations. Thus, as Seligman and Csikszentmihalyi (2000) state, this span of life does not require much negotiation. Brim (1992) regarded middle adulthood as the unexplored territory of human life. Since then, there has been an increase in research in this domain, however quite far from the innovative research developments that have taken place in the other areas of human development

Lachman (2004) pointed out that midlife includes a complex interplay of multiple roles accompanied by several psychological changes. Also, as Jung (1933) pointed out before Lachman, this phase requires several adjustments to negotiate new challenges which are very different from those in the previous stages. Furthermore, this stage also serves as a preparatory phase for the upcoming stages of life (Lachman, 2004).

A very important point to consider is that in middle adulthood, development is no longer considered to be part of the growth process. It is conceived

DOI: 10.4324/9781003568360-3

more as a ratio of gains and losses – gains in terms of enhanced adjustment and mastering the skills of everyday life and the various roles encompassed in it, and also including the fostering of important skills like critical self-reflection, self-transcendence and focusing more on internal growth than on external factors (Dorner et al., 2005).

Psychoanalytic and Object Relation Perspectives on Midlife

Sigmund Freud and Margaret Mahler

Sigmund Freud is the pioneer in several important theoretical fields, one of them being the psychosexual stages of development, where he described five stages: namely oral, anal, phallic, latency and genital. Each of the stages has its onset during various stages of life, and each impacts adult development either in terms of acquisition of healthy patterns or fixation on maladaptive patterns.

Freud often referred himself as 'the conscientious archeologist', whose primarily role was excavating the 'mutilated relics of antiquity'. In this excavation, he completely obliterated the role of the external world. To Freud, it was unconceivable that there might be external contexts which also shape an individual's psyche and which may also lead to healthy positive adult development. His various case studies are an example, where it was observed that other than 'immediate' family, he even excluded members of extended family from the context. Sigmund Freud's core principles mainly focused on childhood, and he surmised that adulthood relied more on the achievements and struggles of childhood, thus supporting his practice of psychoanalysis, which traces current core psychological issues back to infantile origins. Freud's concepts have further been expanded by the separation-individuation theory of Mahler et al. (1975). Even though the theory focused on childhood attachments, their impact continued even during later stages in life.

Mahler is regarded as one of the main contributors to the field of ego psychology, a school of thought which was a continuation of Sigmund Freud's Structural Model (id–ego–superego). Her aim was not to develop a novel theory, but to broaden the scope of pre-existing theories (Mahler, 1952, 1968). Separation-individuation in adulthood manifests itself in the form of recognition of an object without any reference to 'the self' – that is, the object and the self will be regarded as independent (Andelkovic, 2015). It is also reflected in the context of primary relations like spouse, ageing parents, children and grandchildren, colleagues at work and friends. Middle adulthood is characterised by various emotional and developmental challenges which further contribute to the shaping up of different relationships.

During middle adulthood, an individual realises that there needs to be a limiting of expectations. While this limiting may be a painful process for a midlifer, it also leads to the reorganisation of the ego ideal and prioritising of those goals which can be achieved. The painful realisation and other losses can lead to different pathological manifestations, but also to a most complete realisation of one's capacities and a high level of individuation. Pollock (1979) stresses the role of the process of grieving in further development and individuation. Grieving is a universal transformational process which allows for reality to be accepted the way it is – including losses and changes. A successful end of grieving is equal to healing, and it leads to further development and a higher level of satisfaction with life.

Marriage is also an important part of middle adulthood and is also impacted by the separation-individuation process. The relations in the primary family produce, among other things, the inner world of expectations, conscious and unconscious, as well as those which concern the attitude towards other people, and also towards one's partner. Certainly, the relation between partners is only partly formed by internal objects created by introjection or a fantasised mental incorporation of a parent or his/her parts. The mature, balanced marital relation requires that partners become more and more differentiated from the world of internal objects and relations with them in order to be able to invest themselves in a new relation (Kondić & Vidanović, 2011).

Carl Jung

Carl Jung, a Swiss psychiatrist and psychologist, developed his theory not only in the context of childhood, but also extended his understanding to other stages of lifespan including middle adulthood. In fact, Jung was more focused on adulthood than childhood, and he termed middle adulthood as the afternoon of life (Jung, 1933). As early as 1933, Jung stated that the salient features and demands of this phase of life are markedly different from those of the previous stages. It is one of the transitory phases, and hence requires a lot of negotiation with various life challenges.

Considered to be one of the classic models of midlife (Lachman & James, 1997), it emphasises the process of individuation as crucial n middle adulthood (Jung, 1971). Individuation refers to the integration or balancing of all aspects of the psyche (Lachman, 2004). In other words, it includes integration of the conscious and the unconscious (Kelleher, 1992). By psyche, Jung (1933) referred to the conscious ego, personal consciousness and collective unconscious. The collective unconscious consists of archetypes of religious and symbolic themes which have been existing for generations. As an example, Jung stated that there is an amalgamation of the anima (feminine) and animus (masculine) characteristics of the psyche as part of the individuation process. Years of research could not provide conclusive evidence to support this assertion (Lachman, 2004). However, in our everyday life, we have often observed that during middle adulthood, men start taking up household responsibilities which are usually considered feminine practices in a Third World country like India.

Essentially, this quest for integration may not always be a comfortable one, and in some instances may lead to the development of various psychopathology like dissociation, regression and isolation (Storr, 1983).

Erik Erikson, George Valliant and Robert Peck

Erikson views development as a graded process consisting of various life tasks, at different age levels. Each of these tasks has an inherent conflict which if successfully resolved gets successfully transformed into a virtue. These conflicts are usually cumulative across the lifespan and re-emerge later in life if not resolved successfully (Staudinger & Bluck, 2001).

Thus, on one hand, middle adulthood relies on the successful resolution of the tasks at the earlier stages. Other than this, the central theme in midlife is the conflict between generativity versus stagnation. These get unified into themes of nurturing and guiding the next generation. This also includes transmitting values, coaching younger workers or contributing to society in terms of cultural pursuits. In midlife, commitment to others plays a crucial role in promoting wellbeing (McAdams, 2001; McAdams & de St. Aubin, 1998).

Vaillant (1977) added two additional stages which denote middle adulthood. After intimacy and before generativity, he added the phase of career consolidation. This stage symbolises that an individual's personal identity is further broadened to be incorporated as a part of social identity. In other words, the individual's preferred choice of activity gets transformed into their career. This manifests itself in four stages: contentment, compensation, competence and commitment. Successful consolidation of the career will help in the development of career identity. After the stage of generativity comes another substage mentioned by Valliant, known as 'keepers of meaning', which focuses on dissemination of values to society.

Another theorist who critiqued Erikson's theory is Robert Peck (1956, 1968), who believed that in middle adulthood, individuals tend be more preoccupied with self. People must be more accepting of their physical changes. At this stage, they learn to value their cognitive or experiential resources more. Robert Peck has explicitly referred to three stages:

- Ego-differentiation vs work role preoccupation: During this phase, an individual gradually moves towards retirement, redefines and reappraises his/her worth by dedicating him/herself more to societal and cultural pursuits, hence deriving greater satisfaction from this newly achieved role.
- Body-transcendence vs body preoccupation: Middle adulthood is characterised by deterioration of physical health. Individuals who can devote themselves to their moral and societal values experience greater physical and emotional wellbeing. However, Peck believed, this transition usually begins by early adulthood.
- Ego transcendence vs ego preoccupation: This stage is synonymous with Erikson's stage of generativity. Gradually, an individual shifts from fulfilling his/her own desires to making an effort to make society a better place for upcoming generations. The ability to move beyond self-gratification and being more invested towards the betterment of the society as a whole lead to better psychological outcomes.

Bernice Neugarten

Neugarten's most noteworthy concept was that of 'social clocks reflected in age norms' (Ferraro, 2014). She accentuated how age norms and socio-cultural expectations acted as facilitatory or inhibitory factors in adult development. In 1976, Neugarten highlighted the three time spans which differentiated adult development: historical or calendar time, social time and its socially defined expectations, and life or chronological time. Based on that, he stated that with change in historical time, there were changes in social expectations and certain behaviours took more precedence over others in that age span.

Interestingly, a study by Neugarten, Moore and Iowa (1965) found that respondents mentioned age norms for all major events in life, and these age norms served as social controls (Ferraro, 2014). Neugarten (1976) further believed that as individuals pass through each of these age norms, they reformulate their plans and goals of life.

Neugarten (1964, 1966, 1968, 1969, 1970, 1976, 1984, 1986) conducted several studies to understand changes which occur during the years of middle adulthood. Her findings suggested that there are no differences in personality structure across the life span with respect to the personality domains assessed by Neugarten: integrated, defended, passive dependent and independent. Similarly, even with respect to coping strategies, no differences have been found among middle adults.

However, studies also revealed that it was the sense of agency that differentiated healthy midlifers from the rest. This phase was characterised more by introspection and self-reflection (Neugarten, 1964; Lachman, 2004; Ferraro, 2014). Neugarten (1968) also stated that in her interviews, he found that healthy midlifers often reported that they were aware of their competencies and their areas of mastery and considered this a rewarding realisation. She termed this as an 'executive process of personality'. Another interesting finding suggested by Neugarten implied that there was a switching of roles between males and females during middle adulthood. While males became more nurturing and compliant, females became aggressive and defiant (Neugarten & Gutmann, 1958). This stage is also characterised by a lack of concern for social norms. Thus, it is important to note that while new psychological attributes are added in the repertoire of midlifers, many prevailing patterns of functioning also cease of exist.

Daniel Levinson

Levinson was greatly interested in studying human life patterns and how they were organised through various stages. In order to study this process, he collected biographies of 40 men who were grouped based on their occupational categories, prevailing life circumstances, social origins and personal characteristics. In addition to this, secondary data was collected on the lives of these men as described in biographies, autobiographies, poetry, plays and novels

(Levinson, 1977, 1978). While Levinson has given specific descriptions for all age groups, here the focus of the discussion will be on midlifers.

According to Levinson (1977), during the transitory phase to middle adulthood many people start questioning the meaning, value and direction of their lives. Based on the findings for majority of the people, this is a period of moderate or severe stress, when an individual faces tremendous crisis within self as well as in the external world. During this process of reappraisal, individuals often face neurotic problems like anxiety and pathological guilt. These serve as barriers during the transition. During this turmoil, individuals begin to explore various life choices. In the process of this exploration, prevailing structures existing within the individual are challenged, which further makes the course of transition agonising. The social structures in the environment may act as impediments to change, trying to maintain conformity of the individual with the systems that were prevailing during early adulthood.

The progression to midlife becomes difficult because during the preceding years, individuals have given priority to certain aspects of their life at the expense of others which seek immediate expression during this next phase of life. Thus, middle adulthood acts as another step in individuation (Levinson, 1986). During this phase, instead of placing responsibility on the external world, the individual has to accept some responsibility for this and work on motivating him/herself to bring about necessary changes. Very similar to Jung's conceptualisation, all individuals must work on integrating the polarities which usually existed in the earlier phases.

This experience is not same for all individuals. Some individuals have faced so many adversities in the earlier stages that they lack the necessary cognitive or affective resources to create a stable internal structure. Another group of individuals exist who perform their work, social and personal roles effectively but have little or no connection with their internal structures. For the remaining group, they are connected to their internalised structures but have also been able to decipher their values, meanings and directions in life and are working towards achieving them.

Robert Havighurst

Robert Havighurst emphasised on the concept of developmental tasks, which was influenced by Erikson's theory of psychosocial stages. Havighurst (1972) defined a developmental task as the midpoint between two extremes, one of which holds that the child grows best when left alone and the other which maintains the child must learn to grow through restraints imposed by the society. In other words, it is the midway between individual demand and societal demand. A developmental task includes knowledge, skills, attitudes and functions the individual must develop at various stages through personal effort, social expectations and physical maturity. He further stated that each stage is characterised by the need for affection, autonomy and recognition.

Havighurst's theory was a perfect reflection of the biopsychosocial influences on human development.

Each of the specific age ranges have their own developmental tasks. In middle adulthood, the major developmental tasks in the social sphere include achieving a certain level of satisfaction with respect to career, maintaining positive relationships with spouse, aiding teenage children to prepare for the outer world and assisting aged parents. In addition to this, it also encompasses partaking of various social and civic responsibilities. In the biological domain, tasks include accepting physiological changes. The psychological domain includes developing interests inr leisure or pleasurable activities (Staudinger & Bluck, 2001).

While on one hand, these developmental tasks are structured by society, on the other it is the decision of the individual to contribute to the wellbeing of self and others.

Charlotte Buhler

Unlike many other theorists who have viewed midlife only as a challenge, Buhler's conceptualisation considers it as an achievement. Buhler (1968) proposed that the pursuit of creative and leisure activities can be considered an achievement only with respect to its time frame. Pursuit of creative goals contributes to making life more meaningful, and hence enhances satisfaction. However, as mentioned previously, the time frame appears to be of increasing concern in middle adulthood, as it is one of the determining factors of whether an individual will choose leisure or seek creative pursuits. Time frame, Buhler contends, refers to the choice of an individual to live in the past, present or future. Living in the present implies a desire for leisure (Staudinger & Bluck, 2001), whereas there is also an attempt at the harmonious integration of the past and future, which is reflected through efforts of a midlifer to use skills acquired in the past for achievement of goals in the future.

Thus, while middle adulthood brings individuals to a point where their physical maturation is on the verge of decline, it also gives individuals the opportunity to live a more meaningful and fulfilling life through healthy unification of the past and the future.

Finally, the Selective Optimization with Compensation Model of Baltes and Baltes (1990), though primarily used to define successful ageing, can also be applied to midlife. Since with the onset of midlife there occurs a decline in the abilities of midlifers, it is important that midlifers learn to use their abilities optimally by exploiting their strengths in the best possible way which will not only enhance their skills but also compensate for their losses. For example, a woman who likes cooking and tends to feel exhausted can use this skill in the best possible manner by cooking in small amounts every day.

Robert Kegan's Theory of Adult Development

Kegan's (1982, 1995) theory is a comparatively recent theory with a fresh new perspective. Very similar to Piaget's theory, Kegan felt that like children, adults progress through different stages which lead to changes in their perspectives.

Kegan had more of a constructive-developmental perspective, whereby he believed that all individuals actively construct their own world. The essence of the developmental perspective is that Kegan postulated that developmental changes are not only quantitative but also qualitative. He emphasised social, emotional and moral development, which are more qualitative in nature, to support his assertion. Interestingly, the two concepts culminated in explaining that the qualitative changes that occur in individuals during their lifespan development are more of an active process and result due to the meaning individuals give to their environment.

According to Kegan, becoming an adult is suggestive of a process of metamorphosis, whereby individuals progress to a higher stage of development; it means developing an independent sense of self and a gradual transition to developing wisdom and social maturity. It also advances to development of greater self-awareness. This aids individuals in controlling their behaviour and being able to better manage their relationships and their social implications.

Kegan has put forward a very interesting observation that most midlifers fail to perform as high-functioning adults because they are still dependent on their emotions and perceptions of how others think them to be. In this perspective, Kegan has put forward the concept of transformation, which is 'changing the way we know and understand the world' (Morad, 2017).

Upon reflection, this seems akin to the process of re-experiencing the world. Imagine a book that you have read or a movie you saw when you were in high school and you revisit in your midlife; you will observe that there has been a substantial shift in your way of understanding and your perspective.

Kegan believed that transformation is a catalyst for transition to higher stages of development. However, this transitioning requires a subject–object shift. 'Subject' here refers to aspects of our life that control us (emotions, world views, personality traits) and 'object' refers to a situation where we can control an object, and if necessary, we can also detach ourselves from the object.

Thus, transformation and object shift are critical for adult development.

Kegan's Stages of Adult Development typically encompass five stages: two of them are prominent during early childhood and adolescence, and the remaining three are seen in adulthood.

To maintain continuity, the second stage will also be discussed, which is the imperial stage, more commonly found among adolescents. However, Kegan believed that adults fail to ass through this stage. In this stage, an individual is dominated by his/her own needs, interests and agendas. Every relationship a person makes is transactional in nature, as relationships are a way to fulfil their own interests and agendas. There is no focus on internal shared experiences. Their behaviour at this stage is dominated by fear of punishment and not by their values.

The next stage is that of socialised mind, where individuals become highly concerned with the prevailing social system. In this stage, individuals are mostly seeking validation from the external system. They have an inflated sense of responsibility to make sure that they are perceived well by others. In contrast to the earlier stage, individuals develop their own values and beliefs, but those are determined largely by the social system.

The fourth stage is of the self-authoring mind, where individuals develop internal values and meanings and take initiatives to work in accordance with those values and meanings. Interestingly, in this phase individuals choose their desired directions with independent frames of mind. This becomes possible because of their acquired ability to explore their thoughts and feelings as well as to take responsibility for their inner states of mind. However, this state is not characterised by rigidity but by a readiness for negotiation with the changing environment

The fifth and last stage is the interconnected mind. This stage is similar to the Buddhist concept of evolving self (Morad, 2017). It is believed that only 1% of adults reach this stage. Individuals who reach this stage can detach themselves from their thoughts and identities. They have developed multiple self-aspects and are in a constant process of re-inventing themselves. This also indicates their ability to hold multiple thoughts and ideologies.

Thus, summarising the theory, Kegan stated that 'becoming an adult' is not only about acquiring new skills but also about fostering mature and authentic relationships with others. In the higher stages, Kegan has focused on self-authorship, which emphasises redefining our identities, beliefs and sense of self, and this can be instilled by 'practicing curiosity, critical reflection and openness' (Morad, 2017).

While the above narratives provide us with a comprehensive understanding of all the possible theories, it is important to keep in mind that even the most recent theory of midlife dates to 1997. In the last 30 years, the world has undergone tremendous changes. With improvements in employment rules, healthcare schemes, medical facilities and medical infrastructure, the age group conceptualisations have also changed. There have also been changes in the cognitive, social and personality functioning of midlifers. This calls for a need to develop more recent theories to explain the current adaptive styles and functioning of middle adulthood.

References

Anđelković, V. (2015). *Separation-individuation processes in adulthood.* FACTA.

Baltes, P. B., & Baltes, M. M. (1990). Psychological perspectives on successful aging: The model of selective optimization with compensation. In P. B. Baltes & M. M.

Baltes (Eds.), *Successful aging: Perspectives from the behavioural sciences* (pp. 1–34). Cambridge University Press.
Brim, O. B. (1992). *Ambition*. Basic Books.
Bühler, C. (1968). The course of human life as a psychological problem. *Human Development*, *11*(3), 184–200. Retrieved June 27, 2023, from http://www.jstor.org/stable/26761721
Cameron, P. (1969). Age parameters of young adult, middle-aged, old, and aged. *Journal of Gerontology*, *24*(2), 201–202. https://doi.org/10.1093/geronj/24.2.201
Dörner, J., Mickler, C., & Staudinger, U. M. (2005). Self-development at midlife. Lifespan perspectives on adjustment and growth. In S. L. Willis & M. Martin (Eds.), *Middle adulthood: A lifespan perspective* (pp. 277–317). Sage Publications.
Drevenstedt, J. (1976). Perceptions of onsets of young adulthood, middle age, and old age. *Journal of Gerontology*, *31*(1), 53–57. https://doi.org/10.1093/geronj/31.1.53
Erikson, E. H. (1968). *Identity: Youth and crisis*. W W Norton & Company.
Ferraro K. F. (2014). The time of our lives: recognizing the contributions of Mannheim, Neugarten, and Riley to the study of aging. *The Gerontologist*, *54*(1), 127–133. https://doi.org/10.1093/geront/gnt048
Havighurst, R. J. (1972). *Developmental tasks and education*. David McKay.
Jung, C. G. (1933). *Modern man in search of a soul*. Harcourt, Brace.
Jung, C. G. (1971). The stages of life. In J. Campbell (Ed.), *The portable jung*. Viking Press.
Kegan, R. (1982). *The evolving self*. Harvard University Press. https://doi.org/10.2307/j.ctvjz81q8
Kegan, R. (1995). *In over our heads: The mental demands of modern life*. Harvard University Press.
Kelleher K. (1992). The afternoon of life: Jung's view of the tasks of the second half of life. *Perspectives in Psychiatric Care*, *28*(2), 25–28. https://doi.org/10.1111/j.1744-6163.1992.tb00367.x
Kondić, K., & Vidanović, S. (2011). *O deci i roditeljima*. Filozofski fakultet u Nišu.
Lachman, M. E. (2004). Development in midlife. *Annual Review of Psychology*, *55*(1), 305–331. https://doi.org/10.1146/annurev.psych.55.090902.141521
Lachman, M. E., & James, J. B. (1997). Charting the course of midlife development: An overview. In M. E. Lachman & J. B. James (Eds.), *Multiple paths of midlife development* (pp. 1–17). The University of Chicago Press.
Levinson, D. J. (1977). The mid-life transition: A period in adult psychosocial development. *Psychiatry*, *40*(2), 99–112. https://doi.org/10.1080/00332747.1977.11023925
Levinson, D. J. (1978). *The seasons of a man's life*. Knopf.
Levinson, D. J. (1977). The mid-life transition: A period in adult psychosocial development. *Psychiatry*, *40*(2), 99-112.
Levinson, D. J. (1986). A conception of adult development. *American Psychologist*, *41*(1), 3–13. https://doi.org/10.1037/0003-066X.41.1.3
Mahler, M. S. (1952). On child psychosis and schizophrenia: Autistic and symbiotic infantile psychoses. *The Psychoanalytic Study of the Child*, *7*, 286–305.
Mahler, M. S. (1968). *On human symbiosis and the vicissitudes of individuation* (Vol. 1). Infantile Psychosis.
Mahler, M. S., Pine, F., & Bergman, A. (1975). *The psychological birth of the human infant: symbiosis and individuation*. Basic Books.
McAdams, D. P., & de St. Aubin, E. (Eds.). (1998). *Generativity and adult development: How and whywe care for the next generation*. American Psychological Association.
McAdams, D. P. (2001). Generativity in midlife. In M. Lachman (Ed.), *Handbook of midlife development* (pp. 395–443). Wiley.

Morad, N. (2017). How to be an Adult-Kegan's theory of adult development. https://medium.com/@NataliMorad/how-to-be-an-adult-kegans-theory-of-adult-development-d63f4311b553
Neugarten, B. L. (1964). *Personality in middle and late life*. Atherton Press.
Neugarten, B. L., Moore, J. W., & Lowe, J. C. (1965). Age norms, age constraints, and adult socialization. American journal of Sociology, 70(6), 710-717
Neugarten, B. L. (1966). Adult personality: A developmental view. *Human Development, 2*, 61–73.
Neugarten, B. L. (1968). The awareness of middle age. In B. L. Neugarten (Ed.), *Middle age and aging*. University of Chicago Press.
Neugarten, B. L. (1969). Continuities and discontinuities of psychological issues into adult life. *Human Development, 12*, 121–130.
Neugarten, B. L. (1970). Dynamics of transition of middle age to old age. *Journal of Geriatric Psychiatry, 4*, 71–87.
Neugarten, B. L. (1976). Adaptation and the life cycle. *The Counseling Psychologist*, 6, 16–20.
Neugarten, B. L. (1984). Psychological aspects of aging and illness. *Psychosomatics, 25*(2), 123–125.
Neugarten, B. L. (1986). Age in the aging society. *Daedalus, lli*(l), 31–49.
Neugarten, B. L., & Gutmann, D. L. (1958). Age-sex roles and personlaity in middle ages: A thematic apperception study. *Psychological Monographs*, 72 (Whole No. 470).
Peck, R. C. (1968). Psychological developments in the second half of life. In B. L. Neugarten (Ed.), *Middle age and aging* (pp. 88–92). University of Chicago Press.
Peck, R. C. (1956). Psychological developments in the second half of life. In J. E. Anderson (Ed.), *Psychological aspects of aging* (pp. 42–53). American Psychological Association. https://doi.org/10.1037/10032-005
Pollock, G. H. (1979). *Aging or aged: Development or pathology?* Unpublished manuscript.
Seligman, M. E. P., & Csikszentmihalyi, M. (2000). Positive psychology: An introduction. *American Psychologist, 55*(1), 5–14. https://doi.org/10.1037/0003-066X.55.1.5
Shanan, J., & Kedar, H. S. (1980). Phenomenological structuring of the adult lifespan as a function of age and sex. *The International Journal of Aging and Human Development/International Journal of Aging & Human Development, 10*(4), 343–357. https://doi.org/10.2190/kav4-1t3h-mqcp-h2e6
Staudinger, U. M., & Bluck, S. (2001). A view on midlife development from a life-span theory. In M. E. Lachman (Ed.), *Handbook of midlife development* (pp. 3–39). John Wiley & Sons.
Storr, A. (Ed.). (1983). *The essenfial lung*. Princeton University Press.
Vaillant, G. E. (Ed.). (1977). *Adaptation to life*. Little Brown.

3 Midlife from a Philosophical Perspective

Anup Dhar

This chapter builds on my own experiences – or perhaps, non-experiences, absent experiences of midlife. I was never acutely aware of the idea of midlife. I never felt: here *is* midlife. Which age would I call midlife? Is midlife a stage in the biological aging of a subject? Is 45–64 years of age midlife, as has often been suggested? Isn't it too long a range: *19 years* of midlife! What is it a 'mid' to? 'Mid' to current life expectancy? But life expectancy has increased from about 32 years in 1900 to about 71 years in 2021. Between 1901 and 1930, midlife was believed to begin at 35. By 1950, the perception of life and midlife had changed. People were now living longer. The possibility of youth and youthfulness appeared to be extended. Women at 40 were no longer seen as middle-aged. By the 1950s, midlife looked to begin at age 45 and lasted until 64! This was a significant shift from figures in the mid-1850s. What should the figure be *now*? Do we need the concept of midlife any more? Can it be post-fixed by *crisis* any more? Or do we need a more creative and complex take on midlife in particular and life in general? The most important phrase in the previous sentence would be 'life in general'. If life in general and the time of life or the timeline of life (let's call it the *temporal* axis) is conceptualized differently, midlife – as one segment of life – would also be conceptualized differently; or could be seen as nearly redundant. Further, what is midlife along a *spatial* axis and in a spatial sense? Would there be differences in conceptualizations of life and midlife in Europe or in Japan? Or in sub-Saharan Africa? Would *subject positions* – of class, caste, race and gender – affect what would present itself as midlife in a culture? Do we need to *sexuate* the idea of midlife – where *sexuation* refers to being 'unconscious of gender-sexuality'? Would women experience midlife differently? Would a Dalit subject, a black survivor of apartheid, experience midlife differently? Or not at all? Midlife thus requires thinking along three axes:

1. Temporal Axis of Life (one could call it the *temporalization of midlife crisis*);
2. Spatial Axis of Culture (one could call it the *spatialization of midlife crisis*);
3. Subject Positions (one could call it the *subjectivization of midlife crisis*).

DOI: 10.4324/9781003568360-4

In other words, I do not see midlife crisis as either a *given* or as *naturalized* stage of life. I see midlife crisis as open to problematization and as a historical-social process; and not just as a biological or psychological fact. Biology, psychology, sociology, cultural studies,[1] economics and philosophy of life need to come together in a true interdisciplinarity to make sense of midlife crisis.

The Concept of 'Crisis': *Sexuating* Midlife

Let us also reflect for a while on the concept of 'crisis'. Crisis is invoked in economics in the forms of crisis of overproduction in capitalism or financial crisis. Crisis is invoked in medicine: life in crisis as in a myocardial infarction. The term 'crisis' is usually understood as a diagnostic category, whether of a person or of society. Further, does the first glimpse of grey hair symbolize much more than just loss of melanin; does it announce the onset of a deterioration that leads first to old age and ultimately to death? However, 'crisis' in classical Greek (*krísis*) gestured towards political critique, critique of norms or normative dimensions: kind of *putting to crisis* the established paradigm or the normalized. Do we see midlife crisis as a *descriptive designation* of a catastrophe, or as critique of the normalizations of the larger social?

The question of *sexual difference* becomes important here. Erikson's stage pertaining to 'generativity' needs to be *sexuated*. Is midlife a stage of male fatigue and grumpy discontent about the achievements of life? Is it merely about the compromise due to aging that haunts the autonomy and physical strength of the 'manly man'? Is it about the anxiety that pervades the male illusion of vigour and masculinity, as bodies take newer forms (not necessarily begin to *wane*, as is the popular perception). The more that manliness became associated with physicality and power, the greater the threat to a midlife man's sense of mastery. By the end of the 20th century, age-based male emasculation had deepened. Retirement schemes formalized the idea that a man lost power and status as he grew older.

Based on the psychobiographs of 115 women, Sheehy (1976; see Schmidt, 2020) shows how midlife could also be seen as a period of self-fulfilment and creative self-discovery through the dissolution of extant gender roles at the onset of middle age; in women's lives, midlife crisis gestures towards a *critique* of the work-and-life styles of the patriarchal family. So while for men midlife could be an experience of wilting and decline, for women midlife could be the birthing of a new idiom of life that is free from the confines of the patriarchal ideas of duties and obligations, ideas that had ruled the 'daughter-wife-mother' triad in the woman.

Sara Ahmed (2021) connects midlife to the conception of '*living* [at last] a feminist life': 'In the middle of my life ... I left a certain kind of life and embraced a new one.' For Ahmed, the act of rejecting one life – the patriarchal one – and choosing another typifies the feminist critique of traditional lifestyles as the only right choices. In this sense, she argues, 'it is good to think of life as always potentially in crisis'. It is good to keep asking the Socratic question (the Socratic question is also the psychoanalytic question): *who am I; how to live?*'[2]

> Now that I am older …, my life is not a speculative life, or a blueprint for a future life. It's just my life. This oldness is a good feeling – a feeling of nothing more to be decided. What happens now will be something other than the strain of making a decision, or the stress of fighting with nature …. You start life all over again, this time with *yourself. (pg- 179).*

I hence see midlife in terms of the ancient Plotinian (Plōtînos, *c.* 204/205–270 CE) activity of a sculptor, chipping away at related blocks of the marble of self, or accretions, in order to find, as in a new self-becoming. The movement in such practices of the self is thus from a *mirror of being* to a *canvas of becoming*. In the psychoanalytic setting also, the analyst serves as the mirror for the *analysand* (the person in analysis). The analysand sees her motivational, aggressive, nurturant, envious, and erotic architecture (also *arche-texture*) etc. in the analyst-as-mirror-of-self. The invitation to the analysand is to work through the extant architecture and engender self-transformative realignments. The urging in this chapter on midlife is to use the same mirror of self/being as a *canvas of a new be-coming*: as Sara Ahmed does.

Individual Dis-ease as a Symptom of a Larger Social Pathology

This section will be a further reflection on the question of 'crisis'. It will de-pathologize the concept of (midlife) crisis. What is crisis? When is an 'x' seen as crisis? *I see 'individual dis-ease' as a symptom of a larger social (at times cultural) pathology.* I do not pathologize the individual. I hence designate disease as dis-ease, as un-ease, as suffering. For me, individual suffering is a symptom of larger *social pathology*. At times, not just individuals, but larger societies suffer. One can designate it as *social suffering*. Is individual midlife crisis a symptom of larger social pathologies in a neoliberal age, in an age of uncertain and extremely competitive cut-throat job environments, environments that are marked in turn by the hard and cruel logic of output, outcome and target. I hence see midlife crisis – even if it exists in some individuals – as a symptom of a larger social pathology. Without addressing the larger social pathology of the atomization of human beings, of narcissistic attention to self (bordering on self-obsession), of the aggressive teleology of achievement-success, we will not be able to reach an expanded understanding of midlife crisis.

This opens up multiple questions with respect to midlife. Is midlife a biological stage? Is it a psychological stage? Or is it a biopsychosocial stage? Is it a stage of decline? Is it a stage of wilting? Is *senescence* the only way to understand life after 45? Is the idea of 'midlife crisis' a fiction? Is it at all a *depressive crisis* (just like adolescence has been conventionally seen as a psychotic crisis or the crisis of micro-psychosis)? Is what we have hitherto seen as midlife, paradoxically, the *prime of life*? How does one revisit midlife as not being an impossible attempt at preserving younger days? Why preserve? Why remain frozen in younger days? Why not *grow*? Do we need to revisit phrases like ' biological clock is ticking' with respect to recent advances in studies in neuroplasticity? With the discipline of psychology at the doorstep of a new revolution (let's call it the *affective turn*) do we need to rethink midlife – which could be seen as a stage of 'mature affective attunement', even if there are a few facial wrinkles? This chapter will thus offer a counter-hegemonic perspective on midlife. It would also like to argue that it is possible to invert the extant philosophy of midlife through a close reading of, say, Rabindranath Tagore's *Nijer Katha* (imperfectly translated as *My Life* or *Narratives of My Self*) or Gandhi's *My Experiments with Truth*. *Nijer Katha*, for example – at a surface level – is a collection of Tagore's letters. But at a deeper level it is Tagore's *auto-psycho-biograph of midlife*. In this book of letters, Tagore reflects deeply on his own self at age 65. He even seems to suggest that *Jivansmriti* – his *A Book of Memory* (Kakar, 2014) – is not his true autobiography. These letters written at around age 65 *are*. It is in these letters that Tagore explores the architecture of his self; he manages to speak at ease about himself, about the uncanny lanes and bylanes that inhabit the self. Gandhi wrote *My Experiments with Truth* between 1925 and 1929. Gandhi was 56 years old when he started publishing these weekly instalments in his journal *Navjivan*. It would not be out of context to foreground how Gandhi introduced *My Experiments with Truth* (2018, p. 45):

> *it is not my purpose to attempt a real autobiography*. I simply want to tell the story of my numerous experiments with truth, and as my life consists of nothing but those experiments, it is true that the story will take the shape of an autobiography. *But I shall not mind*, if every page of it speaks only of my experiments. I believe, or at any rate flatter myself with the belief, that a connected account of all these experiments will not be without benefit to the *reader*. My experiments in the political field are now known, not only to India, but to a certain extent to the 'civilized' world. For me, they have not much value; and the title of 'Mahatma' that they have won for me has, therefore, even less; often the title has deeply pained me; and there is not a moment I can recall when it may be said to have tickled me. But I should certainly like to narrate my experiments in the spiritual field which are known only to myself, and from which I have derived such power as I possess for working in the political field. If the experiments are really spiritual, then there can be no room for self-praise. they can only add to my humility. the more I reflect and look back on the past, the more vividly do I feel my limitations ... the experiments narrated should be regarded as illustrations, in the light of which everyone may carry on his own experiments according to his own inclinations and capacity.

One can see this as Gandhi's reflection on what we are now designating 'midlife'. He has a balanced view of midlife. He is not overwhelmed by what he has achieved: 'my experiments in the political field are now known, not only to India, but to a certain extent to the "civilized" world. For me, *they have not much value*; and the title of "Mahatma" that they have won for me has, therefore, *even less*.' He is also not overwhelmed by *limitations*: 'if the experiments are really spiritual, then there can be no room for self-praise. they can only add to my humility. The more I reflect and look back on the past, the more vividly do I feel my limitations.' Yet these limitations could serve as 'illustrations, in the light of which everyone may carry on his [or her] own experiments according to his [or her] own inclinations and capacity'. Gandhi also sees the past as the story of numerous experiments *with* truth. He was not conducting experiments to *reach* scientific truth, which is the paradigmatic method in the natural sciences. Gandhi was experimenting with the truths *of* life or the *dharmas* or *dharma-sankats* in life – say, for example, *should* one be violent, even if one were to correct a wrongdoing.

Take the *radical rewriting* of the Bhagvad Gita by Gandhi. What is the fundamental self-doubt or *dharma-sankat* that haunts the text of the psychic in the Bhagvad Gita? The psychic teleology in the Bhagvad Gita has been sparked off by an 'affront to a menstruating woman in the blind king's court of justice', and it is now about to be avenged by the collective of husbands – the Pandavas. However, there is a catch or halt or deferral to this seamless narrative. One of the five husbands – *Arjun* – is haunted by a near-primal doubt that could be so characteristic of the conception of *dharma-sankat* (What should I do? Should I kill? Can I kill?). Not ordinary killing. Can I kill my relatives, my brothers, my teacher Dronacharya, my grandfather Bhisma, especially, even if I am here to avenge the trauma inflicted on 'my' woman? The commonsensical answer would be 'yes, you have to kill' to forestall further harm and auxiliary destruction by a group of marauding men – the Kauravas. Faced with such a *dharma-sankat*, Gandhi's answer, however, would be a resounding *no*: 'satyagraha is essentially a weapon of the truthful. A satyagrahi is pledged to non-violence, and, unless people observe it in thought, word and deed, I cannot offer mass satyagraha.[3] Violence for Gandhi led only to *double destruction*. Destruction of both aggressed and aggressor. Physical death for the aggressed. Moral death for the aggressor. Violence only led to a *radical nothingness*. The *sunyata*, the *void* at the end of the war of Kurukshetra, stands testimony to such an all-consuming nothingness. Midlife had perhaps taken Gandhi to a much deeper reflection on *dharma* and had brought him to an insight (*militant non-violence*, to be precise [Erikson, 1993]) that stood against commonsense defence and legitimization of violence.

Historicizing-culturalizing Midlife

This section of the chapter will first *historicize* the idea of 'midlife'. It will build on the text *Aging by the Book* by Kay Heath (2009) to show how during the Victorian era, midlife (which was hitherto seen as the 'prime of life') was conceptualized as a period of decline in the West. Was there a gender angle to this shift? This was a time when single women were seen to be nearing middle age at 30, mothers in their forties were expected to become sexless, and fortyish men were seen to be in anguish over whether their time for love had gone by. The chapter will argue that our current negative attitude towards midlife springs from Victorian roots (the word 'midlife' first appeared in an English- language dictionary in 1895). The 18th century was an especially crucial period in the 'history of age' because demographic changes such as lengthening lifespan affected definitions of old age. The elderly began to be seen as a separate cohort in the overall population, age came to be defined chronologically rather than by functional capacity and fitness, and the concept of elders as dependents or 'burdens' on society developed, setting the stage for 19th-century pension schemes. In the past, people never kept track of one's exact age; people would round the number to the nearest decade. But with the Enlightenment, more emphasis was placed on record keeping, and ages became known with greater accuracy (see Ottaway, 2008, p. 53). Further, women near the age of menopause, were described with images of lost 'bloom', withering, and fading, past their reproductive prime. Women not only aged into midlife earlier than men in Victorian England, but were also considered elderly sooner (Ottaway, 2008, p. 35).

One hence needs to engage with the concept of 'age' in both philosophy and psychology (and not see age as biological; psychological and psychoanalytical age may be distinctly different from biological age; one may be biologically 50 and yet be childlike psychologically). The chapter thus sees age as not just culturally constructed but as a philosophical concept with psychological roots. Further, is midlife crisis a crisis of the social, and not of the individual? Is midlife pathology a symptom of a larger social pathology, as I have suggested above? Is the subject of midlife in crisis? Or is it society and society's conservatism that puts the subject of midlife in crisis? Does life end at 40, or does it begin at 40? Does one then need to look at midlife *beyond* the standard binarism: decline and rise, end and beginning – which Tagore and Gandhi were trying to do, perhaps, with partial success? This chapter hence foregrounds the importance of the phenomenological turn in our understanding of midlife. In the process, it opens up the axes of embodiment (the 'body-mind') and the difficult task of 'life-writing'. It also argues for the importance of psycho-biographs of midlife – which are psychoanalytic biographs (without, of course, the entrenched ableism and masculinism of Freud and Lacan) – and where the focus is on listening to, communicating and relating with the subject of midlife.[4] Is midlife, then, an uncanny experience of different kinds of en-able-ness? Does a close reading of Tagore's *Nijer Katha* – as suggested above – take us to such a psychobiograph of *midlife en-able-ness* – 'en-able-ness', because I do not see midlife as disable-ness, but as a different kind of en-able-ness?

Midlife *en-able-ness* is missed in many Westernized cultures, primarily because Westernized cultures have become ever more youth-oriented, increasingly devalue ageing, in the process pushing back the years of en-able-ness to earlier stages in the life course. I argue that today's hyper age-consciousness, with its aura of a fate worse than death, is a dogma we have inherited from the Victorians, our predecessors in midlife trauma. Age is universal, a fact of existence for all living things, but one understood differently by each society and era. The idea of midlife hence requires *culturalizing*: 'whatever happens in the body, humans beings are aged by culture first of all' (Schmidt, 2020: 172). While a grandmother's wrinkle in indigenous contexts is interpreted by her granddaughters as a marker of increased status and wisdom, the same wrinkle in hyper-Westernized contexts is read as a sign of loss of youth and a proof of decay. Westernized cultures place great stress on chronological years, and transition from one life stage to another often is discussed in terms of significant birthdays: is one 'over the hill' at 30 or 40 or finally and surely at 50? There is a constant sense of time running out. For men especially, turning 40 meant saying goodbye to impossible dreams, taming and re-channelling the ambition of youth. Nothing could dislodge the stereotype once reserved for men: stalled career, fading youth and listless marriage.

Non-Westernized cultures, however, emphasize other factors. For example, progression through social roles according to community status, including alterations in the lives of one's children, may be more significant than chronological age or biological symptoms (Shweder, 1998, p. xi). Shweder quotes Sudhir Kakar to show how in semi-rural India, one enters the Hindi stage of *burhapa* or abstinence at 50, and when the first child marries, the parents begin a 'psychological transition ... into middle age'. Some may even cease their sexual relationship, because 'It is thought to be polluting and undignified for two generations to copulate under the same roof' (Shweder, 1998, p. xii).

Westernized Indians connected to the circuits of Western academia – socialized into the culture of the discipline of philosophy or psychology – tend to view their own temporal journey in terms of Western ideas of age and ageing, including Western ideas of loss and regret, success and failure, the lives you wanted and the life you have. Western ideas of mortality and finitude, ideas about the temporal structure of human life come to colonize us. We begin to view ourselves in terms of the premium put on youth. One single strand of grey hair or one solitary wrinkle on the face upsets us. Polivka (2000, p. 227), in an article titled 'Postmodern Aging and the Loss of Meaning', quotes Featherstone and Hepworth (1998) to point to, paradoxically, the *end of ageing* (let us call it the optimistic[5] view):

> In fact, they are optimistic about the capacity of biotechnology to slow or even reverse the aging process and create the conditions for a long midlife period extending far into what is now considered old age as we enter a new techno-culture. These developments will make it possible

for 'old' people to take full advantage of the multiple, shifting identities characteristic of postmodern culture, especially those 'old' people with the resources to consume the growing array of medical procedures, technological devices, travel options and cultural goods produced by a high growth, information-based global capitalist economy. According to this perspective, at least implicitly, the aging experience is, in itself, meaningless, so nothing essential is lost in the changes Featherstone/Hepworth describe and endorse. They see greater freedom and room for agency in a greatly lengthened middle age ending in a 'deep' old age, presumably some time past eighty or ninety and older.

Tagore and Gandhi take us beyond this excessively optimistic view as also the ubiquitous view of decline and degeneration to what could be designated as the *reflective phenomenological view of midlife.* For Tagore and Gandhi, midlife is not seen as a life stage. For them, midlife is an existential *question.* When one asks the questions in all earnestness 'Who am I?', 'How should I live?', 'What is the purpose of life?', 'What may I hope for?', one is not just engaging with the question of midlife, but also with the temporality of one's multiple orientations to the past and the future, including one's relation to unrealized possibilities or counterfactuals.

The Mystic Writing Pad of Midlife

Freud's metaphor of the 'mystic writing pad' (Freud, 1923–1925) can offer an interesting way of looking at, making sense of and tolerating the experience of midlife as also setting up an equally interesting way of looking at the relationship between (a) the accumulated traces of the past, including traumatic marks of the past, that cannot be erased but which form a complex and uncanny cartograph and (b) possible new life inscriptions that can be birthed creatively.

The mystic writing pad is a slab of dark brown resin or wax with a worked edging; over the slab is laid a thin transparent sheet; it itself consists of *two* layers which can be detached from each other except at their two ends. The upper layer is a transparent piece of celluloid; the lower layer is made of thin, translucent wax. To make use of the mystic writing pad, one writes up the celluloid portion of the covering sheet which rests on the waxed slab. No pencil or chalk is necessary, since the writing does not depend on material being deposited on the receptive surface.[6] A pointed stylus scratches the surface, and the impressions constitute the 'writing'. At the points which the stylus touches, it presses the lower surface of the waxed work onto the wax slab, and the grooves are visible as dark writing on the otherwise smooth, whitish-grey surface of the celluloid. If one wishes to erase what one has written, all that is necessary is to peel the double covering sheet from the wax slab; the close contact between the celluloid and the wax slab at the places which have been scratched (on which the visibility of the writing depended) is thus brought to an end. The surface is now clear of writing and ready to receive fresh inscriptions. Is midlife such a two-layered moment and experience of life, comprising of (a) the hauntings of past writings or inscriptions and (b) possible present writings or new inscriptions? Does midlife run into crisis because one is haunted by past writings and life looks bereft of possible new writings? The metaphor of the mystic writing pad offers a picture of life that can receive perceptions but retain no permanent trace of them so that the life can act like a clean slate to every new perception while the permanent traces of the excitations which have been received are preserved in 'mnemic systems' lying behind the perceptual systems. Life and midlife is thus endowed with a '*double system* contained in a single differentiated apparatus: a *perceptually available innocence* and an *infinite resource of traces*' and the doubled up process of '*repetition* and *erasure*' (Derrida, 1978, p. 226). Does midlife run into crisis when there is *only* repetition and no erasure? Does midlife run into crisis when there is *only* retention of past traces and no available innocence for the *new*?

The inscriptions *received* on the resin or wax *cannot be lost altogether*; and although such inscriptions would not qualify as legible writing in the ordinary sense of the term, they would still constitute a *script* of the past – albeit an uncanny one. Whenever one is writing, one is writing on the *already written* script, one is *getting written* by the uncanny script of the past, of youth. The new and old, the present and the past, the fresh and the retained have to come to a dialogue to give shape to what Tagore and Gandhi birthed as a *reflective phenomenological view of midlife*, a view that was neither metaphysical about the past nor about the present, about the old nor about the new. *New* writing does not exist: we are written only as we write, by the *legacy* or *past* within us which always already keeps watch over our new writing, be it internal or external. The always already written becomes meaningful only in the context of new writing. The mystic writing pad as metaphor of midlife offers us a Möbius strip of the old and the new, the past and the present.[7]

Notes

1 Neither chronological, biological nor sociological factors alone are sufficient for defining midlife. Only by placing various aspects of midlife within a cultural context can we begin to understand its spectrum of meanings.

2 Philosophy has moved away from the old Socratic questions 'Who am I? How should I live?' The current question of philosophy is mostly focused on the 'nature of the world', or 'what is true' and 'what is false'. It is not directed to the 'self'. Questions are directed towards questions like 'is it a snake or is it a rope?' They are rarely directed to questions like 'Who am I? What are my difficulties and roadblocks? How can I overcome them? How should I live to nurture my creativity?' Philosophy as a 'way of life' (and not a way of knowing the world) has also been seen as *therapia* (see Dhar, 2018 for the turn to *practical* and *transformative* philosophy).

3 '*I had in my speech described Western civilization as being, unlike the Eastern, predominantly based on force.* The questioners pinned me to my faith, and one of them – the captain so far as I recollect – said to me: "supposing the whites carry out their threats, how will you stand by your principle of non-violence?" To which I replied: "I hope god will give me the courage and the sense to forgive them and to refrain from bringing them to law. I have no anger against them. I am only sorry for their ignorance and their narrowness. I know that they sincerely believe that what they are doing today is right and proper. I have no reason therefore to be angry with them' (Gandhi, 2018, p. 319).

4 In 1965, psychoanalyst Elliott Jaques published the essay that coined the phrase: 'Death and the Mid-life Crisis'. In dissecting the crisis, Jaques quotes a patient in his mid-thirties: 'Up till now,' he said, 'life has seemed an endless upward slope, with nothing but the distant horizon in view. Now suddenly I seem to have reached the crest of the hill, and there stretching ahead is the downward slope with the end of the road in sight – far enough away it's true – but there is death observably present at the end.'

5 In 1999, the *Washington Post* ran a special section titled 'Midlife without the Crisis'. In the *New York Times,* the headline was 'New Study Finds Middle Age Is the Prime of Life'.

6 Writing does not depend on material, ink or chalk that is being actually deposited upon the receptive surface. Writing depends on the *impression* the material makes on the receptive surface.

7 The three-dimensional figure of the Möbius strip subverts standard Euclidean experiences of space and the notion of 'inside' and 'outside'. It looks like there are two sides to the Möbius strip, but it has only one. At a particular point of time, at the level of the localized experience of time, there appear to be two sides and the two sides can apparently be distinguished, but when the whole of the strip is traversed, it becomes clear that they are in fact continuous. A shorter temporality offers two experiences of spatiality; a longer temporality offers one. Further, because the two sides are continuous, it is possible to cross over from inside to outside, and from one side to the other. Yet, when one traverses the length of the Möbius strip, it is not possible to pinpoint at which precise point one has crossed over from the inside to the outside or vice versa. The figure does not just problematize binary oppositions but shows how apparently opposed terms – like old and new – could be understood as *mutually constitutive* terms (see Dhar, 2021).

References

Ahmed, S. (2021). *Living a Feminist Life.* Audio CD. https://www.amazon.de/-/en/Sara-Ahmed/dp/B08ZDDSVZ1

Derrida, J. (1978). Structure, sign and play in the discourse of the human sciences. In *Writing and difference* (p. 226). Routledge and Kegan Paul.

Dhar, A. (2018). Melancholy philosophy: Polis-Praxis-Phronesis and the Slave's know-how. In S. B. Das (Ed.), *Abandonment and abjection: Melancholy in philosophy and art.* Aakar Books.

Dhar, A. (2021). The death of depth: Reflections on the religion of politics in India. In Manas Ray (Ed.), *State of democracy in India: Essays on life and politics in contemporary times.* Primus Books.

Erikson, E. H. (1993). *Gandhi's truth: On the origins of militant nonviolence.* W. W. Norton and Company.

Freud, S. (1923–25). A note upon the mystic writing pad. In *The standard edition of the complete psychological works of Sigmund Freud* (Vol. XIX, pp. 225–232)

[A note upon the "Mystic Writing-Pad"' 1940 *The International Journal of Psychoanalysis*, *21*(4), 469–474].
Gandhi, M. K. (2018). *An autobiography or the story of my experiments with truth* (M. Desai, Trans and T. Suhrud, Ed.). Yale University Press.
Heath, K. (2009). *Aging by the book: The emergence of midlife in Victorian Britain*. SUNY Press. Studies in the Long Nineteenth Century.
Kakar, S. (2014). *A book of memory: Confessions and reflections*. Penguin Books India.
Ottaway, S. (2008). *The decline of life: Old age in eighteenth-century England*. Cambridge Studies in Population, Economy and Society in Past Time. Cambridge University Press.
Polivka, L. (2000). Postmodern aging and the loss of meaning. *Journal of Aging and Identity*, *5*, 225–235.
Schmidt, S. (2020). *Midlife crisis: The feminist origins of a Chauvinist Cliché*. The University of Chicago Press.
Shweder, R. A. (Ed.). (1998). *Welcome to middle age!: (And other cultural fictions)*. University of Chicago Press.

4 Midlife through a Sociological Lens

Mallarika Sarkar (Das) and Sritama Chaudhuri

Introducing the Context: Shifts and Continuities in Midlife

Recently, an article published in the *Wall Street Journal* highlighted an intriguing fact – an emerging business industry in America catering to the various needs of midlife (Tergesen, 2023). Since longevity in general has increased, people belonging to various communities and social strata have explored ways of spending their forties, fifties and sixties in a meaningful way. Hence the rise of commercial entrepreneurship to monetise this new chain of demand and supply. Age, health and wellness are interconnected in how individuals make sense of their life, social living, bodies and emotions. With the postponement of death – which now mainly happens in controlled medical environments rather than in the vicinity of one's primary group – the meaning of death has changed (Riley, 1987) along with that the idea of ageing. Scholarship around demographics has found that the overall life expectancy (average years of life) has increased in the majority of the nations over the last century (Vaupel, 2010). Even in the underdeveloped nations of the global South, there has been a steady decline in mortality rates during old age (Rau et al. 2008). Therefore, ways of spending the additional years in good and productive health have become potent topics of discussion among various stakeholders of society. One such deliberation is the rise of research projects on the middle age of human beings. Another such manifestation is the evolving medical attention to the concept of 'delayed ageing' (Kirkwood & Austad, 2000; Miller, 2012). The desire for immortality and the penchant for youth is, however, not a new concept and has remained a dominant theme of every civilisation, religion, mythology and literature. Middle age in this context of longevity and youth falls in the middle, and hence often becomes a component of two extremes – the portal to a long, productive and youthful aging process or a period associated with rumination, introspection and mitigating the perils of the famously phrased 'midlife crisis'. According to Lachman (2004), the term 'midlife' entered public discourse for the first time in 1895 in Funk and Wagnall's standard dictionary. The biological range of midlife and its subjective and psychological perception are still fuzzy. Development is a lifelong process, but surprisingly, not much is known about how midlife develops. Since this field

DOI: 10.4324/9781003568360-5

of inquiry is relatively new, many aspects of midlife are still unexplored. Extensive previous literature has contributed enormously, from childhood and adolescence through old age, but midlife, typically characterised as a transitory and distinct stage of life ranging from age 40 to 65, is often a historically neglected focus of research, 'invisible' years between youth and old age. The reason for lack of interest in enquiring about midlife, as identified by Carpenter and Stockard (2020), was that evidence of physical, mental and emotional development was scant during this period. In addition, the time span for studies of midlife, which lasts almost more than 30 years, is very long in comparison to the time span for studies of youth and age. Therefore, many misconceptions exist about this phase of life, which has led to an uncanny representation of it in public sphere and popular culture. For instance, popular tabloids, cultural stereotyping and colloquial humour often inevitably add the suffix 'crisis' after 'midlife', whereas scholarly research highlights that only a small proportion of people suffer from midlife crisis (Wethington et al., 2005). This unmindful attitude towards midlife may have caused by consideration of those in their middle years as a homogenised group, also known as 'cohort-centrism' (see Riley, 1987, p. 3), and to the fact that there is no uniform consensus on how we define midlife.

This chapter seeks to demystify and de-sanitise midlife. It attempts to contribute to the discourse on midlife development by comprehending the social construction of the middle age life period, a pivotal stage in the life course from a sociological perspective. The chapter underscores the salience of the midlife phase and highlights its diversity compared to other stages of life. The main goal of the chapter is to unfold the internal dynamics of this age cohort being shaped by age and sociocultural factors, to consider midlife as a sociologically constructed and complex phenomenon, and to find out what implications this discourse has on the way it is understood and subjectively experienced. To become adult and to grow old is a natural, inevitable and irreversible process, but often how a person strives to make sense of life in their middle years depends on contexts, experiences and roles. With this objective in mind, particular emphasis is given to the subjective understanding of body image, sexual role during midlife and social representations of middle-aged people in popular culture. The significance of gender, social class and the powerful impact of media and technology in defining middle age are examined further to explore the issue in question. This chapter corroborates the fact that how people 'do' age is directly connected to the theoretical framework of intersectionality. By adopting a sociological approach, grounded in theoretical traditions and empirical approaches, this chapter attempts to fill the existing research gap by offering novel insights and providing a holistic picture of midlife development. In addition, new insights by virtue of its inclusivity and interdisciplinary nature promis to revisit midlife as a pivotal period of the life cycle, as a socially constructed and diverse life period, and may inform policy.

Middle age remains a vital block to the pursuit of healthy living and ageing well. We cannot escape our age, hence it needs our attention. Scholarly and policy consideration of middle age are essential as it is a stage where a matured mind is dealing with bodily changes and functional deterioration on one hand (Pietilä & Ojala, 2011), while possessing many intellectual, emotional, financial and educational ways of mitigating these effects.

The sections that follow strive to unravel the process of ageing, describing middle age in the theoretical context.

Sociological Perspectives of Middle Age and Dominant Narratives

The dominant narratives surrounding middle age are heavily multi-disciplinary, as an exclusive sociological overwiew of the middle-aged cohort is lacking (Maddox, 1979) hence it is an emerging topic of discussion and concern. The sociology of age has been masked by social gerontology due to their overlapping nature. In every social interaction, social process and social change, age has always been an important component but only in recent years have sociologists accorded it importance for rigorous theorisation (Elder, 1975). The Gerontological Society of America was founded in 1945, and thereafter has published its journal committed to theorising on aging (Maddox, 1979). Social gerontology soon followed intersections from various social sciences. However, the study of middle age is not confined in the field of gerontology, as it is shaped by varied theories of society, identity and impression management, modernity and postmodernity, health and wellbeing, and economic consumerism. Among the relevant insightful works of the sociological perspective, some of them are discussed below:

Age as an explanatory variable is employed by one set of sociologists – a bureaucratic convenience. For instance, various societies assign cultural and social significance to chronological age (age 18 for driving, 21 for alcohol consumption, 65 for retirement etc.), which varies from one society to another (Maddox, 1979). The fact that the social meaning of a certain age varies from culture to culture draws sociological attention, as the focus shifts from biological convenience to social group consensus. This seep in the social system allows politics to mingle with the prevalent ageism. This results in standpoint differences, and experience of age becomes a matter of intersectionality, which largely explains why the experience of middle-aged cohorts differ.

Few sociologists find modernisation a key ingredient in how we perceive age. Modernisation here is the infusion of new technology, urbanisation, industrialisation and a new social thinking which influences social structure and social age differentiation (Eisenstadt, 2017). The social meaning and importance of different age groups differ in primitive, industrial and post-industrial societies. For Fischer (1977), the reason for these differences has cultural rather than technological roots. When it comes to middle age, sociological perspective must locate it within the genre of healthy living and quality of life (Higgs et al., 2003a). Because thinking about middle age comes from a place of privilege – a stage post of economic survival, sociologists like, Anthony Giddens (1994), Ulrich Beck (2005) and Zygmont Bauman (2004) focus on the fact that societies have reached a postmaterialist phase where issues concerning economic survival worries are replaced by quality of life. In the contemporary modern society, more attention needs to be given to two pivotal activities – consumption and leisure, which constitute an integral part of healthy living/active ageing (Edwards, 2011). Sociology helps in focusing on these aspects of healthy living and quality of life instead of seeing ageing as merely a process of bodily degeneration (Gelleard & Higgs, 2002).

Middle age has further been subjected to societal policing, as age is an important tool of social control. Social control, in its purest classical sense, refers to the capacity of a social group to regulate itself.

For one school of thought, ageing is much related to the collective change in population composition, structure and behaviour, and in turn, it is about societal change. For Riley (1987), sociology of age strives to see ageing as a process where on one hand people are growing old, and on the other society is going through a process of change as new people are replacing old people in its key institutions. The process of human ageing and social change are interconnected and interdependent as they mutually influence each other. This thought is inspired by Norman Ryder's (1985) work on this cohort as an agent for social change. Sociological research on birth cohorts is predominant as Bengtson et al. (2012, p. 495) elaborate that a social/cultural history is shared by birth cohorts and demonstrates how the features of birth cohorts and events experienced by them combine to affect them in distinct ways, exerting an influence on their behaviours, attitudes, personalities and outcomes throughout the entire life course.

For sociologists, role theory has heavily informed theorisation on life transitions (George, 1993). According to sociologist Linton (1936), status is attached to every social position in the social structure, which determines the role associated with it. An individual's transitioning into middle age can be directly linked to role theory, as middle age may mark an entry or exit from an assigned role (voluntary retirement, for example), which is itself a major life transition with several ramifications (George, 1993). Role theory is an attractive heuristic tool for considering the interconnectedness between age, social structure and individual behaviour. Again, for some sociologists who inspired the constructionist paradigm, like West and Zimmerman (1987) and Goffman (2002), age is about performance and doing an act. In the words of Laz (2003), we cannot avoid the performance of age as long as it a criterion for differentiation.

Subjective Age, Social Identity and Intersectionality

Act according to your age.

(a colloquial phrase)

In many cultures, age has been a matter of performance. People have been acting or performing their age as a given part of their social role expectations (Calassanti, 2003). However, these performances are not always in harmony as there is an incongruence between biological age, subjective age, age identity and societal expectations. Subjective age is defined as the psychological age of an individual – the age one feels (Diehl et al., 2014). Age identity is defined as an individual's subjectivity surrounding their's age and the consequent relatedness with a certain age group (Dolberg & Ayalon, 2018). Age identity also comes with its own age norms, similar-aged social roles, socioeconomic parameters and social expectations (Diehl et al., 2014; Dolberg & Ayalon, 2018). Usually, people don't consciously feel the incongruence in their everyday lived realities. People hardly think of their age daily until and unless they are faced with obstructions in an instance like a certain social expectation of a body image of a younger person not matching with the subjective age of a middle-aged individual; then psychological conflict starts. Also, when collectively society assigns certain professional abilities to biological age, the subjective age may collide and cause a debate amongabout subjective age, societal expectations and social identity (Guellete, 2004). Therefore, the social status and social identity of a particular age becomes tricky, collective in nature and overtly dependent on external factors. Often, research has stated that people who feel younger than their biological age associate themselves with younger age groups and hence have a positive outlook, whereas feeling older may have negative outcomes (Diehl et al., 2014; Barrett & Montepare, 2015). The actualisation of subjective age becomes difficult if societal stigma is attached to it. Dolberg and Ayalon (2018) explain in their case study on Israel's population that the middle-aged cohort is highly associated with negative outcomes due to rising ageist perspectives, growing cases of elder abuse and cultural stereotypes.

The social status and social identity of middle-aged people are highly complex, controversial (Garsatka et al., 2005) and directly linked with intersectionality (Egeland & Gressgård, 2007). By the term 'intersectional', sociologists mean an analytical toolkit to understand how social categories of race, class, gender, caste, religion and region influence the life chances of an individual in terms of advantages and disadvantages, often leading to multiple layers of privilege and disadvantage. Cultural models based out of class, gender and region often influence an individual's perception of ageing along the entire life course. From the point of view of intersectionality, one's age is constructed just like gender via socially constructed role expectations. Empirical research has found that growing old is a highly gendered process, marked with class consciousness and practices (Pietilä & Ojala, 2011). Pietila and Ojala conducted nine in-depth interviews and four focus group discussions on men aged 40-plus and found that their idea of self-worth negotiated and vacillated between the old and young spectrum.

Cultural stereotypes affect both men and women, but the extent of age shaming is higher when it comes to ageing women as their bodily and physical appearances start to change, which feminists have deemed a double standard of ageing (Sontang, 1972; Jackson, 2020). Women are expected to always look good and project their best versions even when they grow old, which reinforces and legitimises sexist and ageist outlooks about women's appearance, including expectations that older women must hide visible signs of ageing via liberal usage of cosmetic surgery, lifestyle changes or application of cosmetics to remain attractive (Kenalemang, 2022). This means that midlife is often associated with an ageless identity. Due to the complexity of the social status of middle-aged women and discrepancies in the knowledge of varied overt and covert symptoms of menopause, much remains unresolved concerning the experiences of pain, distress and personal shame during the menopause transition, often considered to be a major life transition (Nosek et al., 2010). Conclusions highlight experiences of socially and culturally constructed shame and stigma related to the entire experience and discourses on menopause and aging. Alarming results hint towards lack of support from primary social groups as well.

Popular Culture, Social Media and the Cult of 'Active Ageing/ anti-ageing'

Popularly known as 'boomers', the generation born in 1946–1964 revolutionised the social representations of middle-aged cohorts and heavily influenced consumption, leisure and lifestyle choices (Philipson et al., 2008). Much of the popular culture and media representation of the middle-aged lifestyle has been inspired by the life images of boomers, which, sociologically analysed, depict a distinct life course from previous generations (Gilleard & Higgs, 2002). Edmunds and Turner (2005) highlighted that the analysis of UK boomers projected a 'strategic generation in aesthetic, cultural and sexual terms'. This gave rise to sensationalising of the generation in the media. One such idea in vogue is 'staying fit'.

Active ageing, a concept promoted by the World Health Organization, is the process of maximising opportunities for health, participation and security in order to enhance quality of life and wellbeing as people age. This idea has been usurped by popular culture and media and has produced an abundance of projects. Individuals belonging to all genders after age 40 and nearing late old age are now indulging in various health pursuits such as going to gyms, practising yoga, skin botox, and hair and anti-ageing beauty treatments, maintaining an engaged social and community life, following their hobbies and passions, leaving unhealthy partnerships and remarrying, and similar pursuits which all directly and indirectly promote active living and wellness. Television celebrities and social media influencers play a huge role in addressing the overall ageism prevalent in every society. There has been a steady growth of the wellness business, as acquiring the skills of wellness is perceived as a strategy for 'ageing well' among the middle-aged social group as it is largely assumed that older adults devour wellness primarily to postpone signs of ageing (Koskinen et al., 2017). As the earlier section elucidated, the special needs of this contemporary post-materialist era for middle-aged people represent a phenomenon that can be perceived as one of the social milieus in which individuals focus on on their personal ageing experiences and strive to learn the 'wellness skills' they perceive as crucial for an individual's sense of personal care and life management in later years (active third age). To aid this process, there is an emerging technology industry which specialises in delaying ageing.

Sexuality, the Dilemma of 'Body Image' and Social Relationships

The notion that the onset of decline is marked by midlife and that the acceptance of growing limitations is the only plausible way to cope with ageing is generally acceptable as good common sense. Midlife is thrilling because it offers opportunities to people to revisit their most basic assumptions. In this section, we strive to revive the culturally constructed 'dull image' of middle age, focus on social relationships, highlight the active side of midlife, and map it against two vital parameters of healthy living – pleasure and self-realisation (actualisation and fulfilment) (see Higgs et al., 2003b).

There has been colloquial speculation and related biological research about the sexual life of the middle-aged cohort. Much has been written about the sexual health and sexual literacy of early adult populations, but there is a large gap in the sexual health awareness of middle-aged people. Decrease in overall physical agility and sexual intercourse over the ageing process is a natural biological tendency; however, assuming people of middle and later age to be 'asexual' and hence invisible, neglecting their sexual healthcare is a social construct. Gott and Hinchliff (2003) pointed out this vital insight. In the previous section, socially and culturally constructed discrimination related to menopause was discussed, leading to slightly better visibility of women's health concerns owing to menopause. Otherwise, the data is scant on the same topic for both genders. The biggest sociological barrier has been the misconception of lack of sexual life. Kinsey et al. (1998) proved that menopause has never been a significant constraint as the amount of sexual activity persisted consistently among unmarried women aged up to 55 years. Further, research findings shows no drastic change in the sexual functioning of the middle aged population, and it has remained rather constant in the absence of other biological hindrances (George & Weiler, 1981).

In examining how ageing and sexual activity interact, Knox writes that few middle-aged men and women rebel against losing youth and engage in a 'second adolescence', as pointed out by Barbara Waxman. This is why the period around age 40 is sometimes referred to as a precarious age when men in particular tend to look for young women as lovers or second wives. The results can be counterproductive if the younger woman's physical needs are not met, and instead of curbing the man's virility anxiety, the situation may exacerbate it (Merriam, 1978). This age-specific behaviour opens up a further sociological debate about issues relating to primary relations, family and social relations in terms of the relevance of polygamy for an age cohort, faithfulness, divorce, co-parenting of children and the meaning of monogamy for unmarried people in middle age.

The idea of 'body image' plays a crucial role in the overall playfulness of the middle-aged cohort. Body image is a complex phenomenon that requires multi-layered analysis (McCabe & Ricciardelli, 2004). Body image, defined as an amalgamation of the thoughts and feelings an individual nurtures about their body, applies to all genders, may range between positive and negative experiences, and an individual may feel at times positive or negative or a combination of both. Middle-age cohorts often experience severe instances of body image discomfort. There are instances of how body image disturbance can often produce body dissatisfaction (Tiggerman, 2001; 2006) which is often described as the discrepancy between how a person perceives their body image and the ideal body image. As mentioned in the section above, often mass media and popular culture contribute to these feelings, both positively and negatively. A positive instance is celebrities coming out openly and addressing the feelings in open public discourse. Intriguing research has focusesed on the rise of older people in the world of advertisements (Kenalemang, 2022). The research has highlighted the visual sexualisation of older celebrities, which may lead to debate about the individual pangs of 'body shaming'. As Ylänne (2015) opines, the plausible impacts of media portrayals of older adults have been on the rise recently in the field of communication and media studies, as well as in social and cultural gerontology. Unsuitable and erroneous negative depictions tend to reinforce negative stereotypical notions about older people among younger consumers (Gerbner, 1997), potentially reducing older people's self-esteem (Roy, A & Harwood, J, 1997). Positive and varied images are regarded as desirable, especially for older media users, for asserting positive self-identity. In the current century, the visibility and positive portrayal of older adults have indisputably increased in the media, including films and advertisements. Social media platforms like Instagram and TikTok have helped in removing the shyness around 'an ageing body' among many middle-aged cohorts, who openly counter negative body image stereotypes. Empirical research was conducted in China by examining the comments posted by aged TikTok celebrities and by understanding and analysing the dominant themes evident in these popular TikTok accounts. The empirical outcomes reveal that TikTok expedites the social communication of older digital celebrities by fostering a caring and pro-ageing milieu within the realms of digital geography (Yu & Zhao,

2022). Historically, women have faced the negative consequences of body image shaming as there is a particular penchant for female beauty. The topic of men undergoing the process of ageing attracting scholarly attention is a recent development (Thompson, 2008).

When it comes to social relationships, a significant issue the married middle-aged cohort face is their relationship with adult children (Fingerman et al., 2011). Social gerontology has documented that middle-aged cohorts provide support across generations in contemporary families. Most middle-aged adults provide more help to adult children than parents. Middle-aged adults also respond to health crises (e.g., parental disability) and daily needs (educational, marital) in providing intergenerational support. Scholarly studies have shown that individuals hold stereotypes about what is to be achieved by midlife (Krueger et al., 1995). Besides the occurrence of major events, transitions such the increasing caregiving responsibilities for ageing parents and the awareness of self as the bridge between generations are crucial in midlife. Midlife adults tend to view themselves not as the socialised but the socialiser. Neugarten (cited in Lachman, 2004) emphasises the maturity of the individual in the capability for carrying out important roles during midlife.

Middle Age and Workforce Participation

Much of the sociology literature has been devoted to the experiences of retirement with globalised work cultures and highly developed information and communication technologies, which have meant that the nature of work has changed significantly. The work experience and meaning of 'work' have shifted for a lot of employees as the nature of work has become precarious and the diversification of work trajectories has become rampant (Watson, 2017). Higgs et al. (2003b) argue that: retirement is not to be seen as a period of decline, dependency or disengagement, but as a positive choice to renounce work and child-rearing.

Further, in middle age, the work experience becomes complicated as the social landscape of contemporary times is marked by delayed parenthood, family planning and home-based care for the elderly – making it an act of balancing between professional work and intergenerational caregiving (Sawyer & James, 2018). Workforce participation may fluctuate for women. It has been documented that women show complicated patterns of workforce participation in middle age (Majeed et al., 2015). Overall, there has been a substantial increase in the participation of the middle-aged cohort compared to last decade. There exist a multitude of significant sociological, economic, cultural, psychological and demographic reasons why middle-aged managemers and professionals may decide to consider career shifts at midlife. However, a few decades ago, only two out of every 100 executives were expected to plan a fundamental career shift. The scenario changed during the last decade – the middle-aged working cohort are now taking bigger risks, hence this figure has increased to 35% (Holmes & Cartwright,

1993). In 1983, 70% of male full-time workers in the 58–62 age group were loyal to their sole employers. By 2006, half had shifted to a new employers. Career-long employment is no longer dominant, as diversification and risk-taking are on the rise. Owing to the increase in longevity, if the retirement age increases from 63 to 67, it is expected that the majority of men will change jobs at some point after age 50 and work full-time for a new employer (Munnell & Sass, 2008). New requirements for longer productive years are prompting the middle-aged population to think about and 'do' life differently. The previous section elaborated on the various pursuits of healthy living. Social media have also made pursuing hobbies and side hustles as a means for earning a living achievable and lucrative. Often, personal blogs and social media posts inform us that a successful banker has quit a full-time high-paying job in their midforties and is running a successful bakery business. The midlife years therefore appear to be a period of unprecedented opportunity for inner growth.

Conclusion: An Agenda for Policy and Research

Future endeavours surrounding midlife needs to emphasise the diversity in how midlife is experienced across religions, sexual orientation and socioeconomic status. The narrative surrounding midlife needs to unfold the challenges in confronting midlife for minorities, those who identify as LGBT and people in various socioeconomic strata. The full picture of midlife is yet to be unfolded as many questions still remain unaddressed. A promising direction to promote resilience among middle-aged adults is to consider how the varied aspects of everyday life are embedded in the conditions of multiple trajectories over time and space. Thus, a holistic understanding of midlife could have profound consequences.

References

Bauman, Z. (2004). *Work, consumerism and the new poor*. Buckingham: Open University Press.

Barrett, A. E., & Montepare, J. M. (2015). "It's about time": Applying life span and life course perspectives to the study of subjective age. *Annual Review of Gerontology and Geriatrics, 35*(1), 55–77.

Beck, U. (2005). *Risk society*. Sage.

Bengtson, V. L., Elder Jr., G. H., & Putney, N. M. (2012). The life course perspective on ageing: Linked lives, timing, and history. *Adult Lives: A Life Course Perspective*, 9–17.

Carpenter, T., & Stockard, J. (2020). *A decade of change and continuity in midlife*. Cambridge Scholars Publishing.

Diehl, M., Wahl, H. W., Barrett, A. E., Brothers, A. F., Miche, M., Montepare, J. M., & Wurm, S. (2014). Awareness of aging: Theoretical considerations on an emerging concept. *Developmental Review, 34*(2), 93–113.

Dolberg, P., & Ayalon, L. (2018). Subjective meanings and identification with middle age. *The International Journal of Aging and Human Development*, 87(1), 52–76.

Edmunds, J., & Turner, B. S. (2005). Global generations: Social change in the twentieth century. *The British Journal of Sociology*, *56*(4), 559–577.

Edwards, R. D. (2011). Changes in world inequality in length of life: 1970–2000. *Population and Development Review*, 37(3), 499-528.

Eisenstadt, S. N. (2017). *From generation to generation*. Routledge.

Egeland, C., & Gressgård, R. (2007). The "will to empower": Managing the complexity of the others. *NORA—Nordic Journal of Women's Studies*, *15*(4), 207–219.

Elder Jr., G. H. (1975). Age differentiation and the life course. *Annual Review of Sociology*, *1*(1), 165–190.

Fingerman, K. L., Pitzer, L. M., Chan, W., Birditt, K., Franks, M. M., & Zarit, S. (2011). Who gets what and why? Help middle-aged adults provide to parents and grown children. *Journals of Gerontology Series B: Psychological Sciences and Social Sciences*, *66*(1), 87–98.

Fischer, D. H. (1977). *Growing old in America*. Oxford University Press.

Garstka, T. A., Hummert, M. L., & Branscombe, N. R. (2005). Perceiving age discrimination in response to intergenerational inequity. *Journal of Social Issues*, *61*(2), 321–342.

George, L. K. (1993). Sociological perspectives on life transitions. *Annual Review of Sociology*, *19*(1), 353–373.

George, L. K., & Weiler, S. J. (1981). Sexuality in middle and late life: The effects of age, cohort, and gender. *Archives of General Psychiatry*, *38*(8), 919–923.

Gerbner, G. (1997). Gender and age in prime-time television.

Gilleard, C., & Higgs, P. (2002). The third age: Class, cohort or generation? *Ageing & Society*, *22*(3), 369–382.

Giddens, A. (1994). *Beyond left and right*. Polity Press.

Goffman, E. (2002). The presentation of self in everyday life. 1959. Garden City, NY, 259.

Gott, M., & Hinchliff, S. (2003). Barriers to seeking treatment for sexual problems in primary care: a qualitative study with older people. *Family Practice*, *20*(6), 690–695.

Gullette, M. M. (2004). *Aged by culture*. The University of Chicago Press.

Holmes, T., & Cartwright, S. (1993). Career change: Myth or reality? *Employee Relations*, *15*(6), 37–53.

Higgs, P., Hyde, M., Wiggins, R., & Blane, D. (2003a). Researching quality of life in early old age: The importance of the sociological dimension. *Social Policy & Administration*, *37*(3), 239–252.

Higgs, P., Mein, G., Ferrie, J., Hyde, M., & Nazroo, J. (2003b). Pathways to early retirement: Structure and agency in decision-making among British civil servants. *Ageing & Society*, *23*(6), 761–778.

Jackson, M. (2020). 2019 Wilkins–Bernal–Medawar lecture Life begins at 40: The demographic and cultural roots of the midlife crisis. *Notes and Records*, *74*(3), 345–364.

Kenalemang, L. M. (2022). Visual ageism and the subtle sexualisation of older celebrities in L'Oréal's advert campaigns: A multimodal critical discourse analysis. *Ageing & Society*, *42*(9), 2122–2139.

Kirkwood, T. B., & Austad, S. N. (2000). Why do we age? *Nature*, *408*(6809), 233–238.

Kinsey, A. C., Pomeroy, W. B., Martin, C. E., & Gebhard, P. H. (1998). *Sexual behavior in the human female*. Indiana University Press.

Koskinen, V., Ylilahti, M., & Wilska, T. A. (2017). "Healthy to heaven"—Middle-agers looking ahead in the context of wellness consumption. *Journal of Aging Studies*, *40*, 36–43.

Krueger, J., Heckhausen, J., & Hundertmark, J. (1995). Perceiving middle-aged adults: Effects of stereotype-congruent and incongruent information. *The Journals of Gerontology Series B: Psychological Sciences and Social Sciences*, 50(2), 82–93.
Lachman, M. E. (2004). Development in midlife. *Annual Review of Psychology*, *55*, 305–331.
Laz, C. (2003). Age embodied. *Journal of Aging Studies*, 17, 503–519.
Linton, R. (1936). The study of man: An introduction. New York: D. Appleton-Century.
Maddox, G. L. (1979). Sociology of later life. *Annual Review of Sociology*, *5*(1), 113–135.
Majeed, T., Forder, P., Mishra, G., & Byles, J. (2015). Women, work, and illness: A longitudinal analysis of workforce participation patterns for women beyond middle age. *Journal of Women's Health*, *24*(6), 455–465.
Merriam, S. (1978). Middle age: A review of the literature and its implications for educational intervention. *Adult Education*, *29*(1), 39–54.
McCabe, M. P., & Ricciardelli, L. A. (2004). Body image dissatisfaction among males across the lifespan: A review of past literature. *Journal of Psychosomatic Research*, *56*(6), 675–685.
Miller, R. A. (2012). Genes against aging. *Journals of Gerontology Series A: Biomedical Sciences and Medical Sciences*, *67*(5), 495–502.
Munnell, A. H., & Sass, S. A. (2008). *The decline of career employment*. Center for Retirement Research at Boston College.
Nosek, M., Kennedy, H. P., & Gudmundsdottir, M. (2010). Silence, stigma, and shame: A postmodern analysis of distress during menopause. *Advances in Nursing Science*, *33*(3), E24–E36.
Phillipson, C., Leach, R., Money, A., & Biggs, S. (2008). Social and cultural constructions of ageing: The case of the baby boomers. *Sociological Research Online*, *13*(3), 1–14.
Pietilä, I., & Ojala, H. (2011). Acting age in the context of health: Middle-aged working-class men talking about bodies and aging. *Journal of Aging Studies*, *25*(4), 380–389.
Rau, R., Soroko, E., Jasilionis, D., & Vaupel, J. W. (2008). Continued reductions in mortality at advanced ages. *Population and Development Review*, *34*(4), 747–768.
Riley, M. W. (1987). On the significance of age in sociology. *American Sociological Review*, *52*, 1–14.
Roy, A., & Harwood, J. (1997). Underrepresented, positively portrayed: Older adults in television commercials.
Ryder, N. B. (1985). The cohort as a concept in the study of social change. In *Cohort analysis in social research: Beyond the identification problem* (pp. 9–44). Springer New York.
Sawyer, A. M., & James, S. (2018). Are baby boomer women redefining retirement? *Sociology Compass*, *12*(10), e12625.
Sontag, S. (1972). The double standard of aging. *The Saturday Review*, *23*, 29–38.
Tergesen, A. (2023, July 31). *Catering to -our midlife crisis is a growing business*. WSJ. https://www.wsj.com/articles/midlife-crisis-money-business-companies-29dc2273
Thompson, E. H. (2008). Gender matters: Aging men's health. *Generations, 32*, 73–77.
Tiggemann, M. (2001). Effect of gender composition of school on body concerns in adolescent women. *International Journal of Eating Disorders*, *29*(2), 239–243.
Tiggemann, M. (2006). The role of media exposure in adolescent girls' body dissatisfaction and drive for thinness: Prospective results. Journal of social and clinical psychology, 25(5), 523-541
Vaupel, J. W. (2010). Biodemography of human ageing. *Nature*, *464*(7288), 536–542.

Watson, T. (2017). *Sociology, work and organisation*. Taylor & Francis.
Wethington, E., Kessler, R. C., & Pixley, J. E. (2005). *Turning points in adulthood*. na.
West, C., & Zimmerman, D. H. (1987). Doing gender. Gender & society, 1(2), 125-151.
Ylänne, V. (2015). Representations of ageing in the media. In *Routledge handbook of cultural gerontology* (pp. 369–376). Routledge.
Yu, Y., & Zhao, B. (2022). Can TikTok promote a healthier ageing paradigm? A case study of older digital celebrities from China. *Area*, *54*(2), 322–329.

5 Brain, Ageing and Maturity in Middle Adulthood

Masroor Jahan and Ashish Silswal

According to the definition of the *Cambridge English Dictionary*, a 'midlifer' is someone who is middle-aged – i.e., about 45–60 years old. *Encyclopaedia Britannica* states that middle age is arbitarary to some degree and varies from person to person. However, it is commonly stated that middle age lies between the ages of 40 and 60 years, and this is the definition according to the *Collins English Dictionary*. Thus, the general consensus is that a 'midlifer' or a middle aged person is someone who is between the age of 40 and 60 years.

Most of the literature on cognitive development and ageing has either focused on the period from infancy to young adulthood or on old age. Little attention has been given to middle age inspite of the fact that it is a distinct and important stage of life. Advances in research and our understanding of the brain and behaviour have made it quite clear that the seeds of various neuro-psychopathologies and brain diseases are sown years before the onset of symptoms. In future, with more advances in the cognitive neurosciences, we will be able to predict the neurocognitive ageing trajectory more accurately in early stages of life. It might then even be possible to cure various brain diseases with the help of pharmacological and non-pharmacological (psychotherapeutic) means, and more importantly, prevent diseases like Alzheimer's disease, dementia, mild cognitive impairment etc. Midlifers or middle-aged people will the prime target of such interventions. However, lots of research and in-depth understanding of the functioning of brain at midlife will be required to achieve such goals.

The Scope of Studying Brain and Cognitive Functions of Midlifers

Recently, we have seen a lot of rapid advances in uncovering and understanding the mysteries of the brain. This advance in brain science has also increased our understanding of cognitive functioning of people at all ages, including middle age. These advances indicate the brains abilities in terms of neuroplasticity and neurogenesis. Neuroplasticity is the ability of the brain to replenish itself, while neurogenesis is the ability of the brain to regenerate itself. If medical science is able to harness the true potential of neuroplasticity and neurogenesis in future, it might lead to cures for various brain diseases and neuropathologies and even put a halt to cognitive decline in later

DOI: 10.4324/9781003568360-6

stages of life. At present, it is hard to predict what impact our knowledge and understanding of brain will have on cognitive decline that occurs with age, but the future seems bright and promising.

Structural Brain Differences Present in Midlife

Overall, middle-aged adults have decreased structural brain integrity, with decreases in gray and white matter and small increases in tau tangles and amyloid plaques. However, much of the existing research on structural brain changes in middle age is based on cross-sectional studies. Additional longitudinal studies to show trajectories of brain change within individuals, particularly middle-aged adults, would enhance the discipline.

Grey Matter Declines

Several studies have found that grey matter volume decreases with age (Christova & Georgopoulos, 2023), and that cortical thinning is visible by middle age (Salat et al., 2004). The largest amounts of reductions in cortical grey matter have been reported by many in the prefrontal cortex and hippocampus (Salat et al., 2004; Raz et al., 2007), with the hippocampus deteriorating at an increasing pace with age (Raz et al., 2010; Nobis et al., 2019). Shrinkage of the association cortices, cerebellum, caudate and inferior temporal cortex has also been documented (Raz et al., 2005). Nonetheless, detailed investigation of individual trajectories of change has revealed significant individual variability in shrinkage rates, particularly in the lateral prefrontal cortex and cerebellum (Raz et al., 2010). Thus, while reductions are regularly documented on average, specific people may not exhibit this pattern of grey matter reduction in midlife. Individual variances may be caused by disparities in the enrichment and depletion factors that people have encountered.

White Matter Declines

Three methods have been employed to evaluate white matter integrity in middle-aged adults. First, midlife volumetric losses in white matter have been documented, with rapid, non-linear declines beginning in the forties (Ouyang et al., 2021). Prefrontal white matter, like grey matter, tends to change the most in comparison to other regions (Raz et al., 2005). Second, white matter hyperintensities (WMHs), which represent white matter injury, have been found to rise from young adulthood to old age (Roseborough et al., 2022). Third, evidence from diffusion tensor imaging shows that white matter water diffusivity rises with age (Pieciak et al., 2023). As a result, converging evidence suggests that some white matter deterioration occurs even in middle age.

β-amyloid Plaques and Neurofibrillary Tangles

The build-up and spread of β-amyloid plaques in the brain has been said to be an important characteristic of Alzheimer's disease (AD) (Hillen, 2019).

Many research studies have also suggested that substantial deposition of β-amyloid plaques is required, but that on its own it is not sufficient to develop Alzheimer's disease. Autopsy data suggest that a small percentage of cognitively healthy people also have amyloid plaques, and amyloid deposition has even been found postmortem in some healthy middle-aged individuals (Braak & Braak, 1991, 1997). Recently, the ability to image amyloid deposition in vivo has been available, and current evidence on middle-aged adults suggests that amyloid deposition increases dramatically between the ages of 30 and 89 years in cognitively normal people (Rodrigue et al., 2012). Greater levels of β-amyloid have been linked to poor episodic memory (Souto et al., 2021), abnormal neuronal activity during memory encoding (Kennedy et al., 2012), and dementia development (Volicer, 2020). Build-up of amyloid plaques in the brain is a slow process and it takes years to accumulate. This has led many researchers to speculate that amyloid deposition in the brain begins in midlife (Jack et al., 2013). This speculation has been supported by various autopsy reports. However, it is not yet very clear, and more research is needed to find out the association between midlife amyloid deposition and cognitive impairment or dementia.

Alzheimer's disease has also been characterised by the buildup of of tau neurofibrillary tangles across the neocortex (Braak & Braak, 1991, 1997). When autopsies are performed on patients suffering from Alzheimer's disease or mild cognitive Impairment, tau tangles are found in their brains (Guillozet et al., 2003), and the degree of tau deposition is substantially linked with decline in cognitive functioning and disease severity (Horie et al., 2020). Furthermore, autopsy data show that the initial focal deposits of neurofibrillary tangles can be discovered as early as age 25, with approximately 50% of people exhibiting these localized neurofibrillary tangles by age 55 (Braak et al., 2011). According to Rabin et al. (2022), tau tangles and cognitive deterioration are facilitated by the interaction between neuritic amyloid plaques and cerebral amyloid angiopathy. However, very little is known regarding the long-term impact of decreased tau levels on cognition throughout the lifespan. The recent development of new ligands that allow in vivo tau positron emission tomography (PET) imaging will allow scientists to explore the association between midlife tau levels and current and future cognitive health in greater depth. The newly developed tau PET imaging will allow scientists to investigate the interactions between amyloid, tau and dementia, as well as whether these are useful indicators in midlife.

Brain Structures That Are Relatively Preserved in Midlife

Despite broad recognition of age-related structural brain deterioration, not all neuronal structures are impacted equally. It has been found that the hippocampus exhibits significant age-related reductions even in midlife (Raz et al., 2005); on the other hand, primary sensory cortices such as the primary visual cortex have been found to be quite stable and have not shown significant deterioration with age (Raz et al., 2005; Salat et al., 2004). It has also been noticed that there is marked variability in the rate of deterioration in different brain structures. Various explanations for this observation have been proposed. One of the prime reasons is the possibility that brain degradation mirrors the developmental sequence of brain maturation (i.e., first in, last out; Ribot's law).

Neural Activity Patterns in Midlife

Literature on functional imaging talks about an interesting finding. There are research projects that report that when exposed to verbal material, left-lateralized activation is seen in young adults; on the other hand, bilateral patterns of neural activity are seen in the dorsolateral prefrontal cortex of older adults (Reuter-Lorenz & Cappell, 2008). This pattern is found in numerous tasks and is also found in the parietal cortices (Huang et al., 2012). According to the scaffolding theory of ageing and cognition (STAC) hypothesis, older people's recruitment of the extra hemisphere is a compensatory mechanism for maintaining cognitive function in the face of structural deterioration.

The age at which the shift from left-lateralized to bilateral activity happens during verbal encoding and working memory tasks is an intriguing and relevant subject about which little is known. According to the STAC model, the age at which individuals demonstrate a bilateral pattern may be a predictor of neural frailty, with those demonstrating earlier bilateral recruitment potentially experiencing higher rates of future cognitive decline. The findings of the Betula Aging Study support this notion. Pudas et al. (2014) predicted activation in the bilateral hippocampus and left inferior frontal gyrus during a word encoding test using both midlife memory performance and change in memory performance from middle to old age. According to the findings, memory performance in middle age predicted twice as much variance in functional data as memory change data predicted. The findings give solid evidence that middle-aged cognition and brain function can be used to predict future brain health. Because of its longitudinal structure and very early use of neuroimaging, the Betula dataset is expected to be a valuable resource in resolving these difficulties. However, limited cross-sectional data on this topic suggest that the age at which neural activity variations are identified varies depending on both the task type and the engaged brain networks.

Cognition in Midlife

While we sometimes equate ageing with cognitive deterioration (because of how the media portrays it), ageing does not always imply a deterioration in cognitive abilities. In fact, as we age, our tacit knowledge grows, our inductive reasoning ability increases, our verbal memory improves, our vocabulary expands, and other forms of practical thinking and skills also improve.

The Seattle Longitudinal Study (SLS) is one of the important studies that have focused on the cognitive abilities of adults. The study began in 1956 and study revealed some important aspects of the cognitive abilities of midlifers. Schaie and Willis have described the findings of these studies in the following words: 'We have generally shown that reliably replicable average age decrements in psychometric abilities do not occur prior to age 60, but that such reliable decrement can be found for all abilities by 74 years of age' (Schaie & Willis, 2010). Thus, according to them, cognitive decline begins by the sixth decade, and this deterioration increases progressively over time. On the other hand, Singh-Manoux et al. argued that significant losses in cognitive abilities can begin as early as age 45 (Singh-Manoux et al., 2012a). Many researchers have stated that individuals in middle age should take care of their cognitive health along with their physical health at this stage of life as both are linked to a great extent. Ignoring cognitive health will lead to deterioration of cognitive functioning, which will have an impact on both mental health and physical health. On the other hand, good physical health will act as a protective factor against cognitive deterioration in old age.

Another important source of longitudinal research data on midlife is the Midlife in the United States Studies (MIDUS). These studies began in 1994 and supported the notion that midlife is not completely stable and there are declines of different degrees in some cognitive as well as physical abilities. Decline has been observed in processing speed, often known as fluid intelligence. Physiological declines have been observed in lung capacity of midlifers as well as their muscle mass. However, these loses are compensated by expansion in knowledge and expertise as well as better emotional regulation. The authors of the study also proposed that the severity and extent of cognitive decline at this age can be reduced by continued cognitive focus and cognitive exercise.

Differences Present in Core Cognitive Abilities in Midlife

Middle age is often marked by modest reductions in fluid processing and increases in crystallized knowledge and experience (see, e.g., Lachman et al., 2014). Middle-aged adults are in the transition phase between young adulthood and old age, and their cognitive performance may be at its peak. Although they have had some reductions in fluid abilities, these declines have been quite mild, and middle-aged adults experience tremendous expansion in their knowledge base, which is anticipated to provide significant support to daily cognitive function. Indeed, research from the workplace suggests that people reach their career optimum in their fifties (Helson & Soto, 2005), perhaps because they have optimal levels of cognitive capacity as well as world knowledge and experience.

What follows is a summary of what is known about midlife cognition, emphasizing where variations are identified between longitudinal and cross-sectional research, each of which have their strengths and disadvantages. Because of re-test and dropout effects, longitudinal studies are likely to underestimate decline (see, e.g., Salthouse, 2009), but cross-sectional studies may overestimate age-related differences due to cohort effects and the inability to detect within-person change. This, combined with a wide variety of individual variances (see, e.g., Willis & Schaie, 2005), creates a complicated picture of midlife cognition. Furthermore, a study by Hartshorne and Germine (2015) found that different cognitive skills peak at different ages, with evidence for specific peaks occurring in midlife. As a result, cognitive developments are not homogeneous over the lifespan.

Processing Speed

Many longitudinal and cross-sectional studies show that processing speed decreases from adolescence to middle age to old age (Willis & Schaie, 1999; Park et al., 2002; Salthouse, 2009). MIDUS found fewer variations in processing speed between middle-aged and younger persons, but increased losses after age 65 (Soederberg Miller & Lachman, 2000). Thus, while processing speed reduces with age, midlife declines are not as severe as late-life declines.

Executive Functioning

Executive functioning deficits have also been seen in middle age. Middle-aged adults had poorer executive performance on novel experimental tasks than their younger counterparts (Garden et al., 2001; MacPherson et al., 2002). According to the limited longitudinal evidence available, only a minority of individuals demonstrate detectable midlife executive declines. The SLS specifically tested verbal fluency at ages 46, 53 and 60, and only 20% of participants experienced reductions; 69% remained steady; and 11% improved (Willis & Schaie, 2005). However, it must be noted that in longitudinal designs, repeated testing could mask some decline. Thus, whereas cross-sectional evidence implies that middle-aged people have more trouble performing higher-level mental manipulations like inhibiting, updating and shifting quickly and effectively, longitudinal data imply that the changes are more modest.

Working Memory

The results of cross-sectional data on working memory ability at midlife have mixed findings. Park et al. (2002) discovered decreases in line span, letter rotation, reading span and computation span as people moved from young to middle ages. Nonetheless, in a later investigation, middle-aged people performed similarly to younger adults on operation span and letter-number sequencing (Park et al., 2013). The disparity in these findings could be related to task difficulty differences, such as simple span activities naking fewer cognitive demands than sophisticated working memory tasks, or to differences in the sample being tested. Longitudinal evaluations of working memory in midlife are less common. Hultsch et al. (1992) demonstrated a three-year longitudinal deterioration in complex span tasks in a middle-aged adult population. Another longitudinal study found midlife reductions in listening span, although this decline was only seen in people with poor vascular health (Raz et al., 2007).

Episodic Memory

In comparison to young adults, middle-aged adults exhibit both deficits and improvements in episodic memory. Willis and Schaie (1999) discovered a peak in verbal memory at midlife, whereas Zelinski and Burnight (1997) found no longitudinal change in episodic list recall. Cross-sectional studies, on the other hand, have repeatedly demonstrated losses in episodic memory with age, even in middle age (Park et al., 2002; Mitchell & Bruss, 2003). The gap between cross-sectional and longitudinal findings could be attributed to both significant individual variability in memory ability and severe retest effects on memory tasks. First, Willis and Schaie (2005) discovered that 31% of their subjects deteriorated, 53% remained stable and 16% improved on delayed recall tests from ages 46 to 53 to 60. Second, retest effects on memory tasks are prevalent (Salthouse, 2009). Nonetheless, even when practice effects are taken into account, other research project have revealed no longitudinal decreases in midlife episodic memory (Ronnlund et al., 2005).

Implicit Memory

In midlife, implicit memory appears to be stable. There were no age differences between younger, middle-aged and old-aged people in cross-sectional implicit tests of word-fragment completion, word-stem completion and picture-fragment identification (Mitchell & Bruss, 2003). Additionally, similar patterns were found among young, midlife and old-aged people when behavioural and electrophysiological correlates of repetition priming were analysed (Hamberger & Friedman, 1992). Hultsch et al. (1992) found no deterioration in word-stem completion after three years, which appears to be consistent with these findings.

Spatial Processing

According to the Seattle Longitudinal Study, peak levels of spatial processing on mental rotation tasks were observed around midlife (Willis & Schaie, 1999). This finding was supported by the fact that 30–36-year-olds had increased spatial abilities on figure and object rotation 16 years later (Zelinski & Burnight, 1997). However, cross-sectionally, middle-aged people had inferior spatial processing than younger ones (Salthouse, 2009).

Reasoning

When it comes to reasoning performance in middle age, the results are mixed. Cross-sectional data show both stability (Soederberg Miller & Lachman, 2000) and deterioration (Salthouse, 2009). Willis and Schaie (1999) syudied peak inductive reasoning performance in midlife, and Zelinski and Burnight (1997) explored reasoning stability in persons aged 30–36 after 16 years. Nonetheless, longitudinal midlife reductions in fluid reasoning have been observed (Raz et al., 2007).

Problem Solving

Research on interpersonal problem solving ability shows that older people have more effective ways of dealing with social and emotional problems than younger people (Blanchard-Fields, 2007). There is no evidence that older people perform worse than their younger counterparts in occupational contexts (Park & Gutchess, 2000). However, there is some cognitive decline in midlife. Thus, to compensate for the loss or deterioration of such cognitive abilities, older workers use more effective strategies and more efficient tactics than their younger counterparts. Also, they rely more on their knowledge and experience, which further helps them in solving problems.

Social and Emotional Processing

According to some cross-sectional evidence, the ability to recognize emotions and make moral decisions is intact in midlife (MacPherson et al., 2002), and social reasoning increases with age (Spenser et al., 2020). However, Heidrich and Denney (1994) found that social problem solving abilities increased from ages 20 to 40, but then deteriorated. These discrepancies could be explained by the degree to which the social and emotional activities required fluid skills. Additional research should look into the causes of these disparities, as well as longitudinal midlife trajectories of social and emotional processing.

Crystallized Knowledge

Both longitudinal and cross-sectional studies show that crystallized intelligence remains stable or increases in middle age (Rönnlund et al., 2005; Park et al., 2013; Hartshorne & Germine, 2015), with middle-aged adults possessing high levels of semantic memory and general world knowledge. Middle-aged individuals, for example, have been demonstrated repeatedly to have superior vocabulary to younger people (Soederberg Miller & Lachman, 2000; Park et al., 2002). Continuing on this path, middle-aged adults can have a smaller vocabulary than older adults (Park et al., 2002). Nonetheless, middle-aged adults have higher levels of fluid processing than older adults, which may compensate for the gap in crystallized information.

Midlifers in Education

It is clear that some aspects of cognition deteriorate with age. For example, working memory and processing speed are not as efficient as they are in youth. However, losses in the efficiency of these abilities are compensated by using higher-order cognitive strategies. These strategies may consist of memory methods such as mnemonics, remembering by summarizing or by comparing concepts. Unlike young learners, older learners rely less on rote memorization (Lachman, 2004).

Older learners take more time to learn new material; however, once learned, it stays in their memory for long periods of time and they are less likely to forget it. Adult learners have the tendency to look for relevance and meaning in whatever they are learning. This is one of the reasons why adults find it difficult to learn material that is meaningless to them or they are not familiar with. Whenever they are given something to learn or they have to store something in their memory, they ask themselves, "Why is this important?" Older adults are task-oriented learners who want to structure their activities around problem solving.

Everyday Functioning

In real-world activities, middle-aged adults appear to have minimal deficits. Baltes et al. (1995), for example, demonstrated good performance on existential life planning and life management tasks up to the age of 80 years. Furthermore, Garden et al. (2001) discovered that middle-aged adults schedule and plan real-life tasks and errands more successfully than younger ones, breaching fewer task rules. This higher daily functioning is mirrored in their peak levels of work performance (Helson & Soto, 2005). On the other hand, Denney and Pearce (1989) discovered that everyday problem solving reduced around the age of 40 in tasks that relied more heavily on fluid processing. Overall, middle-aged persons perform well in everyday tasks when they can draw on their knowledge and experiences. However, additional longitudinal studies of everyday functioning in midlife are required to make more solid conclusions.

Does Cognition in Middle Age Predict Future Cognitive Function?

Several research projects have begun to investigate the influence of midlife cognition on future cognitive performance. Willis and Schaie (2005) found that midlife performance on delayed recall and word fluency predicted cognitive deterioration in old age. Furthermore, early midlife cognitive abnormalities may be a sign of preclinical dementia progression, as LaRue and Jarvik (1987) discovered that midlife cognitive deficiencies predicted dementia 20 years later. Data from the Lothian Birth Cohort showed that intelligence at age 11 was connected with improved cognition at age 79, but childhood mental ability was not related to the rate of late-life cognitive decline from 79 to 83 (Gow et al., 2008).

Additionally, according to Salthouse and Soubelet, within-individual variability in cognitive abilities at the time of initial testing may serve as a good predictor of the cognitive abilities the person will have in future. They also stated that it seems that within-individual variability is actually a better predictor of pathological changes than changes that are a part of the normal ageing process. In their research they found that those older adults who had greatest three- to four-year longitudinal decline in their cognitive abilities showed most variability in cognitive abilities at the time of initial testing (Salthouse & Soubelet, 2014).

Factors That Affect Brain Health

Brain health can be affected by many factors. Some of these are biological in nature, while others are contextual or based on the lifestyles of people. Thus, factors affecting brain health are classified as biologically based factors and contextually based lifestyle factors.

Biological Factors That Affect Brain Health

There are numerous biological factors that can influence brain form and function. The emphasis here is on biological factors in midlife that influence current and future cognitive and neurological performance. It is crucial to highlight, however, that certain factors interact with one another (e.g., people with poor vascular health may be more likely to develop diabetes, obesity and hypercholesterolemia).

Genes

Many researchers link the apolipoprotein E type 4 (APOE ε4) allele with poor cognitive abilities and the development of Alzheimer's disease in later stages of life (Raulin et al., 2022). The APOE ε4 allele is said to be linked with decline in some cognitive abilities such as spatial memory and visual spatial attention in midlife (Greenwood et al., 2014). Blair et al. (2005) stated that presence of the APOE ε4 allele is associated with cognitive deterioration that happens during midlife. White matter volume reductions were also reported in APOE ε4 carriers who were also homozygous TT for the cholinergic receptor gene CHRNA (Espeseth et al., 2006). Furthermore, when compared to older people, middle-aged persons with these genetic traits had significantly slower response times for invalid signals on a Posner attention task, indicating that these genetic differences had the greatest impact on attention during midlife. Furthermore, functional neuroimaging measurements revealed altered brain activation in APOE ε4 carriers in comparison to non-carriers, with evidence for both increases and decreases in activation. Filippini et al. (2009) discovered that juvenile APOE ε4 carriers showed higher brain activity during memory encoding and abnormally enhanced default mode activity at rest than non-carriers, implying that altered neural activity may persist until midlife. Furthermore, APOE ε4 carriers had reduced neural activation during a semantic categorization test in a sample of middle-aged adults (Lind et al., 2006). Individuals with particular genetic predispositions have shown changes in cognition, brain structure and neural function even in midlife.

Vascular Health

A common risk factor for impaired cognition and brain health is poor vascular health, which includes hypertension, atherosclerosis and arterial stiffness. Midlife hypertension has been linked to slower processing speed (Sun et al., 2020), poor block design (Elias et al., 2004) and faster WMH progression (Raz et al., 2007; Debette et al., 2011). High systolic blood pressure during middle age also contributes to poor brain health. Those who have high systolic blood pressure during midlife have greater chances of developing WMHs after ten years (Swan et al., 1998), as well as reduced cognitive performance 26 years later (Launer et al., 1995). Finally, neuroimaging studies during a two-back task found that middle-aged persons with poor vascular health, metabolic syndrome or increased arterial stiffness exhibited lower parietal and frontal brain activation (Haley, 2014).

Glucose Tolerance and Diabetes Mellitus

Impaired glucose tolerance at midlife can be one of the factors that may lead to deterioration in some important cognitive abilities and poor brain health. Diabetes that has its onset in midlife is associated with a loss in verbal fluency and processing speed (Blair et al., 2005), as well as a more rapid rise in temporal horn volume, which indicates hippocampal atrophy (Debette et al., 2011). Furthermore, middle-aged persons with poor glucose tolerance had a higher drop in regional blood flow to the frontal, parietal and temporal cortices than people with normal glucose tolerance (Thambisetty et al., 2013). Diabetes in midlife has been linked to an increased risk of mild cognitive impairment (You et al., 2021), all types of dementia (Dove et al., 2021), Alzheimer's disease (Yamada et al., 2003) and vascular dementia (Yamada et al., 2003) in later stages of life.

Weight

Obesity in middle age has also been linked to decreased executive function, visuomotor skills and memory (Debette et al., 2011). According to Singh-Manoux et al. (2012b), people with midlife obesity and metabolic abnormalities experienced the fastest deterioration in cognition after ten years. Furthermore, despite controlling for age, gender, education, blood pressure and diabetes, higher midlife body mass index (BMI) was related with inferior episodic memory (Cournot et al., 2006). Sabia et al. (2008), for example, indicated that being fat or underweight in early adulthood, early midlife or late midlife was associated with worse cognition in late midlife. After controlling for cardiovascular risk factors, obesity around the age of 40 years was linked to later-life cognition, whereas obesity around the age of 60 was not, showing that midlife obesity was more important. There are also weight-related structural alterations. In a middle-aged sample, for example, BMI was found to be independently linked with decreased brain volume (Ward et al., 2005).

Cholesterol

High cholesterol in middle age, like other risk factors, has been associated to cognitive impairment (Blair et al., 2005). High cholesterol during middle age has been found to be a significant risk factor for mild cognitive impairment (Yaffe et al., 2020). A research found found that midlifers who had elevated levels of cholesterol had reduced activation of the left inferior parietal lobe, right superior frontal gyrus and right middle frontal gyrus during a two-back task (Gonzales et al., 2011).

Depression

Persistent symptoms of depression in middle age appear to impair cognitive and neurological function. Extensive midlife depressive symptoms, in particular, were linked to lower late midlife memory, reasoning, vocabulary and fluency (Singh-Manoux et al., 2010). Furthermore, patients with major depressive disorder in midlife activated the hippocampus and anterior cingulate cortex less than controls during episodic encoding (Bremner et al., 2004). Thus, psychobiological mental health issues such as depression appear to alter cognition and brain function in midlife and later life. The directionality of the impacts, however, is uncertain, as altered brain and cognitive function may contribute to the development of a variety of mental health problems.

Lifestyle Factors That Affect Brain Health

Controllable and uncontrolled lifestyle factors, like biological factors, influence cognitive and brain health. Unlike biological variables, these lifestyle factors reflect personal preferences and societal impacts on daily life. While large longitudinal studies on lifestyle factors have not exclusively examined middle-aged individuals, decreases in lifestyle engagement in physical, social and cognitive activities predicted decreases in verbal speed, episodic memory and semantic memory in samples of both middle-aged and older adults (Small et al., 2012; Lachman et al., 2014). Thus, everyday involvement has been demonstrated to play a significant role in cognitive ageing; however, Small et al. (2012) noted that declines in cognitive abilities can also lead to decreasing lifestyle engagement.

Socioeconomic Status

People with low socioeconomic status (SES) who do not have equal access to certain enrichment elements (such as higher education), may face more daily stress and may have less time for leisure. As a result, low SES may reduce the impact of protective variables while exacerbating the impact of risk factors. For example, Singh-Manoux et al. (2008) discovered that atherosclerosis was linked with poor cognitive abilities only in those individuals who belonged to the lower strata of socioeconomic status. Thus it can be said that socioeconomic status of a person has the ability to influence the individual's risk of cognitive deterioration during midlife.

Education and Intellectual Engagement

It has been found that higher levels of education and intellectual activities can protect a person's cognitive abilities against cognitive decline due to ageing (Reuter-Lorenz & Park, 2014). An interesting fact is that education is most strongly linked with cognitive abilities during midlife itself (Mortensen et al., 2014). Thus, higher educational status and greater cognitive engagement of midlifers will protect them against age-related deterioration of cognitive abilities in later life. On the other hand low, educational levels and low engagement in cognitive tasks may lead to cognitive decline in later stages of life (Lachman et al., 2010).

Beliefs

Personal beliefs have also been connected to cognitive and functional differences. Middle-aged adults who believed that they had greater control over their cognitive abilities performed better in tests of reasoning abilities (Soederberg Miller & Lachman, 2000). Furthermore, higher perceived cognitive impairment was associated with lower frontal activity during a working memory task (Haley et al., 2011). While the findings of these studies are intriguing, the direction of causality is questionable because individual belief styles may be based on self-observed cognitive performance.

Social Engagement

Better cognition is connected with increased social engagement, and lower cognition is associated with social withdrawal (Small et al., 2012). Seeman et al. (2010) found that those with higher levels of social interaction had better executive function and episodic memory in a sample of adults aged 35–85. Maintaining social relationships appears to promote cognitive health even in midlife.

Stress

Stress and cognition in humans have an inverted-U connection, with moderate stress related with better cognition and excessive stress associated with poor cognition (Lupien et al., 2009). Greater levels of self-reported daily stress were consistently connected to lower performance on a complex episodic memory test that required executive functioning. The findings are consistent across different age groups. Midlifers who reported high levels of stress performed similarly to those who were 40 years older but reported low levels of stress.

Exercise

It has been found that indulging in some sort of physical activity or exercise during middle age will lead to better cognitive abilities and brain health, and it will also provide protection from cognitive deterioration in later stages of life (Erickson et al., 2022). A research project found that middle-aged individuals who were involved in higher levels of physical activity also had better executive control on a flanker task than middle-aged individuals who had low levels of physical activity (Hillman et al., 2006). Research has also shown that regular physical exercise has the ability to improve various cognitive abilities such as attention, higher executive functions, processing speed and memory (Randolph & Randolph, 2013). Physical activity during midlife has also been associated with larger brain volume and increased grey matter, particularly in the frontal lobes (Rovio et al., 2010). Thus, increased physical exercise and activity in midlife appear to boost overall cognition and help to maintain the structure of the brain.

Diet

Dietary variations have also been connected to cognitive health. Consumption of high saturated fat is linked to poor cognitive abilities. On the other hand, consuming high amounts of polyunsaturated fat does not cause cognitive impairment and is associated with better semantic memory (Eskelinen et al., 2008). Processing speed is negatively impacted by low levels of vitamin D in elderly as well as middle-aged people (Lee et al., 2009). Similarly, a vitamin-rich, low-fat diet may improve cognitive performance.

Sleep

Pain can have a negative impact on the amount and quality of sleep in middle-aged and elder people. It is difficult for a person to sleep if they are suffering from chronic pain. Also, pain can cause disruption of sleep many times in the middle of the night. Thus, a person suffering from pain may wake up not feeling refreshed even after sleeping for adequate amount of time. People who suffer from chronic pain have a sleep debt of about 42 minutes, and those with acute pain have a sleep debt of about 14 minutes. Stress and overall bad health are also important contributors to less overall sleep and low quality of sleep. Midlifers with low life satisfaction take longer to fall asleep than those who feel more satisfied with their life. There are various causes of sleep deprivation in midlife. Anxiety, day-to-day concerns and hassles and midlife challenges can lead to sleep deprivation in this age group. In middle-aged women, menopause can have a negative impact on their sleep duration and quality. Having children at home can also have an impact on sleep. Infants and toddlers have a tendency to disturb their parents' sleep, especially in the middle of the night. Inexperienced parents especially have a lot of concern for their children, and this negatively impacts the amount and quality of their sleep. This is truer if the responsibility for rearing a child falls on one particular parent. On the other hand, having a partner and sharing the responsibilities of rearing a child with them can lead to better sleep amount and quality.

According to most experts, having and undisturbed six to eight hours of sleep at night leads to better cognition. Sleeping less than six hours or more than eight hours can have a negative impact on a person's cognition. According to Randolph and Randolph (2013), middle-aged and elderly people who slept for more than eight hours or less than six hours each night had lower levels of cognitive abilities than those who slept for of six to eight hours each night. They found that middle-aged and elderly people who slept for six to eight hours each night had better reasoning abilities, semantic fluency and vocabulary (Randolph & Randolph, 2013).

Too little sleep can lead to a lot of negative impacts on an individual's physical as well as mental health. Physical complaints are common in people who sleep less as they are not able to provide adequate rest to their bodies. Lack of sleep can also lead to emotional problems in midlifers, reducing their emotional regulation and frustration tolerance abilities. Prolonged sleep deprivation can also have a negative impact on the immune system and might increase the risk of infections and diseases (Ferrie et al., 2007). Poor sleeping habits can also lead to changes in weight (especially obesity), impairment in memory and increase in blood pressure (Ferrie et al., 2007). Lack of sleep in middle age has also be said to be associated with various forms of cancers like colon cancer and breast cancer. Sleep deprivation is also associated with heart diseases and type 2 diabetes. It is said that lack of sleep is a stressful situation which leads to increases in the stress hormone of cortisol, which further keeps the body in an alert and aroused state, thereby keeping blood pressure high. Sleep is also linked with long life. It has been found that elderly people with better sleeping habits lived longer than those with poor sleeping habits (Dew et al., 2003). Growth hormone is secreted during deep sleep and leads to acceleration of protein synthesis, breakdown of fat for energy, and cell division. Thus, if there is sleep deprivation, there will be reduced release of growth hormone, reduced amounts of energy and reduced cell division. This will lead to reduced ability of the body to repair the wear and tear of everyday life. This will be reflected as signs of ageing.

In middle adulthood, sleep problems can also decrease glucose functioning. Glucose functioning is directly linked to metabolic health and diabetes risk. Middle-aged people are at a greater risk of suffering from diabetes. This risk is further enhanced by irregular sleeping patterns. Irregular sleep leads to irregular exposure to light, which can disturb the biological clock or circadian rhythm of a person. Disturbed circadian rhythm negatively affects glucose metabolism and energy homeostasis, which further lead to increased risk of diabetes and other health issues.

Smoking

Smoking in midlife has been linked to decreasing brain volume and an increased risk of WMH (Debette et al., 2011). Smokers exhibited poorer cognitive ability in midlife and a faster rate of deterioration five years later (Randolph & Randolph, 2013). As a result, smoking in midlife may hasten cognitive and neurological deterioration.

Alcohol

Alcohol has an effect on the brain via slowing or inhibiting communication between brain cells. Slurred speech, foggy memory, tiredness, and dizziness can result. Alcohol can also cause altered balance and coordination by affecting the cerebellum. Research has shown that chronic alcoholism can also lead to memory impairments. Also, long-term alcohol abuse can lead to disruption of emotional and social aspects of one's life. An alteration in body temperature in long alcoholics is also common. However, one can prevent these things by abstaining from alcohol or drinking in moderation. It is also true that as people age, they are at a greater risk of suffering from negative effects of alcohol than they would have been at a younger age. A similar dose of alcohol will have a greater negative impact on a middle-aged or older person than it will have on a younger person. Thus, midlifers should be more concerned about the detrimental effects of alcohol than their younger counterparts. In addition, several medications might be hazardous when taken with alcohol.

Some investigators have found a U-shaped relationship between consumption of alcohol during middle age and the probability of having mild cognitive impairment in later stages of life. On the other hand, some researchers found that only those alcoholics who had the apolipoprotein e4 allele had a greater risk of suffering from dementia at later stages in life (Chosy et al., 2022).

Social Isolation and Loneliness

Social isolation and loneliness also have a negative impact on mental health and cognitive abilities of a person during midlife. Middle-aged people who suffer from loneliness are at a greater risk of developing dementia in later stages of life, and lack of social activity during midlife can lead to poor cognitive functions in later stages of life. Being socially isolated and lonely during midlife is linked to poor cognition, with depression acting as a putative mediator between loneliness and poor cognition (Cardona & Andrés, 2023). According to several studies, the relationship between social isolation, loneliness and cognitive decline may be bidirectional.

Brain Injuries

Midlifers are also vulnerable to falls, automobile accidents and other events that might result in injury to the brain. Alcohol, psychotropic drugs and some medications can have a negative impact on a person's ability to drive safely, increasing the risk of an accident and brain injury. Motor vehicle accidents and occupational accidents are common in midlifers. These accidents can lead to brain injury, which may lead to loss of cognitive functions, temporarily or permanently.

Predicting Future Cognition

Individual differences in brain health at midlife must be understood in order to predict future cognitive ageing trajectories or to diagnose neuropathology. Continued research into individual differences in enrichment and depletion factors at middle age will help us understand how many different factors influence cognition early on and how deterministic they are of brain function and health. Overall, it is obvious that midlife cognitive neuroscience is complicated. Some cognitive capacities peak in middle age, while others begin to diminish. Some neural networks change between young adulthood and middle age, while others remain unchanged and are quite stable until old age. Furthermore, there are numerous individual differences. More research is needed to continue unravelling the subtle features of the complex and varied middle-aged brain, as brain health and function at midlife may prove to be a useful predictor of future cognition and illness.

Conclusion

Our brains undergo a multitude of changes as we age. Some of these changes are typical and anticipated, while others may indicate a concern. Many studies on cognitive ageing have mostly focused on the elderly. However, factors influencing brain form and function have long-term consequences that build throughout a lifetime. Middle age is frequently regarded as a time of little or no cognitive change. Midlife, on the other hand, is a time when many people begin to detect changes in their cognitive ability and overall brain function. A reduction in cognitive capacities is one of the most visible changes that many people face in their forties. This can be exhibited as forgetfulness, trouble concentrating or reduced processing speed. People in their forties and fifties frequently complain about their mental capacities, such as the fact that their minds don't function as quickly as they once did, that they are easily distracted and that they can't remember things like they used to. While these changes are natural and to some extent expected, there are a variety of variables that may lead to more serious cognitive decline, such as chronic stress, poor sleep, sedentary lifestyle, changes in brain chemistry and hormone balance. However, the middle-aged mind retains many of its youthful abilities and even develops some new ones. The human brain appears to be able to rewire itself well into middle age, taking decades of events and behaviours into consideration. There is an on-going potential for plasticity, reorganization and capacity preservation. We can also take various steps in order to take care of our cognitive health during midlife. Taking such steps will reduce the changes of any deterioration that may occur in later stages of life.

References

Baltes, P. B., Staudinger, U. M., Maercker, A., & Smith, J. (1995). People nominated as wise: A comparative study of wisdom-related knowledge. *Psychology and Aging*, *10*(2), 155–166.

Blair, C. K., Folsom, A. R., Knopman, D. S., Bray, M. S., Mosley, T. H., & Boerwinkle, E. (2005). APOE genotype and cognitive decline in a middle-aged cohort. *Neurology*, *64*(2), 268–276.

Blanchard-Fields, F. (2007). Everyday problem solving and emotion. *Current Directions in Psychological Science*, *16*(1), 26–31.

Braak, H., & Braak, E. (1991). Neuropathological stageing of Alzheimer-related changes. *Acta Neuropathologica*, *82*(4), 239–259.

Braak, H., & Braak, E. (1997). Frequency of stages of alzheimer-related lesions in different age categories. *Neurobiology of Aging*, *18*(4), 351–357.

Braak, H., Thal, D. R., Ghebremedhin, E., & Del Tredici, K. (2011). Stages of the pathologic process in alzheimer disease: Age categories from 1 to 100 years. *Journal of Neuropathology & Experimental Neurology*, *70*(11), 960–969.

Bremner, J. D., Vythilingam, M., Vermetten, E., Vaccarino, V., & Charney, D. S. (2004). Deficits in hippocampal and anterior cingulate functioning during verbal declarative memory encoding in midlife major depression. *American Journal of Psychiatry*, *161*(4), 637–645.

Cardona, M., & Andrés, P. (2023). Are social isolation and loneliness associated with cognitive decline in ageing? *Frontiers in Aging Neuroscience*, *15*, 1075563.

Chosy, E. J., Edland, S., Launer, L., & White, L. R. (2022). Midlife alcohol consumption and later life cognitive impairment: Light drinking is not protective and APOE genotype does not change this relationship. *PLoS One*, *17*(3), e0264575.

Christova, P., & Georgopoulos, A. P. (2023). Changes of cortical gray matter volume during development: A Human Connectome Project study. *Journal of Neurophysiology*, *130*(1), 117–122.

Cournot, M., Marquié, J. C., Ansiau, D., Martinaud, C., Fonds, H., Ferrières, J., & Ruidavets, J. B. (2006). Relation between body mass index and cognitive function in healthy middle-aged men and women. *Neurology*, *67*(7), 1208–1214.

Debette, S., Seshadri, S., Beiser, A., Au, R., Himali, J. J., Palumbo, C., Wolf, P. A., & DeCarli, C. (2011). Midlife vascular risk factor exposure accelerates structural brain aging and cognitive decline. *Neurology*, *77*(5), 461–468.

Denney, N. W., & Pearce, K. A. (1989). A developmental study of practical problem solving in adults. *Psychology and Aging*, *4*(4), 438–442.

Dew, M. A., Hoch, C. C., Buysse, D. J., Monk, T. H., Begley, A. E., Houck, P. R., Hall, M., Kupfer, D. J., & Reynolds, C. F. (2003). Healthy older adults' sleep predicts all-cause mortality at 4 to 19 years of follow-up. *Psychosomatic Medicine*, *65*(1), 63–73.

Dove, A., Shang, Y., Xu, W., Grande, G., Laukka, E. J., Fratiglioni, L., & Marseglia, A. (2021). The impact of diabetes on cognitive impairment and its progression to dementia. *Alzheimer's & Dementia*, *17*(11), 1769–1778.

Elias, P. K., Elias, M. F., Robbins, M. A., & Budge, M. M. (2004). Blood pressure-related cognitive decline. *Hypertension*, *44*(5), 631–636.

Erickson, K. I., Donofry, S. D., Sewell, K. R., Brown, B. M., & Stillman, C. M. (2022). Cognitive aging and the promise of physical activity. *Annual Review of Clinical Psychology*, *18*(1), 417.

Eskelinen, M. H., Ngandu, T., Helkala, E., Tuomilehto, J., Nissinen, A., Soininen, H., & Kivipelto, M. (2008). Fat intake at midlife and cognitive impairment later in life: A population-based CAIDE study. *International Journal of Geriatric Psychiatry*, *23*(7), 741–747.

Espeseth, T., Greenwood, P. M., Reinvang, I., Fjell, A. M., Walhovd, K. B., Westlye, L. T., Wehling, E., Lundervold, A., Rootwelt, H., & Parasuraman, R. (2006). Interactive effects of APOE and CHRNA4 on attention and white matter volume in healthy middle-aged and older adults. *Cognitive, Affective, & Behavioral Neuroscience*, *6*(1), 31–43.

Ferrie, J. E., Shipley, M. J., Cappuccio, F. P., Brunner, E., Miller, M. A., Kumari, M., & Marmot, M. G. (2007). A prospective study of change in sleep duration: Associations with mortality in the Whitehall II cohort. *Sleep*, *30*(12), 1659–1666.

Filippini, N., MacIntosh, B. J., Hough, M. G., Goodwin, G. M., Frisoni, G. B., Smith, S. M., Matthews, P. M., Beckmann, C. F., & Mackay, C. E. (2009). Distinct patterns of brain activity in young carriers of the *APOE* -ε4 allele. *Proceedings of the National Academy of Sciences*, *106*(17), 7209–7214.

Garden, S. E., Phillips, L. H., & MacPherson, S. E. (2001). Midlife aging, open-ended planning, and laboratory measures of executive function. *Neuropsychology*, *15*(4), 472–482.

Gonzales, M. M., Tarumi, T., Eagan, D. E., Tanaka, H., Biney, F. O., & Haley, A. P. (2011). Current serum lipoprotein levels and fMRI response to working memory in midlife. *Dementia and Geriatric Cognitive Disorders*, *31*(4), 259–267.

Gow, A. J., Johnson, W., Pattie, A., Whiteman, M. C., Starr, J., & Deary, I. J. (2008). Mental ability in childhood and cognitive aging. *Gerontology*, *54*(3), 177–186.

Greenwood, P. M., Espeseth, T., Lin, M.-K., Reinvang, I., & Parasuraman, R. (2014). Longitudinal change in working memory as a function of APOE genotype in midlife and old age. *Scandinavian Journal of Psychology*, *55*(3), 268–277.

Guillozet, A. L., Weintraub, S., Mash, D. C., & Mesulam, M. M. (2003). Neurofibrillary tangles, amyloid, and memory in aging and mild cognitive impairment. *Archives of Neurology*, *60*(5), 729.

Haley, A. P. (2014). Vascular functions and brain integrity in midlife: Effects of obesity and metabolic syndrome. *Advances in Vascular Medicine*, *2014*, 1–7.

Haley, A. P., Eagan, D. E., Gonzales, M. M., Biney, F. O., & Cooper, R. A. (2011). Functional magnetic resonance imaging of working memory reveals frontal hypoactivation in middle-aged adults with cognitive complaints. *Journal of the International Neuropsychological Society*, *17*(5), 915–924.

Hamberger, M., & Friedman, D. (1992). Event-related potential correlates of repetition priming and stimulus classification in young, middle-aged, and older adults. *Journal of Gerontology*, *47*(6), P395–P405.

Hartshorne, J. K., & Germine, L. T. (2015). When does cognitive functioning peak? The asynchronous rise and fall of different cognitive abilities across the life span. *Psychological Science*, *26*(4), 433–443.
Heidrich, S. M., & Denney, N. W. (1994). Does social problem solving differ from other types of problem solving during the adult years? *Experimental Aging Research*, *20*(2), 105–126.
Helson, R., & Soto, C. J. (2005). Up and down in middle age: Monotonic and nonmonotonic changes in roles, status, and personality. *Journal of Personality and Social Psychology*, *89*(2), 194–204.
Hillen, H. (2019). The Beta Amyloid Dysfunction (BAD) hypothesis for Alzheimer's disease. *Frontiers in Neuroscience*, *13*, 1154.
Hillman, C. H., Motl, R. W., Pontifex, M. B., Posthuma, D., Stubbe, J. H., Boomsma, D. I., & de Geus, E. J. C. (2006). Physical activity and cognitive function in a cross-section of younger and older community-dwelling individuals. *Health Psychology*, *25*(6), 678–687.
Horie, K., Barthélemy, N. R., Sato, C., & Bateman, R. J. (2020). CSF tau microtubule binding region identifies tau tangle and clinical stages of Alzheimer's disease. *Brain*, *144*(2), 515–527.
Huang, C.-M., Polk, T. A., Goh, J. O., & Park, D. C. (2012). Both left and right posterior parietal activations contribute to compensatory processes in normal aging. *Neuropsychologia*, *50*(1), 55–66.
Hultsch, D. F., Hertzog, C., Small, B. J., McDonald-Miszczak, L., & Dixon, R. A. (1992). Short-term longitudinal change in cognitive performance in later life. *Psychology and Aging*, *7*(4), 571–584.
Jack, C. R., Knopman, D. S., Jagust, W. J., Petersen, R. C., Weiner, M. W., Aisen, P. S., Shaw, L. M., Vemuri, P., Wiste, H. J., Weigand, S. D., Lesnick, T. G., Pankratz, V. S., Donohue, M. C., & Trojanowski, J. Q. (2013). Tracking pathophysiological processes in Alzheimer's disease: An updated hypothetical model of dynamic biomarkers. *The Lancet Neurology*, *12*(2), 207–216.
Kennedy, K. M., Rodrigue, K. M., Devous, M. D., Hebrank, A., Bischof, G. N., & Park, D. C. (2012). Effects of beta-amyloid accumulation on neural function during encoding across the adult lifespan. *NeuroImage*, *62*(1), 1–8.
La Rue, A., & Jarvik, L. F. (1987). Cognitive function and prediction of dementia in old age. *The International Journal of Aging and Human Development*, *25*(2), 79–89.
Lachman, M. E. (2004). Development in midlife. *Annual Review of Psychology*, *55*(1), 305–331.
Lachman, M. E., Agrigoroaei, S., Murphy, C., & Tun, P. A. (2010). Frequent cognitive activity compensates for education differences in episodic memory. *The American Journal of Geriatric Psychiatry*, *18*(1), 4–10.
Lachman, M. E., Teshale, S., & Agrigoroaei, S. (2014). Midlife as a pivotal period in the life course. *International Journal of Behavioral Development*, *39*(1), 20–31.
Launer, L. J., Masaki, K., Petrovitch, H., Foley, D., & Havlik, R. J. (1995). The association between midlife blood pressure levels and late-life cognitive function. The Honolulu-Asia aging study. *JAMA*, *274*(23), 1846–1851.
Lee, D. M., Tajar, A., Ulubaev, A., Pendleton, N., O'Neill, T. W., O'Connor, D. B., Bartfai, G., Boonen, S., Bouillon, R., Casanueva, F. F., Finn, J. D., Forti, G., Giwercman, A., Han, T. S., Huhtaniemi, I. T., Kula, K., Lean, M. E. J., Punab, M., Silman, A. J., & Vanderschueren, D. (2009). Association between 25-hydroxyvitamin D levels and cognitive performance in middle-aged and older European men. *Journal of Neurology, Neurosurgery & Psychiatry*, *80*(7), 722–729.
Lind, J., Persson, J., Ingvar, M., Larsson, A., Cruts, M., Van Broeckhoven, C., Adolfsson, R., Bäckman, L., Nilsson, L.-G., Petersson, K. M., & Nyberg, L. (2006).

Reduced functional brain activity response in cognitively intact apolipoprotein E ε4 carriers. *Brain*, *129(5)*, 1240–1248.
Lupien, S. J., McEwen, B. S., Gunnar, M. R., & Heim, C. (2009). Effects of stress throughout the lifespan on the brain, behaviour and cognition. *Nature Reviews Neuroscience*, *10*(6), 434–445.
MacPherson, S. E., Phillips, L. H., & Della Sala, S. (2002). Age, executive function, and social decision making: A dorsolateral prefrontal theory of cognitive aging. *Psychology and Aging*, *17*(4), 598–609.
Mitchell, D. B., & Bruss, P. J. (2003). Age differences in implicit memory: Conceptual, perceptual, or methodological? *Psychology and Aging*, *18*(4), 807–822.
Mortensen, E. L., Flensborg-Madsen, T., Molbo, D., Fagerlund, B., Christensen, U., Lund, R., Osler, M., & Avlund, K. (2014). The relationship between cognitive ability and demographic factors in late midlife. *Journal of Aging and Health*, *26*(1), 37–53.
Nobis, L., Manohar, S. G., Smith, S. M., Alfaro-Almagro, F., Jenkinson, M., Mackay, C. E., & Husain, M. (2019). Hippocampal volume across age: Nomograms derived from over 19,700 people in UK Biobank. *NeuroImage: Clinical*, *23*, 101904.
Ouyang, Y., Cui, D., Yuan, Z., Liu, Z., Jiao, Q., Yin, T., & Qiu, J. (2021). Analysis of age-related white matter microstructures based on diffusion tensor imaging. *Frontiers in Aging Neuroscience*, *13*, Article 664911.
Park, D. C., & Gutchess, A. H. (2000). Cognitive aging and everyday life. In D. C. Park & N. Schwarz (Eds.), *Cognitive aging: A primer* (pp. 217–232). Psychology Press.
Park, D. C., Lautenschlager, G., Hedden, T., Davidson, N. S., Smith, A. D., & Smith, P. K. (2002). Models of visuospatial and verbal memory across the adult life span. *Psychology and Aging*, *17*(2), 299–320.
Park, H., Kennedy, K. M., Rodrigue, K. M., Hebrank, A., & Park, D. C. (2013). An fMRI study of episodic encoding across the lifespan: Changes in subsequent memory effects are evident by middle-age. *Neuropsychologia*, *51*(3), 448–456.
Pieciak, T., Guillem París, Beck, D., Maximov, I. I., Tristán-Vega, A., Rodrigo de Luis-García, Westlye, L. T., & Aja-Fernandez, S. (2023). Spherical means-based free-water volume fraction from diffusion MRI increases non-linearly with age in the white matter of the healthy human brain. *NeuroImage*, *279*, 120324–120324.
Pudas, S., Persson, J., Nilsson, L.-G., & Nyberg, L. (2014). Midlife memory ability accounts for brain activity differences in healthy aging. *Neurobiology of Aging*, *35*(11), 2495–2503.
Rabin, J. S., Nichols, E., Renaud La Joie, Aslanyan, V., Priya Palta, Dams-O'Connor, K., Kumar, R. G., George, K. M., Satizábal, C. L., Schneider, J. A., Pa, J., & Brickman, A. M. (2022). Cerebral amyloid angiopathy interacts with neuritic amyloid plaques to promote tau and cognitive decline. *Brain*, *145*(8), 2823–2833.
Randolph, J. S., & Randolph, J. J. (2013). *Modifiable lifestyle factors and cognition through midlife* (pp. 25–55). Springer EBooks.
Raulin, A.-C., Doss, S. V., Trottier, Z. A., Ikezu, T. C., Bu, G., & Liu, C.-C. (2022). ApoE in Alzheimer's disease: Pathophysiology and therapeutic strategies. *Molecular Neurodegeneration*, *17*(1), Article No. 72.
Raz, N., Ghisletta, P., Rodrigue, K. M., Kennedy, K. M., & Lindenberger, U. (2010). Trajectories of brain aging in middle-aged and older adults: Regional and individual differences. *NeuroImage*, *51*(2), 501–511.
Raz, N., Lindenberger, U., Rodrigue, K. M., Kennedy, K. M., Head, D., Williamson, A., Dahle, C., Gerstorf, D., & Acker, J. D. (2005). Regional brain changes in aging healthy adults: General trends, individual differences and modifiers. *Cerebral Cortex*, *15*(11), 1676–1689.

Raz, N., Rodrigue, K. M., Kennedy, K. M., & Acker, J. D. (2007). Vascular health and longitudinal changes in brain and cognition in middle-aged and older adults. *Neuropsychology, 21*(2), 149–157.

Reuter-Lorenz, P. A., & Cappell, K. A. (2008). Neurocognitive aging and the compensation hypothesis. *Current Directions in Psychological Science, 17*(3), 177–182.

Reuter-Lorenz, P. A., & Park, D. C. (2014). How does it STAC up? Revisiting the scaffolding theory of aging and cognition. *Neuropsychology Review, 24*(3), 355–370.

Rodrigue, K. M., Kennedy, K. M., Devous, M. D., Rieck, J. R., Hebrank, A. C., Diaz-Arrastia, R., Mathews, D., & Park, D. C. (2012). Amyloid burden in healthy aging: Regional distribution and cognitive consequences. *Neurology, 78*(6), 387–395.

Rönnlund, M., Nyberg, L., Bäckman, L., & Nilsson, L.-G. (2005). Stability, growth, and decline in adult life span development of declarative memory: Cross-sectional and longitudinal data from a population-based study. *Psychology and Aging, 20*(1), 3–18.

Roseborough, A. D., Saad, L., Goodman, M., Cipriano, L. E., Hachinski, V. C., & Whitehead, S. N. (2022). White matter hyperintensities and longitudinal cognitive decline in cognitively normal populations and across diagnostic categories: A meta-analysis, systematic review, and recommendations for future study harmonization. *Alzheimer's & Dementia, 15*, e12501.

Rovio, S., Spulber, G., Nieminen, L. J., Niskanen, E., Winblad, B., Tuomilehto, J., Nissinen, A., Soininen, H., & Kivipelto, M. (2010). The effect of midlife physical activity on structural brain changes in the elderly. *Neurobiology of Aging, 31*(11), 1927–1936.

Sabia, S., Kivimaki, M., Shipley, M. J., Marmot, M. G., & Singh-Manoux, A. (2008). Body mass index over the adult life course and cognition in late midlife: the Whitehall II Cohort Study. *The American Journal of Clinical Nutrition, 89*(2), 601–607.

Salat, D. H., Buckner, R. L., Snyder, A. Z., Greve, D. N., Desikan, R. S. R., Busa, E., Morris, J. C., Dale, A. M., & Fischl, B. (2004). Thinning of the cerebral cortex in aging. *Cerebral Cortex, 14*(7), 721–730.

Salthouse, T. A. (2009). When does age-related cognitive decline begin? *Neurobiology of Aging, 30*(4), 507–514.

Salthouse, T. A., & Soubelet, A. (2014). Heterogeneous ability profiles may be a unique indicator of impending cognitive decline. *Neuropsychology, 28*(5), 812–818.

Schaie, K. W., & Willis, S. L. (2010). The Seattle longitudinal study of adult cognitive development. *ISSBD Bulletin, 57*(1), 24–29.

Seeman, T. E., Miller-Martinez, D. M., Stein Merkin, S., Lachman, M. E., Tun, P. A., & Karlamangla, A. S. (2010). Histories of social engagement and adult cognition: Midlife in the U.S. study. *The Journals of Gerontology Series B: Psychological Sciences and Social Sciences, 66B*(Supplement 1), i141–i152.

Singh-Manoux, A., Akbaraly, T. N., Marmot, M., Melchior, M., Ankri, J., Sabia, S., & Ferrie, J. E. (2010). Persistent depressive symptoms and cognitive function in late midlife. *The Journal of Clinical Psychiatry, 71*(10), 1379–1385.

Singh-Manoux, A., Britton, A., Kivimaki, M., Guéguen, A., Halcox, J., & Marmot, M. (2008). Socioeconomic status moderates the association between carotid intima-media thickness and cognition in midlife: Evidence from the Whitehall II study. *Atherosclerosis, 197*(2), 541–548.

Singh-Manoux, A., Czernichow, S., Elbaz, A., Dugravot, A., Sabia, S., Hagger-Johnson, G., Kaffashian, S., Zins, M., Brunner, E. J., Nabi, H., & Kivimaki,

M. (2012a). Obesity phenotypes in midlife and cognition in early old age: The Whitehall II cohort study. *Neurology*, *79*(8), 755–762.
Singh-Manoux, A., Kivimaki, M., Glymour, M. M., Elbaz, A., Berr, C., Ebmeier, K. P., Ferrie, J. E., & Dugravot, A. (2012b). Timing of onset of cognitive decline: Results from Whitehall II prospective cohort study. *BMJ*, *344*(4), d7622–d7622.
Small, B. J., Dixon, R. A., McArdle, J. J., & Grimm, K. J. (2012). Do changes in lifestyle engagement moderate cognitive decline in normal aging? Evidence from the Victoria longitudinal study. *Neuropsychology*, *26*(2), 144–155.
Soederberg Miller, L. M., & Lachman, M. E. (2000). Cognitive performance and the role of control beliefs in midlife. *Aging, Neuropsychology, and Cognition*, *7*(2), 69–85.
Souto, J. J., Silva, G. M., Almeida, N. L., Shoshina, I. I., Santos, N. A., & Fernandes, T. P. (2021). Age-related episodic memory decline and the role of amyloid-β: A systematic review. *Dementia & Neuropsychologia*, *15*(3), 299–313.
Spenser, K., Bull, R., Betts, L., & Winder, B. (2020). Underpinning prosociality: Age related performance in theory of mind, empathic understanding, and moral reasoning. *Cognitive Development*, *56*, 100928.
Sun, D., Thomas, E. A., Launer, L. J., Sidney, S., Yaffe, K., & Fornage, M. (2020). Association of blood pressure with cognitive function at midlife: A Mendelian randomization study. *BMC Medical Genomics*, *13*(1), 121.
Swan, G. E., DeCarli, C., Miller, B. L., Reed, T., Wolf, P. A., Jack, L. M., & Carmelli, D. (1998). Association of midlife blood pressure to late-life cognitive decline and brain morphology. *Neurology*, *51*(4), 986–993.
Thambisetty, M., Beason-Held, L. L., An, Y., Kraut, M. A., Metter, J., Egan, J. M., Ferrucci, L., O'Brien, R., & Resnick, S. M. (2013). Impaired glucose tolerance in midlife and longitudinal changes in brain function during aging. *Neurobiology of Aging*, *34*(10), 2271–2276.
Volicer, L. (2020). Physiological and pathological functions of beta-amyloid in the brain and alzheimer's disease: A review. *Chinese Journal of Physiology*, *63*(3), 95.
Ward, M. A., Carlsson, C. M., Trivedi, M. A., Sager, M. A., & Johnson, S. C. (2005). The effect of body mass index on global brain volume in middle-aged adults: A cross sectional study. *BMC Neurology*, *5*, 23.
Willis, S. L., & Schaie, K. W. (1999). Intellectual functioning in midlife. In S. L. Willis & J. D. Reid (Eds.), *Life in the middle: Psychological and social development in middle age* (pp. 233–247). Academic Press.
Willis, S. L., & Schaie, K. W. (2005). Cognitive trajectories in midlife and cognitive functioning in old age. In S. L. Willis & M. Martin (Eds.), *Middle adulthood: A lifespan perspective* (pp. 243–275). Sage Publications, Inc.
Yaffe, K., Bahorik, A. L., Hoang, T. D., Forrester, S., Jacobs, D. R., Lewis, C. E., Lloyd-Jones, D. M., Sidney, S., & Reis, J. P. (2020). Cardiovascular risk factors and accelerated cognitive decline in midlife: The CARDIA study. *Neurology*, *95*(7), e839–e846.
Yamada, M., Kasagi, F., Sasaki, H., Masunari, N., Mimori, Y., & Suzuki, G. (2003). Association between dementia and midlife risk factors: The radiation effects research foundation adult health study. *Journal of the American Geriatrics Society*, *51*(3), 410–414.
You, Y., Liu, Z., Chen, Y., Xu, Y., Qin, J., Guo, S., Huang, J., & Tao, J. (2021). The prevalence of mild cognitive impairment in type 2 diabetes mellitus patients: A systematic review and meta-analysis. *Acta Diabetologica*, *58*(6), 671–685.
Zelinski, E. M., & Burnight, K. P. (1997). Sixteen-year longitudinal and time lag changes in memory and cognition in older adults. *Psychology and Aging*, *12*(3), 503–513.

PART II

The Experience of the Intra- and Interpersonal Spaces

Some Crucial Insights

6 Attachment, Intimacy and Close Relationships in Midlife

Poulomi Bhar, Sweta Sah and Subrata Dasgupta

Attachment refers to the emotional bond that we form with our significant others. Intimacy refers to the deep emotional connection we feel with our close friends and family members. Close relationships provide us with love, support and a sense of belonging. They can also help us to cope with stress and difficult life events. Intimacy is more than just physical in nature; it also entails psychological closeness. According to research, having a single confidante – a person with whom we can be authentic and whom we can trust by not exploiting our secrets and vulnerabilities – is more important to happiness than having a large social network (Taylor, 2010). Midlife is a time of significant change and transition. Many people experience changes in their careers, their relationships and their health. These changes can put a strain on our close relationships. Usually after marriage in young adulthood, the marital quality remains high and couples have abundant time for themselves to devote all their resources to each other. As the marriage progresses, after few years of parenting, there is some evidence for a regression to a hedonic set-point: that is, most individuals have a set happiness point or level, and both good and bad life events – marriage, bereavement, unemployment, births and so on – have some effect for a period of time; but over many months, they will return to that set-point. One of the best studies in this area is that of Luhmann et al. (2012), who report a gradual decline in subjective wellbeing after a few years, especially in the component of affective wellbeing. In some cases, adverse events obviously have an effect on subjective wellbeing and happiness, and these effects can be stronger than the positive effects of being married (Lucas, 2005). Also, there is another phenomenon through which midlife challenges can be aggravated: empty nest syndrome. This involves feelings of sadness, anxiety and loss that some parents and caregivers feel when their grown children move out of the home.

Empty nest syndrome is not a medical or psychiatric health condition, but it can lead to mental health issues, such as depression and anxiety. However, the symptoms are not always negative: in some cases, a sense of relief and excitement about a new episode of having me/we time can also be part of the empty nest experience. Also, children may sometimes return

DOI: 10.4324/9781003568360-8

to the family for renewed support after a difficult launch into adulthood; these are described as "boomerang children". Altogether, these factors can create midlife crisis, which sums up the overall emotional, physical and social conflicts as middle-aged adults face a developmental transition (Kim et al., 2014). However, midlife can also be a time of great personal growth and transformation. As we age, we may become more secure in our attachments, more intimate with our loved ones, and more appreciative of our close relationships. A recent study indicates that our close connections during our middle years of life are influenced by a variety of factors, including our attachment style, gender and life experiences. Attachment style is one of the most important predictors of the quality of our close relationships. Securely attached individuals tend to have more satisfying and stable relationships than insecurely attached individuals. They are more likely to trust their partners, to feel comfortable expressing their emotions and to resolve conflict in a constructive way. Gender also plays a role in the quality of our close relationships in midlife. Women value intimacy in relationships more than men do, and they also tend to communicate their emotions more than men do. Conversely, males value independence in relationships more than women do, and they have a tendency to be more physically affectionate. Life experiences also shape the quality of our close relationships in midlife. Individuals with experience of trauma or loss in their lives may have difficulty forming or maintaining close relationships.Attachment theory provides a useful framework for understanding the development and maintenance of close relationships in midlife. According to attachment theory, our early relationships with our primary caregivers shape our attachment style, which in turn influences our expectations and behaviours in our adult relationships.

One hypothesis of human social-emotional development is attachment theory. According to John Bowlby (1969, 1973, 1980), human infants are born with an "attachment behavioural system" that helps them to maintain proximity to the primary attachment figure. Attachment behaviours include crying, reaching, smiling and crawling. Attachment behaviour is evolutionary adaptive behaviour, according to Bowlby, because it has protected us from predators in our "environment of evolutionary adaptiveness". Additionally, he has alluded to the potential for the infant to pick up certain survival skills from its attachment figure or figures (Bowlby, 1969/1989). The infant forms a mental image of these relationships based on consistent interaction with its attachment figures. These mental images are what Bowlby (1973, 1980) called "internal working models", highlighting their dynamic ("working") character (see also Crittenden, 1990). The models get increasingly sophisticated as cognitive capacity rises. One-year-old infants' internal working models of attachment relationships and individual differences in attachment behaviour were originally identified by Mary Ainsworth (Ainsworth, et al., 1978). Three forms of attachment were identified by Ainsworth et al. (1978): anxious-ambivalent (C), anxious-avoidant (A) and secure (also known as

B). A fourth category, anxious-disorganized (D), has been identified through subsequent study (Main & Solomon, 1986, 1990).

Dominant Attachment Styles (Secure, Avoidant, Anxious and Disorganized Style) Developed in Childhood and their Interplay in Midlife

In childhood, parents typically serve as the primary attachment figures for a child, but as adolescence unfolds, attachment shifts toward other figures. Within partner relationships, individuals develop behavioral patterns based on their learned attachment styles. Consequently, both the parental–filial bond and the couple relationship share fundamental aspects, constituting forms of attachment. Adulthood witnesses the pursuit of new attachment figures, driven by social and sexual maturation, making partner relationships conducive to attachment development. The adult attachment system operates by seeking proximity early in a relationship and influencing partner selection through internal working models. Dysfunctional attachment can induce stress and anxiety. However, the healthiness of couple bonds varies based on the attachment styles within the relationship. Couples, as distinct social entities from families, serve various functions in society and adhere to societal and historical norms and expectations.

In early adulthood (ages 20–40), individuals may engage in intimate relationships that are often transient. During middle adulthood (ages 40–65), couple dynamics commonly involve conflicts arising from the dual responsibilities of caring for both children and ageing parents. As the years progress, children marry and move out, leaving the nest empty. It is widely recognized that individuals with secure attachments typically experience higher levels of satisfaction and engagement in their relationships, whereas those with insecure attachments tend to exhibit greater dissatisfaction. Insecure attachment styles often correlate with ineffective affective communication; individuals with anxious attachments may resort to defensive aggression when resolving conflicts, while those with avoidant attachments tend to avoid conflict resolution altogether. Additionally, attachment styles influence attitudes, emotions and behavioural strategies within relationships; for instance, individuals with anxious attachments often perceive more conflict, leading to increased stress and diminished relationship quality due to a loss of closeness and satisfaction.

Brennan et al. (1998) and; Karantzas et al. (2010) discovered two primary dimensions concerning adult attachment patterns. One key aspect, termed attachment-related anxiety, reflects individuals' concerns about their partners' availability, responsiveness and attentiveness. Those scoring high on this dimension tend to worry about these aspects, while those scoring low feel more secure in their partners' responsiveness. The second significant aspect is attachment-related avoidance, which pertains to individuals' preferences regarding reliance and openness with others. Those scoring high on this dimension are less inclined to depend on others or open up, whereas those scoring low are more comfortable with intimacy and mutual dependency. A typical secure adult exhibits low scores on both dimensions.

This pattern is also reflected in the four-category model of adult attachment, provided by Bartholomew and Horowitz (1991). This model represents the four attachment styles – secure, fearful-avoidant, dismissing-avoidant and preoccupied – in a two-dimensional space, anchored by the dimensions of attachment anxiety and avoidance.

Recent studies on adult attachment have uncovered intriguing complexities regarding the interplay between avoidance and defence. While some avoidant adults, often termed fearful-avoidant adults, struggle with adjustment despite their defensive tendencies, others, known as dismissing-avoidant adults, exhibit adaptive use of defensive strategies. For instance, in an experimental scenario where adults discussed the prospect of losing their partner, Fraley and Shaver (1997) observed that dismissing individuals (those high in attachment-related avoidance but low in attachment-related anxiety) showed similar physiological distress levels, measured via skin conductance, as other individuals. However, when instructed to suppress their thoughts and feelings, dismissing individuals effectively complied. They managed to deactivate their physiological arousal to some extent and reduce their focus on attachment-related thoughts. In contrast, fearful-avoidant individuals were less successful in suppressing their emotions.

The Conventional versus Contemporary Explanation of Attachment: Incorporating New Views and Ideas into the Traditional Framework

Recent research is challenging Bowlby's belief that early attachment patterns serve as blueprints for adult relationships. While adult attachment styles may partially stem from early experiences, these experiences do not entirely dictate whether individuals will develop secure or insecure attachment bonds in adulthood (Fraley & Roisman, 2018). Despite receiving supportive caregiving during childhood, many individuals still exhibit insecurity in their adult relationships. Conversely, some individuals with less-than-ideal caregiving experiences grow into relatively secure adults. Therefore, ongoing efforts in adult attachment research aim to comprehend the dynamics of attachment changes over time and the factors influencing continuity and change.

Hence, contemporary perspectives are honing in on two primary themes. Firstly, early experiences are viewed not as singular predictors of later adult and midlife relationships, but rather as laying the groundwork for optimal psychological wellbeing (Sroufe et al., 2005). According to this perspective, each developmental stage offers an opportunity for attachment styles to evolve. For instance, supportive caregiving from parents may equip children with the skills necessary for success in other social relationships. These interpersonal experiences can aid in navigating the transitions into early adulthood and midlife. Recent observations by social psychologists suggest that the "relatively stable anchor" of early attachment styles can be recalibrated in response to significant life events and adult circumstances (Willis, 2011). Research has also shown that pivotal life changes, such as becoming a parent, can create contexts that disrupt attachment patterns (Simpson et al., 2007). Therefore, this viewpoint posits that certain contexts maintain attachment patterns while others facilitate change. This marks a significant departure from traditional views in attachment research, which assert that early experiences entirely determine adult interpersonal functioning (Duck, 1994).

Additionally, modern research trends reveal that attachment styles are not uniform; they exhibit differentiation and hierarchy. When individuals encounter experiences that deviate from their expectations, they might not simply revise or update their mental representations of themselves and their close relationships (known as internal working models, as Bowlby termed them); instead, they may develop new representations to incorporate those unique experiences. Consequently, some adults may simultaneously maintain insecure working models regarding their parental relationships while holding secure working models regarding their romantic partners.

Collins and Read (1994) foresaw the significance of this differentiation in their exploration of attachment's hierarchical structure. They proposed that, beyond overarching representations of attachment, individuals also form specific representations tailored to particular relational categories (such as relationships with parents or peers).

Types of Intimacy and Their Reflection in Midlife Relationships

Intimacy leads to stronger relationships, which can provide many health benefits, such as sharpening one's memory, hastening recovery from illness, and strengthening the immune system. There is also a strong connection between intimacy and mental health. Being intimate with a partner can raise self-esteem. Being fully accepted by another human being, regardless of how you feel or what you believe in can make one feel better and more secure about oneself. Enhanced self-acceptance, in turn, boosts confidence to reveal more of who you are, further deepening connection with a partner. Greater self-esteem can also reduce stress and relieve anxiety, improving overall psychological wellbeing and enhancing quality of life.

1) Emotional intimacy: Emotional intimacy is based on trust and respect. In an emotionally intimate relationship, an adult can let their guard down and freely share innermost feelings without fear of being judged. You know you can be open because you're in a safe space where you can simply be yourself. You are secure knowing that your significant other has your best interests in mind when they speak up. At the same time, you are also protective of them and are careful not to have offensive manners, even as you are able to express your emotions.

2) Experiential or physical intimacy: While sex can make you more comfortable with each other, deepen your connection and allow yourselves to be more affectionate, it is only one component of physical intimacy. Physical or experiential intimacy is built on shared experiences. It can involve spending time with each other and doing things together, such as taking vacations, watching movies or going for walks in the park. Or it can refer to the use of the sense of touch to draw closer, like when you snuggle or kiss. Velotti (2021) suggested that more touching can build a stronger relationship. And it doesn't have to be a prelude to sex (nor a replacement for it). For instance, holding hands with your partner is a non-sexual physical act that can help you feel like you're in better harmony with that person.
3) Spiritual intimacy: Spiritual intimacy means being familiar with and having an understanding of your partner's spiritual beliefs. Although sharing common religious beliefs can make it easier for both of you to discuss spiritual questions and be transparent about your struggles, divergent beliefs should not keep you from developing spiritual intimacy. Similar to other kinds of intimacy, respect plays a crucial role in spiritual intimacy, as suggested by Adamczyk and Segrin (2018). When you value your partner's individuality, you also respect their right to choose their religious beliefs. This also means listening more and being more considerate in speaking.
4) Intellectual intimacy: Whereas emotional intimacy involves being able to freely share your emotions, intellectual intimacy is having the confidence to express your ideas or thoughts with your significant other. This, too, is hinged on mutual respect, where both parties in a relationship will not cancel each other out over differing views. Instead, you hold your significant other's opinions highly. You can also amiably discuss with them despite your contrasting positions. You can even use your opposing views to enrich each other's knowledge and stimulate critical and creative thinking. Intellectual intimacy will get increasingly important as people age and become less physically capable or energetic to connect with their partners through sex.

The above-mentioned types of intimacy are present in midlife relationships, and these intimacies have a strong connection between the different types of attachment styles as secure attachment style will have all the above-mentioned intimacies strongly in midlife.

Types of Close Ties in Midlife: Romantic Relationships, Friendships and Family Relationships

The words "relationship" or "close tie" can refer to a variety of social interactions, and they vary according to the resources they get (Internal or external) that in turn strengthen the relationship and serve the wellbeing of the partners involved. With this resource, they can confront and manage different stressors, both individually and as a couple.

Friends are a good substitute for family and acquaintances in all age groups. Friends provide a change of pace from daily routines as well as support, direction and guidance. Friendship plays a central part and is the greatest source of support in middle age (Schmidt et al., 2023). Despite the demands of job, school and family, many young adults are able to keep up at least some connections; for middle-aged individuals, however, maintaining friendships becomes more challenging. Having additional time for socializing is frequently rare in this period because life duties are at an all-time high. Middle-aged people may therefore have fewer pals than their newlywed and retired peers. However, quality always wins out over number when it comes to friendships. Indeed, some of the closest ties between friends are formed and nourished during middle adulthood rather than young adulthood.

Love evolves with time, and by middle adulthood these changes could be noticeable. Three elements make up the ideal adult form of love: desire, intimacy and commitment. This type of love is known as complete love. As intimacy and commitment increase, desire often wanes in middle-aged couples. Put another way, a lot of middle-aged people end up in marriages that are characterized by compassionate love, which is intimate and dedicated but not passionate. However, a relationship that has lost its sexual component need not stay that way, nor do these modifications require the end of a long-term relationship. As a matter of fact, a lot of middle-aged couples discover successful strategies for strengthening their bond, rekindling their desire, being more emotionally intimate and boosting communication. These perceptions of love are positively related to marital satisfaction (Yoo & Joo, 2022), and it can be really astonishing how much understanding develops between two people over time.

Apart from traditional heterosexual partnerships, the previously stated availability of external resources has changed the landscape for same-sex partnerships and queer relationships in the last two decades (Rostosky & Riggle, 2017). In fact, it has been seen that those in same-sex relationships sometimes have stronger attachment to their partners as primary attachment figures of adulthood than heterosexuals (Diamond & Dube, 2002).

Family relationships are enduring and consequential for wellbeing across the life course, and it is needless to mention that they are of immense weight in midlife also (especially during the phases of midlife crisis, they can act as places of relief). In fact, it is well established that family relationships of any kind – marital, intergenerational or sibling ties – have an important influence on wellbeing (Thomas & Umberson, 2017).

Challenges to Close Relationships in Midlife: Aging and Health Concerns – Fitting into the New Role of Caregiver, Maintaining a Satisfying Marital Relationship, Empty Nest Syndrome and Loss of Loved Ones

As in any other developmental life stage, middle age has its own challenges, and resolution patterns vary across individuals.

In the early stages of life, an infant stays close to the attachment figure in times of danger. The exploratory behaviour system offers a framework for growth and development as the child becomes older, and they start to move further away from their caregiver, but still the caregiver retains the function of "safe haven" in times of distress. This process of exploration and individuation evolves over time, and while entering early adulthood, a sense of autonomy is usually established. As in the present chapter our emphasis is on midlife, we will focus on the themes that loom large for middle-aged adults: monitoring and taking responsibility for aged parents while simultaneously providing care to adolescent or younger children (Perrig-Chiello & Hoeoflinger, 2005). How responsibly this caregiving is provided, depends on "intergenerational solidarity" (Silverstein & Bengston, 1997). The term "solidarity" means the amount of cohesion among family members. Literature on intergenerational solidarity indicates that aged parents and their adult children retain an affectional bond and it is related to reduced relationship stress in middle adulthood, thus decreasing the midlife crisis.

Another array of research suggests that contemporary family relationships are diverse, fluid and often unresolved, thus family relationships of midlife are characterized not only by intergenerational solidarity, but also by "intergenerational ambivalence" (Connidis & McMullin, 2002). This indicates that an individual experiences both feelings of affection and resentment, loyalty and distress toward a parent, and such ambivalence is reported to be increased if there is childhood experience of tensions between dependency and autonomy motivation in both parent and child. Solidarity literature does not fully capture the range of emotions experienced by people in close relationships of midlife. It is the intergenerational ambivalence perspective that suggests that it is normal to have an ebb and flow of affectional bonds over time, especially in midlife when adults experience age-graded changes in care-seeking and caregiving role reversals due to ageing of parental attachment figures. For middle-aged adults, parents retain their positions as their attachment figures (which may be primary or not; if marital partners serve fulfilling attachment needs, they may replace the parents and become primary attachment figures), which is a continuation of the old dyad. Also, a new role of caregiver emerges as the parents are now infirm and dependent, so the middle-aged adult needs to step up and provide care. Thus, the middle-aged adult is now faced with a crisis or challenge – the challenge of role reversal, the transition from middle-aged child to middle-aged caregiver (Diehl et al., 1998) – and the flow of attachment security is reversed, which may lead to midlife crisis if not dealt with in a balanced way.

A significant challenge of midlife is to maintain a bona fide marital relationship with the spouse. The term "marital satisfaction" describes the overall favourability each spouse feels in their marriage (Roach et al., 1981). It is often viewed as an individual's interpretation of the overall quality of the marriage or the person's happiness with the marriage. As has been generally observed, marital satisfaction follows a U-shaped pattern, with the highest satisfaction in early phases of marriage, declining with childbirth and parenting (due to increased responsibilities), and increasing again in later life when finances usually stabilize and childcare responsibilities end. Not all marriages are stable, and middle adults do not exhibit immunity to problems in relationships. Many marriages end in divorce, and there can be many reasons for the dissolution of relationships: some cannot handle the stress, demands and conflicts of a relationship, and in other cases the spouses may change and grow in different directions. Long-term relationships (the ones in middle adulthood as it usually involves adolescent offsprings and considerable length of marriage) rarely end because of difficulties with just one of the partners; conflicts or problems, whatever the issues, usually involve both partners. On the contrary, among many factors of successful companionship, it is essential to have a balanced blend of an effective communication pattern, intimacy, commitment, admiration, mutual emotional support and both considering each other as a best friend. If these conditions are shared, midlife can be an opportunity for renewal, because with maturity comes a deeper understanding of love, patience and the significance of genuine connection.

Middle age is also a time when chronic or serious health conditions in one member of a couple or in both can occur, and they typically bring with them the demands of caregiving. Caring for a diseased spouse is a well-known stressor, and it has many associated adverse effects, both psychological and physical (Burton et al., 2003). Also, to see a loved one's suffering often takes a toll on spouse caregivers that can contribute to the negative toll on them and can trigger a range of negative emotions, including distress, sadness and frustration. Managing these emotions is an important task for both spouse caregivers and their ill partners.

Another phenomenon of midlife causing crisis is empty nest syndrome. It is feeling a lack of purpose in life or emotional stress in response to all the children leaving home or getting busy in their own lives, leaving little time for parents. It can have a group of symptoms, including depression, loneliness and low self-esteem. It strongly relates to parents' wellbeing (Coleman et al. 1989).

Another common attachment-related crisis of adulthood and especially midlife is dealing with the bereavement of parental loss – the ultimate separation from a primary attachment figure of childhood. In some cases, there is the loss of the marital partner, and when this happens it creates an enormous effect as middle age is the time when couples usually reunite in terms of emotional closeness as childcare responsibilities tend to decrease. The loss of a parent, which is an usual phenomenon of midlife, usually creates intense grief reactions, and these reactions are often conflicted because of the intergenerational ambivalence mentioned earlier – thus, such loss episodes stir up a host of unresolved and deeply embedded mixed emotions. Midlife marital relationships play a role as a moderator variable here. It has been seen that the death of a parent can change the relational quality with a marital partner in both positive and negative ways. A fulfilling marital relationship can serve as the greatest source of support at this juncture; if this happens, it actually strengthens the marital relationship further (Moss & Moss, 1984), but if not, it can have a deleterious effect on the relationship, which in turn increases both the partners' negative behaviours toward each other (Umberson et al., 2006).

Another area where the midlife crisis unfolds has been seen in gender role changes during midlife. Women are likely to go through a period of self-reflection as they shift from serving the needs of others (especially if their dependent children are now independent) to moving towardaddressing their own needs. In heterosexual relationships, during this time, women can start to expand their sense of self by reclaiming their autonomy and assertiveness, while men do so by reclaiming the more relational part of themselves. Same-sex or queer relationships, however, do not have this pressure of traditional gender roles, but they continuously confront stigma. So same-sex partners who have survived a few adult years in partnership now experience midlife expansion of self not in terms of changed gender roles, but around those areas of self that have so far been neglected, denied and muted in fear of internally or externally expressed homophobia, thus setting stage for enhancing resilience.

Understanding the Indian Perspective

Midlife can bring about a lot of changes and losses, such as deteriorating health, retirement, caring for aged parents and taking on unanticipated responsibilities for adult children or grandchildren. Suicide rates rise as people get older. Depression and substance misuse are common, yet they are frequently misdiagnosed and untreated. There is minimal indication that men and women deal differently with midlife crises. According to a study by Hazra et al. (2023) both men and women undergo midlife crisis. Over 50% of men and 36.1% of women said they were going through a midlife crisis. People experiencing a midlife disaster might additionally show off a number of the subsequent feelings and behaviours:

- Dissatisfaction in a relationship: A person may need to change their relationship's language, feel bored with sex, or drastically change their sexual inclinations.

- Obsessive care about one's appearance: An individual can reduce or cure the signs and symptoms of ageing by wearing clothing that makes them look "younger", eating a specific diet, exercising consistently, or using cosmetics or therapies. It may also be difficult for the individual to comprehend who they have become.
- Occupational dissatisfaction: A person going through a midlife crisis may feel bitter and green with envy of younger coworkers, particularly those who appear to be on their way up, and may want to stop working or take a sabbatical from their responsibilities.
- Emotional pain: A person may feel melancholy or empty (particularly for long periods of time), be irritable or quick to anger, regularly think about mortality, question spiritual beliefs, act recklessly, or overuse drugs and alcohol in an attempt to break free from inner turmoil.
- People experience anger at this stage because they are irritated by the problems of midlife or their incapacity to manage those challenges.

Rawat et al. (2020), studied the Midlife Crisis "Her" Experience. The goal of the study was to see if there was a difference in India between the mental state of middle-aged professional and on-working women. The dimensions under study were anxiety, depression and stress. Only differences in depression levels featured in the results. Non-working women were more likely to have a midlife crisis.

Bouncing Back from Midlife crisis: The Importance of Intimate, Close Relationships in Midlife and How to Maintain Them

Close relationships are integral to any individual's subjective ell being and physiological functioning, and research in this field shows that there is increased risk of dementia and cognitive decline, susceptibility to vascular disease, and increased mortality in those who feel isolated and alone. However, loneliness cannot be defined by mere physical absence of others or people living a solitary existence; it can be felt when surrounded by many others, but still the individual perceives discrepancies in interacting with others and a lack of social support. Someone may have expansive close relationships and still feel a dearth of emotional satisfaction in their life.

In addition to middle-aged parents spending more time, money and energy taking care of their adult children, they are also increasingly taking care of their own ageing and ailing parents. Middle-aged people are sometimes referred to as "the sandwich generation" (in the sense that they are both taking care of and responsibility for adult/adolescent children as well as aged, ailing parents) (Dukhovnov & Zagheni, 2015), and obviously this increases their levels of stress. Research has clearly indicated that conflict between partners is a major factor leading to lower subjective wellbeing (Gere & Schimmack, 2011). Not only marital problems but negative relationships of any kind are linked to ineffective social support (Reblin et al., 2010) and are great sources of stress (Holt-Lunstad et al., 2007). Thus, only close and emotionally fulfilling relationships can provide immunity to negative feelings and depression in this scenario. Maintaining a healthy relationship demands ongoing care; it is built on the foundation of trust, dependability, reasonable expectations, active listening and connecting with empathy, optimism and genuine caring. It also requires respecting each person's needs while establishing a physical, emotional and psychological connection, which are essential components of a healthy partnership.

Conclusion

To sum up, this chapter has focused on midlife and its dynamics in terms of close relationships, their complex interplay during middle adulthood and how the cognitive-affective-motivational schemas known as attachment styles are responsible for variations in relationship satisfaction and intimacy. These factors were addressed from different perspectives, and we tried to review the existing notions of attachment in compariison with recent research in terms of whether childhood attachment is the primary factor, or a blend of social, environmental, cognitive and other personal factors lead to individual differences in relationship satisfaction in midlife, thus creating either an atmosphere of satisfaction and fulfilment or frustration and hopelessness, leading to midlife crisis.

References

Adamczyk, K., & Segrin, C. (2018). Relationship status and romantic loneliness in Polish and U.S. Young Adults [Data set, Computer software and study materials]. OSF Repository.

Ainsworth, M. D. S., Blehar, M. C., Waters, E., & Wall, S. (1978). *Patterns of attachment A psychological study of the strange situation*. Erlbaum.

Bartholomew, K., & Horowitz, L. M. (1991). Attachment styles among young adults: A test of a four-category model. *Journal of Personality and Social Psychology, 61*(2), 226–244. https://doi.org/10.1037/0022-3514.61.2.226

Bowlby, J. (1969). *Attachment and loss Vol l Attachment*. Basic Books.

Bowlby, J. (1973). *Attachment and loss Vol 2 Separation anxiety and anger*. Basic Books

Bowlby, J. (1980). *Attachment and loss Vol 3 Sadness and depression*. Basic Books.

Bowlby, J. (1969/1989). *Attachment and loss Vol l Attachment*. Penguin.

Brennan, K. A., Clark, C. L., & Shaver, P. R. (1998). Self-report measurement of adult romantic attachment: An integrative overview. In J. A. Simpson & W. S. Rholes (Eds.), *Attachment theory and close relationships* (pp. 46–76). Guildford Press.

Burton, L. C., Zdaniuk, B., Schulz, R., Jackson, S., & Hirsch, C. (2003). Transitions in spousal caregiving. -*The Gerontologist, 43*(2), 230–241.

Coleman, L. M., Antonucci, T. C., Adelmann, P. K., & Crohan, S. E. (1989). Empty nest, cohort, and employment in the well-being of midlife women. *Sex Roles, 20*(3–4), 173–189.

Connidis, I. A., &McMullin, J. A. (2002). Sociological ambivalence and family ties: A critical perspective. *Journal of Marriage and Family*, *64*(3), 558–567.

Crittenden, P. M. (1990). Internal representational models of attachment relationships. *Infant Mental Health Journal, 11*, 259–277.

Diamond, L. M., & Dubé, E. M. (2002). Friendship and attachment among heterosexual and sexual-minority youths: Does the gender of your friend matter?. *Journal of Youth and Adolescence, 31*, 155-166.

Diehl, M., Elnick, A. B., Bourbeau, L. S., & Labouvie-Vief, G. (1998). Adult attachment styles: Their relations to family context and personality. *Journal of Personality and Social Psychology, 74*(6), 1656.

Duck, S. (1994). Attaching meaning to attachment. *Psychological Inquiry, 5*, 34–38.

Dukhovnov, D., & Zagheni, E. (2015). Who takes care of whom in the United States? Time transfers by age and sex. *Population and Development Review, 41*(2), 183–206.

Fraley, R. C., & Roisman, G. I. (2018). The development of adult attachment styles: Four lessons. *Current Opinion in Psychology, 25*, 26–30.

Fraley, R. C., & Shaver, P. R. (1997). Adult attachment and the suppression of unwanted thoughts. *Journal of personality and social psychology*, 73(5), 1080.

Gere, J., & Schimmack, U. (2011). A multi-occasion multi-rater model of affective dispositions and affective well-being. *Journal of Happiness Studies, 12*, 931–945.

Holt-Lunstad, J., Uchino, B. N., Smith, T. W., & Hicks, A. (2007). On the importance of relationship quality: The impact of ambivalence in friendships on cardiovascular functioning. *Annals of Behavioral Medicine, 33*(3), 278–290.

Karantzas, G. C., Feeney, J. A., & Wilkinson, R. (2010). Is less more? Confirmatory factor analysis of the attachment style Questionnaires. *Journal of Social and Personal Relationships, 27*(6), 749–780. https://doi.org/10.1177/0265407510373756

Kim, E. Y., Jang, M. Y., & Jung, E. Y. (2014). The effects of subjective health status, climacteric symptoms and coping behaviours of office workers men on midlife crisis. *Korean Journal of Stress Research, 22*, 77–86.

Lucas, R. E. (2005). Time does not heal all wounds: A longitudinal study of reaction and adaptation to divorce. Psychological science, 16(12), 945-950.

Luhmann, M., Hofmann, W., Eid, M., & Lucas, R. E. (2012). Subjective well-being and adaptation to life events: a meta-analysis. *Journal of personality and social psychology, 102*(3), 592.

Main, M., & Solomon, J. (1986). Discovery of an insecure-disorganized/disonented attachment pattern. In T. B. Brazelton & M. W. Yogman (Eds.), *Affecnve development m mfancy* (pp. 95–124). Ablex Publishing Corporation.

Main, M., & Solomon, J. (1990). Procedures for identify infants äs disorganized/disconented during the Ainsworth strange situation. In M. T. Greenberg, D. Cicchetti, & E. M. Cummmgs (Eds.), *Attachment m the preschool years theory, research, and intervention* (pp. 121–160). University of Chicago Press.

Moss, M. S., & Moss, S. Z. (1983–84). The impact of parental death on middle aged children. *Omega: Journal of Death and Dying, 41*, 65–75.

Perrig-Chiello, P., & Hoepflinger, F. (2005). Aging parents and their middle aged children: Demographic and psychosocial challenges, *European Journal of Aging*, 2, 183–191.

Rawat, S., Yadav, A., & Gohar, M. (2020). An epidemiological study to assess unmet needs for family planning among married women in an urban slum area of Mumbai. International Journal of Community Medicine and Public Health, 7(11), 4493.

Reblin, M., Uchino, B. N., & Smith, T. W. (2010). Provider and recipient factors that may moderate the effectiveness of received support: Examining the effects of relationship quality and expectations for support on behavioral and cardiovascular reactions. *Journal of Behavioral Medicine, 33*, 423–431.

Roach, A. J., Frazier, L. P., & Bowden, S. R. (1981). The marital satisfaction scale: Development of a measure for intervention research. *Joournal of Marriage & Family*, *43*(3), 537–546.
Rostosky, S. S., & Riggle, E. D. (2017). Same-sex relationships and minority stress. *Current Opinion in Psychology*, *13*, 29–38.
Schmidt, M. E., Pellicciotti, H., & Long, R. M. (2023). An exploration of friendship and well-being in established adulthood and midlife. *Journal of Adult Development*, *30*, 53–63. https://doi.org/10.1007/s10804-022-09421-8
Silverstein, M., &Bengston, V. L. (1997). Intergenerational solidarity and the structure of adult child-parent relationships in American families. *Americal Journal of Sociology, 103*, 429–460.
Simpson, J. A., Collins, W. A., Tran, S., & Haydon, K. C. (2007). Attachment and the experience and expression of emotions in romantic relationships: A developmental perspective. *Journal of Personality and Social Psychology, 92*(2), 355–367.
Sroufe, L. A., Egeland, B., Carlson, E. A., & Collins, W. A. (2005). *The development of the person: The Minnesota study of risk and adaptation from birth to adulthood*. Guilford.
Taylor, M. G. (2010). Capturing transitions and trajectories: the role of socioeconomic status in later life disability. *Journals of Gerontology Series B: Psychological Sciences and Social Sciences*, *65*(6), 733-743.
Thomas, P. A., Liu, H., & Umberson, D. (2017). Family relationships and well-being. *Innovation in Aging, 1*(3), igx025. https://doi.org/10.1093/geroni/igx025
Umberson, D., Williams, K., Powers, D. A., Liu, H., & Needham, B. (2006). You make me sick: Marital quality and health over the life course. *Journal of Health and Social Behavior*, *47*, 1–16. http://dx.doi.org/10.1177/002214650604700101
Velotti, P., Zobel, B. S., Rogier, G., & Tambelli, R. (2021). Exploring relationships: A systematic review on intimate partner violence and attachment. *Frontiers in Psychology, 9,* 1166. https://doi.org/10.3389/fpsyg.2018.01166
Willis, J. T. (2011). Investigating interpersonal attachment as a function of romantic status. The University of Texas at San Antonio.
Yoo, G., & Joo, S. (2022). Love for a marriage story: The association between love and marital satisfaction in middle adulthood. *Journal of Child and Family Studies, 31*, 1570–1581. https://doi.org/10.1007/s10826-021-02055-6

7 Attachment in Workspace and Midlife

Deepshikha Ray

Work as a Relational Context in Middle Adulthood

"Middle age" has been defined by the *Collins English Dictionary* and *Oxford English Dictionary* as a period in life between "young" and "old" age, and is approximately analogous to the age range 40/45–60/65 years. Psychologists also refer to this age as "midlife" and "middle adulthood" (Lachman, 2004; Toothman & Barrett, 2011; Srivastava et al., 2003). However, research also suggests that the age margins of middle adulthood are not definable in absolute terms (Helson et al., 2006; Toothman & Barrett, 2011) and vary as a function of culture, personal and social contexts (Toothman & Barrett, 2011).

Modern understanding of individual psychosocial development focuses not only on how individuals engage with relationships and community, but also how they create identities and meaning through vocational engagement (Erikson, 1968). Formal vocation/occupation often involves a structured environment, with people (employees) having shared goals, interests and values, and as a result employees develop a sense of collective identity. Structured employment acts as a source of financial sustenance. But it also engenders the development of new skills and relationships (with co-workers), and thereby becomes a core aspect of our self-appraisal. Also, human beings are never passive recipients of external inputs. Instead, human employees and their personalities also actively shape the work environment. In fact, some researchers believe that in the process of adapting to the demands of the job, such as conscientiously completing assigned tasks, attuning to others' needs to minimize conflict etc., adult employees also undergo modifications in personality (Hogan & Roberts, 2004; Schooler et al., 2004). However, according to Ryff and Essex (1992), the extent to which job environment-induced behavioural changes become an individual's dispositional pattern depends on the extent to which the individual is suffused into their job role.

According to Bowen et al. (2011), work/employment is an important developmental context, and more specifically, when longevity has increased, accompanied by changes in the labour market and family structure, it is becoming important to understand the role played by employment in shaping psychosocial adaptation in adults, particularly middle-aged and older adults.

DOI: 10.4324/9781003568360-9

Attachment Styles and Work Experience

Attachment theories, mostly based on the work of Bowlby (1973) and Ainsworth (1978), propose that human beings have an innate tendency to seek proximity or forge an enduring emotional bond with a caregiver (parent) to enhance their prospects of survival, and depending on the manner in which such tendencies are responded to, an individual develops a relatively permanent pattern of bonding with other individuals across their lifespan (Fraley & Brumbaugh, 2004; Fraley & Shaver, 2008). Although research into attachment styles originally predominated in the sub-discipline of developmental psychology, gradually it became obvious that working models of attachment developed on the basis of early parent–child interaction continue to influence interpersonal experiences in adulthood such as romantic relationships and leader–follower relationships (Troth & Miller, 2000), the latter making the study of attachment styles relevant in workplace settings. Leader–follower dynamics are similar to the dynamics of parent–children relationships, but other facets of human attachment styles which are apparent in the workplace are job satisfaction and trust in co-workers. According to Sutin et al. (2009), relationships in the workplace are influenced by each individual employee's unique perspective on relationships mediated by their personal experience of trust, communication and care in interpersonal relationships.

Freud (1961) first espoused the idea that leaders are somewhat like "proxy father-figures", and this led to a series of research projects examining the relationship between adult attachment styles, childhood experiences and perception of leaders (Kahn & Kram, 1994; Bresnahan & Mitroff, 2007). Bernstein (2014) also proposed that experiences of attachment and separation and the accompanying emotions have an impact on relationships within organizations, and particularly relationships with authority figures (leaders). According to Wright and Prerone (2008), the attachment style of an individual employee not only influences their efficacy in dealing with occupational relationships, but also indirectly affects their career efficacy. In a similar vein, individuals with secure attachment have been more frequently found to be effective in leadership roles in an organization, probably because they can generate more trust in interpersonal relationships and their attitudes toward the workplace and co-workers are more acceptable (Harms, 2011).

Hazan and Shaver (1990) proposed that adult behaviour in a work situation can be considered analogous to the exploratory behaviour of children against the backdrop of a securely attached relationship with the caregiver; in the context of the adult in a workplace, the existing interpersonal attachments provide the necessary security base. In the same way as secure attachment fosters emotional regulation in the context of interpersonal relationships, adult attachment styles will also have an impact on relationships with and reactions to co-workers and the work environment. Hazan and Shaver (1990) obtained findings that substantiate the theoretical claim, in that securely attached employees reported greater levels of job satisfaction, relationship satisfaction with co-workers, job security and satisfaction with their appraisals. Also, in comparison to securely attached personnel, workers with insecure attachment reported being unacknowledged in the workplace, being anxious about possible rejection by co-workers, lower levels of job satisfaction, and increased absenteeism due to illness (Hazan & Shaver, 1990; Sumer & Knight, 2001). Hardy & Barkham (1994) also examined the association between interpersonal attachment styles and difficulties experienced in the workplace. They found that lower levels of job satisfaction, poor relationships with co-workers, and less autonomy and appreciation in a job are more frequently present in individuals with anxious and avoidant attachment styles. Similarly, Joplin et al. (1999) observed that that individuals with avoidant attachment style more frequently reported experiencing poorer physical and psychological health. In a similar vein, secure attachment has been found to be associated with improved self-reported health in nurses (Simmons, 2003). According to Tziner et al. (2014), co-workers with secure attachment, in comparison to their insecure counterparts, report increased job satisfaction, better relationships with colleagues, less anxiety related to failure in the job etc. It is reasonable to believe that just as securely attached individuals are capable of forming supportive relationships with their colleagues, anxious/avoidantly attached individuals will have a tendency to be pessimistic about relationships with colleagues, have poor job satisfaction, and may also be less able to disengage from negative emotions which can contribute to stress and burnout (Gillath et al., 2005).

According to Maslach et al. (1997), "job burnout" is a work-related stressful condition characterized by chronic exhaustion and a lack of professional efficacy or a reduced sense of accomplishment, accompanied by psychological distancing from work through manifestation of cynicism. Research has systematically attributed job burnout to disturbed interpersonal relationships with colleagues and/or supervisors (Day & Leiter, 2014), and reduction in job burnout has been found to be associated with improvements in relationships with co-workers (Leiter et al., 2012). Attachment styles of employees have also been found to predict job burnout and job satisfaction. For example, Ronen & Mikulincer (2012) reported that managers with insecure attachment experienced more job burnout and less job satisfaction. In a similar study, Littman-Ovadia et al. (2013) found that job autonomy mediated the relationship between avoidant attachment and performance.

Attachment-related negative emotions intensify the demanding nature of social encounters because anxiously attached individuals experience negative emotions during social interactions as well as while thinking about the consequences of social interactions. It is obvious that in such situations with predominant anxiety, job performance takes a back seat (Bohlmeijer et al., 2010). Attachment-induced anxiety can make social relationships in the workplace problematic and/or distant, which may further impair an employee's ability to experience a collective sense of accomplishment of their professional efficacy.

Organizational Commitment, Work Centrality and Work Experiences

According to Rousseau (1998), employees often personify the organization by using terms such as "we", and this tendency reflects an attempt to create a sense of identification with the organization. Levenson et al. (1962) proposed the term "anthropomorphization" to refer to employees' attribution of human-like qualities to the organization. The fact that employees often have this subjective experience of being in a relationship with their organization has been documented in research by O'Reilly and Chatman (1986) and Peterson and Martin (1996). The psychological processes underlying an individual employee's psychological bond with their organization are (i) identification with the ethos of the organization, (ii) instrumental involvement for extrinsic rewards and (iii) internalization of organizational values (Kelman, 1958; O'Reilly & Chatman, 1986). According to Smith et al. (1983), it is critical for an organization to have employees who are psychologically attached to it in order to enhance "organizational citizenship" behavior such as cooperation, altruism etc., which, in turn, improves the efficacy of an organization (Katz, 1964).

Kielhofner (2008) opined that "occupational identity" refers to self-awareness as a worker, which includes their occupational interests, competencies and goals, which can be considered as one of the central components of identity that exerts a significant impact on individuals' self-definition and wellbeing (Bowling et al., 2010). Some researchers have also conceptualized occupational identity as one of the core components of general identity (Kroger, 2007; Skorikov & Vondracek, 2007). Organizational commitment can be defined as the psychological attachment of an employee to the organization (Walsh, k., & Taylor, M., 2002). Some theorists (Meyer et al., 2002) have conceived of three types of organizational commitment: (i) affective commitment, which indicates the employee's emotional attachment to the organization and its goals, (ii) continuance commitment, which reflects a cognitive process or a sublime understanding between the employee and the organization based on the costs of leaving the job, and (iii) normative commitment, which relates to feelings of obligation towards the organization. Research has consistently demonstrated that organizational commitment enhances employee productivity (Wagner, 2007; Parry, 2008) as well as the employee's attitude toward seeking a change of job (Riketta, 2002; Rynes, 2004). Several studies have identified age of the employee to be a crucial factor that determines organizational commitment. For example, Riketta (2002), on the basis of his meta-analysis, found that age of the employee and organizational tenure are significantly associated with organizational commitment. It can be assumed that as the age of the employee and time spent in the organization increase, employees tend to adapt to and identify more with organizational values (Hinrichs, 1964). In another study, Cakinberk et al. (2011) observed that identification with the organization is higher in employees who are well over 30 years old in comparison to young adults. Similarly, Khanifar et al. (2012) and Mosadeghrad and Ferdosi (2013) reported that senior and older employees are more committed to their organizations. These findings are also supported by Kumar et al. (2016), who found that organizational commitment is significantly higher among employees with an organizational tenure of more than 15 years, implying that organizational commitment is greater in middle-aged workers.

The relationship between an employee and their organization can also be conceptualized in terms of "psychological contracts" between an employee and the organization. Rousseau (1995) defined the psychological contract as employees' perceptions about the mutual written and unwritten obligations between them and their organizations. In general, psychological contracts positively influence attitudes towards the job and job performance (Bal et al., 2008; Zhao et al., 2007). However, individual differences play an important role in the perception or appraisal of psychological contracts. For example, according to Bal et al. (2008) and Schalk et al. (2010), with increases in age, employees tend to be more benevolent toward their organizations and perceive more personal obligations toward them. According to organizational psychologists, there are primarily two types of psychological contracts within the organizational setup: "transactional contracts" and "relational contracts". As these terms suggest, transactional contracts refer to short-term contracts with financial aspects, and relational contracts signify mutually agreeable aspects of the relationship in a job setup (Rousseau & Parks, 1993). Vantilborgh et al. (2015) showed in their research that age is negatively correlated with transactional contracts, suggesting that with increases in age, employees tend to lose interest in monetizable elements of organizational relationships in comparison to socio-emotional aspects of the relationships. But in a similar study, Bal and Kooji (2011) found that the relationship between age and psychological contracts is moderated by another concept: "work centrality". Walsh and Gordon (2008) defined "work centrality" as "individual beliefs regarding the degree of importance that work plays in their lives". This means that persons with high work centrality have a stronger identification with their job role and appraise their work as a significant aspect of their life. Research (Judge et al., 2005; Xanthopoulou et al., 2009) has made it evident that individuals with high work centrality are more willing to work out relational contracts with their organization because they are interested in investing valuable emotional and time resources in the organization and work. The research findings of Armstrong-Stassen and Schlosser (2008) also substantiate the proposition that older workers with high work centrality are more prone to develop relational contracts. Rousseau (2001) also proposed that older workers have more stable psychological contracts with their organizations. Older workers also reported less negative emotions and loss of organizational commitment after breaches of psychological contracts (Bal et al., 2013).

Intersection of Gender and Job Roles in Middle Adulthood

Gender stereotypes are preconceived ideas that attribute specific characteristics to all the members of a gender (Money, 1955). For instance, men are often believed to have natural leadership qualities or aptitudes in science subjects, or women are conceived to be good in caretaking jobs and in jobs that require spontaneous communication. The roots of gender stereotypes can be traced back to patriarchy-induced gendered division of labour and gendered socialization fostered by family and other social institutions (Ruble et al., 2007). There is no denying the fact that gender-related barriers and biases are on the decline, and there have been increases in the implementation of policies promoting gender equality in various countries of the world. However, gender stereotypes and patriarchal mindsets continue to exist in society and negatively impact women's career progression (Tabassum & Nayak, 2021). According to the International Business Report (IBR, 2020), only 29% women occupy senior management positions worldwide, and the World Economic Forum (2017) found that an average gender gap of 32% continues to be present in the domains of economic participation and opportunity, educational attainment, health and survival, and political empowerment.

Gender Roles in Middle Adulthood

One of the most intriguing aspects of progression into middle adulthood is "gender shift", which is a transition from conventional manners of lifestyle and meaning-making related to gender stereotypes. This is manifested as a wish/need to explore those aspects of being a "male" or a "female" which were not hitherto explored due to the constraints imposed by traditional gender roles. Gilligan (1993), in this context, proposed that during midlife, women try to reclaim "their voices". Huyck (1999) investigated gender stereotypes in middle-aged males and females (who were parents to young adult offspring). The results from personal interviews clearly displayed that most of the participants (both male and female), though aware of conventional gender roles, expressed ambivalent attitudes toward them. Also, a majority of the participants (both male and female) reported that in the wake of midlife, they had progressed beyond their gender-stipulated roles. For example, about 17% of middle-aged men said that they preferred to work in the kitchen or that they didn't like watching a game of football, and 26% of middle-aged women said that they indulged in gender-incongruent activities like carpentry or watching sports. Similarly, 30% of men reported that they were emotional and sensitive, whereas 28% of women reported that they were outspoken and did not prefer to rely on men. These findings substantiate the notion that in midlife, gender becomes "bimodal", or in other words, men and women tend to become more "androgynous".

These findings may also have implications for individuals opting for non-conventional career options in their middle adulthood irrespective of whether they have thrived in their previous job roles. It is believed that in middle adulthood, individuals often resort to a review of their life after spending a substantial part of it in apparently successful yet personally unfulfilling pursuits. According to Shultz (2003), middle adulthood is characterized by an increasing trend to actively seek out non-traditional career paths. Vogelsang et al. (2018) examined emotional wellbeing of individuals after late life/midlife career changes and found that such changes, despite the associated challenges, lead to greater emotional wellbeing.

Gender Stereotypes in Jobs and the Glass Ceiling Effect

Although many occupations have become gender-neutral in recent times (e.g., the job of a firefighter is not restricted to men) and significant milestones have been reached in the organizational sector regarding promotion of and legislation for equal opportunities for women and men, women are still a minority with respect to organizational positions that require decision making.

Middle adulthood is expected to represent the middle stage of an individual's work life (Kanfer & Ankerman, 2004), and can be conceptualized by the presence of mastery in the job role one performs and feelings of engagement with the job (McEvoy & Blahna, 2001). However, such a straightforward logic does not apply to women employees in the advanced stages of their career. There is enough research to suggest that there are disparities in the promotion rate between men and women and that women are scarcely represented in senior management positions (Dambrin & Lambert, 2012). Various studies in different parts of the world (Al-Manasra, 2013; Ghorbani & Tung, 2007; Napasri & Yukongdi, 2015; Yang & Konrad, 2011) indicate that prevailing perceptions of the superiority of males exclude females from leadership (managerial positions), which in turn acts as a barrier to progression of women's careers. For example, Broadbridge and Fielden (2018). reported that women occupied only 16% of positions on the executive committees of large Belgian companies. Also, there is substantive research in support of the presence of gender stereotypes in organizational leaders and how they bias selection and career advancement decisions related to women (Koch et al., 2015; Cuddy et al., 2015; Heilman, 2001). The "glass ceiling" is a term which symbolizes a variety of barriers faced by women and by minorities as they seek to improve their employment status. Morrison et al. (1992) described the glass ceiling as a transparent barrier that keeps women from rising above a certain level in organizations. Often, the dominant organizational culture is "gendered" in the sense that senior managers are overwhelmingly men. As a result, the organizational culture encompasses and promotes a "masculine" notion of leadership characterized by conventional views of a man – i.e., men embody independence, authority, competitiveness etc., values which are in tandem with the qualities of a leader (Broadbridge & Hearn, 2008; Koenig et al., 2011). Such gender stereotypes contribute to the phenomenon of the glass ceiling, whereby women are considered less potent and committed to the roles of senior managers, which in turn, adversely affects their recruitment and/or promotion (Van Vianen & Fisher, 2002).

Laufer (2005) proposed that unique needs of women might predispose them to create a "self-imposed glass ceiling". For example, women may choose not to opt for certain prestigious positions/jobs as their demands are at odds with their family responsibilities, and in spite of economic independence, women endorse traditional gender roles and family values. This brings us to the concept of "work–family conflict", which can be defined as a type of inter-role conflict in which the demands and responsibility of a formal job and family interfere with each other (Netemeyer et al., 1996). The lack of support from organizations such as childcare support services and maternity leave arrangements may intensify the problems experienced by working women in their effort to balance work and family roles (dual roles) and attain senior positions in jobs reflecting their years of service (in middle adulthood). As stated earlier, to resolve such conflicts, women may choose to work in low-profile jobs or jobs that allow for part-time employment or breaks in tenure, which help them combine job and family responsibilities (Akpinar-Sposito, 2013). These choices seriously jeopardize the chances of a woman employee in her midlife achieving career progression in comparison to her male counterparts. Middle-aged women employees are also often less flexible regarding geographical mobility in pursuit of career advancement/promotion because of their dual roles, particularly related to child-rearing, leading to interruptions in their careers (Pochic, 2005; Bender & Pigeyre, 2008). Thus, women, even when they have advanced considerably in terms of age, are at a disadvantage with respect to choice of job, salary and prestige (Baxter & Wright, 2000).

The phenomenon of the glass ceiling may diminish women's self-appraisal in terms of self-esteem, self-efficacy and optimism and discourage them from seeking and obtaining promotions (Tran, 2014). As Downes et al. (2014) put it, "women also internalize negative evaluations and stereotypes by those in the majority to the point where they limit themselves and turn down opportunities for advancement due to the fear that they will not succeed".

Conclusion

Middle adulthood is a critical stage of life during which individuals are expected to fulfill dichotomous role responsibilities of taking care of their children as well as their elderly parents while striking a difficult balance between the needs and aspirations of different generations. However, contrary to conventional views on middle adulthood, contemporary perspectives view this stage of life through a more optimistic lens: middle-aged people are considered as more autonomous in terms of control over their lives in general, and finances and obligations in particular. In middle adulthood, working individuals are generally more confident in their job roles because of experience and the fact their roles are more consolidated. Also, new-found freedom from childcare roles (as the children grow up) can give middle-aged individuals a fresh new perspective on their lives and interpersonal relationships, particularly relationships with their partners.

Occupational status and roles are critical sources of identity for individuals in all stages of life, including middle adulthood. However, commitment to job roles, organizational values, relationships with co-workers and job satisfaction are related to an individual's perspective on their relationships, and their attitudes and values are shaped by their past interpersonal experiences. This brings up the issue of adult attachment styles which go beyond influencing and predicting the quality of personal relationships in adults and also mediate workplace relationships in terms of attitudes toward co-workers (seniors, peers and subordinates).

Gender stereotypes, being ubiquitous in their influence, also have an impact on the job roles and occupational identities of middle-aged women. Despite substantial improvement in attitudes toward women, women still lag behind in leadership status and pay packages in comparison to their male peers. Often, because of internalization of social stereotypes, there is a self-imposed restriction on achieving success by women.

However, women have often been said to reclaim their identity during middle adulthood by looking beyond gender stereotypes and the social constraints related to such stereotypes.

References

Ainsworth, M. D. S. (1978). The bowlby-ainsworth attachment theory. *Behavioral and Brain Sciences*, *1*(3), 436–438.

Akpinar-Sposito, C. (2013). Career barriers for women executives and the Glass Ceiling Syndrome: The case study comparison between French and Turkish women executives. *Procedia-Social and Behavioral Sciences*, *75*, 488–497.

Al-Manasra, E. A. (2013). What are the "glass ceiling" barriers effects on women career progress in Jordan? *International Journal of Business and Management*, *8*(6), 40.

Armstrong-Stassen, M., & Schlosser, F. (2008). Benefits of a supportive development climate for older workers. *Journal of Managerial Psychology*, *23*(4), 419–437.

Bal, P. M., & Kooij, D. (2011). The relations between work centrality, psychological contracts, and job attitudes: The influence of age. *European Journal of Work and Organizational Psychology*, *20*(4), 497–523.

Bal, P. M., De Cooman, R., & Mol, S. T. (2013). Dynamics of psychological contracts with work engagement and turnover intention: The influence of organizational tenure. *European Journal of Work and Organizational Psychology*, *22*(1), 107–122.

Bal, P. M., De Lange, A. H., Jansen, P. G., & Van Der Velde, M. E. (2008). Psychological contract breach and job attitudes: A meta-analysis of age as a moderator. *Journal of Vocational Behavior*, *72*(1), 143–158.

Baxter, J., & Wright, E. O. (2000). The glass ceiling hypothesis: A comparative study of the United States, Sweden, and Australia. *Gender & Society*, *14*(2), 275–294.

Bender, A. F., & Pigeyre, F. (2008). *Les carrières des femmes* (No. hal-00756087).

Bernstein, R. E., Tenedios, C. M., Laurent, H. K., Measelle, J. R., & Ablow, J. C. (2014). The eye of the begetter: Predicting infant attachment disorganization

from women's prenatal interpretations of infant facial expressions. *Infant Mental Health Journal*, *35*(3), 233–244.
Bohlmeijer, E., Prenger, R., Taal, E., & Cuijpers, P. (2010). The effects of mindfulness-based stress reduction therapy on mental health of adults with a chronic medical disease: a meta-analysis. *Journal of psychosomatic research*, 68(6), 539-544.
Bowen, C. E., Noack, M. G., & Staudinger, U. M. (2011). Aging in the work context. In Handbook of the *psychology of aging*, 263–277. Academic Press.
Bowlby, J. (1973). Attachment and loss. Volume II. Separation, anxiety and anger. In *Attachment and loss. volume II. Separation, anxiety and anger* (pp. 429-p). The Hogarth Press and the Institute of Psycho-Analysis.
Bowling, N. A., Eschleman, K. J., Wang, Q., Kirkendall, C., & Alarcon, G. (2010). A meta-analysis of the predictors and consequences of organization-based self-esteem. *Journal of Occupational and Organizational Psychology, 83*(3), 601–626.
Bresnahan, C. G., & Mitroff, I. I. (2007). Leadership and attachment theory. *American Psychologist, 62*(6), 607–608.
Broadbridge, A., & Hearn, J. (2008). Gender and management: New directions in research and continuing patterns in practice. *British Journal of Management*, *19*(s1), 38–49.
Broadbridge, A. M., & Fielden, S. L. (2018). *Research handbook of diversity and careers*. Edward Elgar Publishing.
Çakinberk, A., Derin, N., & Demirel, E. T. (2011). Shaping of organizational identification by organizational commitment: Example of private education institutions in Malatya and Tunceli. *İşletme Araştırmaları Dergisi*, *3*(1), 89–121.
Cuddy, A. J., Wilmuth, C. A., Yap, A. J., & Carney, D. R. (2015). Preparatory power posing affects nonverbal presence and job interview performance. *Journal of Applied Psychology*, *100*(4), 1286.
Dambrin, C., & Lambert, C. (2012). Who is she and who are we? A reflexive journey in research into the rarity of women in the highest ranks of accountancy. *Critical Perspectives on Accounting*, *23*(1), 1–16.
Day, A., & Leiter, M. P. (2014). The good and bad of working relationships: Implications for burnout. In M. P. Leiter, A. B. Bakker, & C. Maslach (Eds.), *Burnout at work* (pp. 56–79). Psychology Press.
Downes, M., Hemmasi, M., & Eshghi, G. (2014). When a perceived glass ceiling impacts organizational commitment and turnover intent: The mediating role of distributive justice. *Journal of Diversity Management (JDM)*, *9*(2), 131–146.
Erikson, E. H. (1968). Identity youth and crisis (No. 7). WW Norton & company.
Fraley, R. C., Brumbaugh, C. C., Rholes, W. S., & Simpson, J. A. (2004). A dynamical systems approach to conceptualizing and studying stability and change in attachment security. In W. S. Rholes & J. A. Simpson (Eds.), *Adult attachment: Theory, research, and clinical implications* (pp. 86–132). Guilford Publications.
Freud, S., & Freud, E. L. (1961). Letters of Sigmund Freud, 1873–1939. *(No Title)*.
Ghorbani, M., & Tung, R. L. (2007). Behind the veil: An exploratory study of the myths and realities of women in the Iranian workforce. *Human Resource Management Journal*, *17*(4), 376–392.
Gillath, O., Bunge, S. A., Shaver, P. R., Wendelken, C., & Mikulincer, M. (2005). Attachment-style differences in the ability to suppress negative thoughts: Exploring the neural correlates. *Neuroimage*, *28*(4), 835–847.
Gilligan, C. (1993). *In a different voice: Psychological theory and women's development*. Harvard University Press.
Hardy, G. E., & Barkham, M. (1994). The relationship between interpersonal attachment styles and work difficulties. *Human Relations*, *47*(3), 263–281.

Harms, P. D. (2011). Adult attachment styles in the workplace. *Human Resource Management Review*, *21*(4), 285–296.
Hazan, C., & Shaver, P. R. (1990). Love and work: An attachment-theoretical perspective. *Journal of Personality and Social Psychology*, *59*(2), 270.
Heilman, M. E. (2001). Description and prescription: How gender stereotypes prevent women's ascent up the organizational ladder. *Journal of Social Issues*, *57*(4), 657–674.
Helson, R. M., George, L. G., & John, O. P. (2009). Challenge episodes over middle age: A person-centered study of aging well in poor health. *Journal of Research in Personality*, 43(3), 323-334
Hinrichs, J. R. (1964). Communications activity of industrial research personnel. *Personnel Psychology*.
Hogan, R., & Roberts, B. W. (2004). A socioanalytic model of maturity. *Journal of Career Assessment*, 12(2), 207-217.
Huyck, M. H. (1999). Gender roles and gender identity in midlife. In *Life in the middle* (pp. 209–232). Academic Press.
IBR. (2020). *Women in business 2020: Putting the blueprint into action*. Grant Thornton Report (pp. 1–7). https://www.grantthornton.global/globalassets/1.-memberfirms/global/insights/women-in-business/2020/women-inbusiness-2020_report.pdf
Joplin, J. R., Nelson, D. L., & Quick, J. C. (1999). Attachment behavior and health: Relationships at work and home. *Journal of Organizational Behavior*, *20*(6), 783–796.
Judge, T. A., Bono, J. E., Erez, A., & Locke, E. A. (2005). Core self-evaluations and job and life satisfaction: The role of self-concordance and goal attainment. *Journal of Applied Psychology*, *90*(2), 257.
Kahn, W. A., & Kram, K. E. (1994). Authority at work: Internal models and their organizational consequences. *Academy of Management Review*, *19*(1), 17–50.
Kanfer, R., & Ackerman, P. L. (2004). Aging, adult development, and work motivation. *Academy of Management Review*, *29*(3), 440–458.
Katz, D. (1964). The motivational basis of organizational behavior. *Behavioral Science*, *9*(2), 131–146.
Kelman, H. C. (1958). Compliance, identification, and internalization: Three processes of attitude change. *Journal of Conflict Resolution*, *2*(1), 51–60.
Khanifar, H., Nazari, K., Emami, M., & Soltani, H. (2012). Impacts corporate social responsibility activities on company financial performance. *Interdisciplinary Journal of Contemporary Research in Business*, *3*(9), 583–592.
Kielhofner, G. (2008). Introduction to the model of human occupation. *Model of Human Occupation, Theory and Application*, 1–9.
Koch, A. J., D'Mello, S. D., & Sackett, P. R. (2015). A meta-analysis of gender stereotypes and bias in experimental simulations of employment decision making. *Journal of Applied Psychology*, *100*(1), 128.
Koenig, A. M., Eagly, A. H., Mitchell, A. A., & Ristikari, T. (2011). Are leader stereotypes masculine? A meta-analysis of three research paradigms. *Psychological Bulletin*, *137*(4), 616.
Kroger, J. (2007). Why is identity achievement so elusive? *Identity: An International Journal of Theory and Research*, *7*(4), 331–348.
Kumar, P., Mehra, A., Inder, D., & Sharma, N. (2016). Organizational commitment and intrinsic motivation of regular and contractual primary health care providers. *Journal of Family Medicine and Primary Care*, *5*(1), 94.
Lachman, M. E. (2004). Development in midlife. *Annu. Rev. Psychol.*, *55*(1), 305-331.
Laufer, D., Silver, D. H., & Meyer, T. (2005). Exploring differences between older and younger consumers in attributions of blame for product harm crises. *Academy of Marketing Science Review*, 2005, 1.

Leiter, M. P., Day, A., Oore, D. G., & Spence Laschinger, H. K. (2012). Getting better and staying better: Assessing civility, incivility, distress, and job attitudes one year after a civility intervention. *Journal of Occupational Health Psychology*, *17*(4), 425.
Levinson, H., Price, C. R., Munden, K. J., Mandl, H. J., & Solley, C. M. (1962). *Men, management, and mental health*. Harvard University Press.
Littman-Ovadia, H., Oren, L., & Lavy, S. (2013). Attachment and autonomy in the workplace: New insights. *Journal of Career Assessment*, *21*(4), 502–518.
Maslach, C., Jackson, S. E., & Leiter, M. P. (1997). *Maslach burnout inventory*. Scarecrow Education.
McEvoy, G. M., & Blahna, M. J. (2001). Engagement or disengagement? Older workers and the looming labor shortage. *Business Horizons*, 44(5), 46-46.
Meyer, J. P., Stanley, D. J., Herscovitch, L., & Topolnytsky, L. (2002). Affective, continuance, and normative commitment to the organization: A meta-analysis of antecedents, correlates, and consequences. *Journal of Vocational Behavior*, *61*(1), 20–52.
Money, J. (1955). Hermaphroditism, gender and precocity in hyperadrenocorticism: Psychologic findings. *Bulletin of the Johns Hopkins Hospital*, *96*(6), 253–264.
Morrison, A. M. (1992). New solutions to the same old glass ceiling. *Women in Management Review*, *7*(4), 15–19.
Mosadeghrad, A. M., & Ferdosi, M. (2013). Leadership, job satisfaction and organizational commitment in the healthcare sector: Proposing and testing a model. *Materia Socio-Medica*, *25*(2), 121.
Napasri, T., & Yukongdi, V. (2015). A study of Thai female executives: Perceived barriers to career advancement. *Review of Integrative Business and Economics Research*, *4*(3), 108.
Netemeyer, R. G., Boles, J. S., & McMurrian, R. (1996). Development and validation of work–family conflict and family–work conflict scales. *Journal of Applied Psychology*, *81*(4), 400.
O'Reilly, C. A., & Chatman, J. (1986). Organizational commitment and psychological attachment: The effects of compliance, identification, and internalization on prosocial behavior. *Journal of Applied Psychology*, *71*(3), 492.
Parry, J. (2008). Intention to leave the profession: Antecedents and role in nurse turnover. *Journal of Advanced Nursing*, *64*(2), 157–167.
Pochic, S. (2005). Faire carrière: l'apport d'une approche en terme de genre. *Formation Emploi. Revue française de sciences sociales*, *91*, 75–93.
Riketta, M. (2002). Attitudinal organizational commitment and job performance: a meta-analysis. *Journal of Organizational Behavior: The International Journal of Industrial, Occupational and Organizational Psychology and Behavior*, *23*(3), 257–266.
Ronen, S., & Mikulincer, M. (2012). Predicting employees' satisfaction and burnout from managers' attachment and caregiving orientations. *European Journal of Work and Organizational Psychology*, *21*(6), 828–849.
Rousseau, D. M. (1995). *Psychological contracts in organizations: Understanding written and unwritten agreements*. Sage Publications.
Rousseau, D. M. (1998). The'problem'of the psychological contract considered. *Journal of Organizational Behavior*, *19*, 665–671.
Rousseau, D. M. (2001). Schema, promise and mutuality: The building blocks of the psychological contract. *Journal of Occupational and Organizational Psychology*, *74*(4), 511–541.
Rousseau, D. M., & McLean Parks, J. (1993). The contracts of individuals and organizations. *Research in Organizational Behavior*, *15*, 1–1.

Ruble, D. N., Taylor, L. J., Cyphers, L., Greulich, F. K., Lurye, L. E., & Shrout, P. E. (2007). The role of gender constancy in early gender development. *Child Development*, *78*(4), 1121–1136.
Ryff, C. D., & Essex, M. J. (1992). The interpretation of life experience and well-being: The sample case of relocation. *Psychology and aging*, 7(4), 507.
Rynes, S. L. (2004). Where do we go from here? Imagining new roles for human resources. *Journal of Management Inquiry*, *13*(3), 203–213.
Schalk, R., Van Veldhoven, M., De Lange, A. H., De Witte, H., Kraus, K., Stamov-Roßnagel, C., & Zacher, H. (2010). Moving European research on work and ageing forward: Overview and agenda. *European Journal of Work and Organizational Psychology*, *19*(1), 76–101.
Schooler, C., Mulatu, M. S., & Oates, G. (2004). Occupational self-direction, intellectual functioning, and self-directed orientation in older workers: Findings and implications for individuals and societies. *American Journal of Sociology*, 110(1), 161-197.
Shaver, P. R., & Fraley, R. C. (2008). Attachment, loss, and grief: Bowlby's views and current controversies. In J. Cassidy & P. R. Shaver (Eds.), *Handbook of attachment: Theory, research, and clinical applications* (2nd ed., pp. 48–77). The Guilford Press.
Shultz, K. S. (2003). Bridge employment: Work after retirement. In G. A. Adams & T. A. Beehr (Eds.), *Retirement: Reasons, processes, and results* (pp. 214–241). Springer.
Simmons, J. (2003). Balancing performance, accountability and equity in stakeholder relationships: Towards more socially responsible HR practice. *Corporate Social Responsibility and Environmental Management*, *10*(3), 129–140.
Skorikov, V. B., & Vondracek, F. W. (2007). Vocational identity. In V. B. Skorikov & W. Patton (Eds.), *Career development in childhood and adolescence* (pp. 143–168). Brill.
Smith, C., Organ, D. W., & Near, J. P. (1983). Organizational citizenship behavior: Its nature and antecedents. *Journal of Applied Psychology*, *68*(4), 653.
Srivastava, S., John, O. P., Gosling, S. D., & Potter, J. (2003). Development of personality in early and middle adulthood: Set like plaster or persistent change?. *Journal of personality and social psychology*, 84(5), 1041.
Sumer, H. C., & Knight, P. A. (2001). How do people with different attachment styles balance work and family? A personality perspective on work–family linkage. *Journal of Applied Psychology*, *86*(4), 653.
Sutin, A. R., Costa, P. T., Miech, R., & Eaton, W. W. (2009). Personality and career success: Concurrent and longitudinal relations. *European Journal of Personality*, *23*(2), 71–84.
Tabassum, N., & Nayak, B. S. (2021). Gender stereotypes and their impact on women's career progressions from a managerial perspective. *IIM Kozhikode Society & Management Review*, *10*(2), 192–208.
Toothman, E. L., & Barrett, A. E. (2011). Mapping midlife: An examination of social factors shaping conceptions of the timing of middle age. *Advances in Life Course Research*, 16(3), 99-111
Tran, T. T. T. (2014). *Identifying the existence of the glass ceiling and examining the impact on the participation of female executives in the Vietnamese banking sector* (Master's thesis). Unitec Institute of Technology.
Troth, A., & Miller, J. (2000). Attachment links to team functioning and leadership behavior. In M. Sheehan, S. Ramsay, & J. Patrick (Eds.), *Transcending boundaries: Integrating people, processes and systems* (pp. 385–392). Griffith University.
Tziner, A., Ben-David, A., Oren, L., & Sharoni, G. (2014). Attachment to work, job satisfaction and work centrality. *Leadership & Organization Development Journal, 35*, 555–565.

Vantilborgh, T., Dries, N., De Vos, A., & Bal, P. M. (2015). The psychological contracts of older employees. In P. M. Bal, D. Kooij, & D. Rousseau (Eds.), *Aging workers and the employee-employer relationship* (pp. 107–127). Springer.
Van Vianen, A. E., & Fischer, A. H. (2002). Illuminating the glass ceiling: The role of organizational culture preferences. *Journal of Occupational and Organizational Psychology*, *75*(3), 315–337.
Vogelsang, E. M., Shultz, K. S., & Olson, D. A. (2018). Emotional well-being following a later life career change: The roles of agency and resources. The International Journal of Aging and Human Development, 87(4), 327-346
Wagner, J. (2007). Exports and productivity: A survey of the evidence from firm-level data. *World Economy*, *30*(1), 60–82.
Walsh, K., & Gordon, J. R. (2008). Creating an individual work identity. *Human Resource Management Review*, *18*(1), 46–61.
Walsh, K., & Taylor, M. (2002). Reframing organizational commitment within a contemporary careers framework. Cornell University, Center for Hospitality Research.
Wright, S. L., & Perrone, K. M. (2008). The impact of attachment on career-related variables: A review of the literature and proposed theoretical framework to guide future research. *Journal of Career Development*, *35*(2), 87–106.
Xanthopoulou, D., Bakker, A. B., Demerouti, E., & Schaufeli, W. B. (2009). Reciprocal relationships between job resources, personal resources, and work engagement. *Journal of Vocational Behavior*, *74*(3), 235–244.
Yang, Y., & Konrad, A. M. (2011). Understanding diversity management practices: Implications of institutional theory and resource-based theory. *Group & Organization Management*, *36*(1), 6–38.
Zhao, H. A. O., Wayne, S. J., Glibkowski, B. C., & Bravo, J. (2007). The impact of psychological contract breach on work-related outcomes: A meta-analysis. *Personnel Psychology*, *60*(3), 647–680.

8 Midlife and Parenthood

Rudrani Chatterjee and Zainab Ahmed

How we go about defining midlife parenthood is a challenge. Are we to talk in terms of the age of the parents or the children or take both into account, or do we talk in terms of social roles and statuses. The course of human development is complex and contingent on many factors at an individual and environmental level.

In terms of evolution of the socio-relational context, parenthood has been a cherished part of living. The longing to hold and nurture a created extension of ourselves is an expression of joyfulness and hope. Let us explore the nuances of this relationship from the vantage point of socio-relational evolution.

i) Parental role: Children grow up and (mostly) cease to remain children. A parent is a parent before the child comes, and remains one even after the child leaves the nest. The parental role, then, is full of ambiguity. A parent is an authority figure, but not quite; a friend, but not quite; a role model, but not quite; a caregiver, but not only so. Mostly viewed as the "arch-enemies" of adolescents or "superheroes" of children, parents have quite a roller-coaster ride in the name of parenting. The parental role demands changes with the developmental stages of the child. What is "nurturing" parental behaviour to a child of five years can become "overprotective", if not modified, to a child of 11 years. The relationship of the parent and child, like any other, is intertwined. To the child, a parent is a pillar of support and dependence, and a point of security and certainty in an unfamiliar world. The child fulfils the parents' need to nurture and nudge, to foster growth, to exert influence, to feel a unique sense of meaning, purpose and worthiness in being responsible for a living' other – somewhat reminiscent of their own vulnerable selves and unlived dreams.

Classically, the parental role perspective (Scott & Alwin, 1989) distinguishes between the parenting experience of mothers and fathers, in that mothers of toddlers experience greater distress by virtue of the demands and hence stress of their maternal roles than their paternal counterparts (Nomaguchi & Milkie, 2003; Umberson et al., 1996). This complies with the gendered role

DOI: 10.4324/9781003568360-10

perspective which held that the socio-emotional salience and psychological rewards associated with parental roles meant more to women. It was thus implied that parenthood and the emotional investments made therein had much to do with women's "self-hood". However, a generational perspective might help us put this observation into some context.

ii) Change in the parenting experience with changing times: Parenting practices have caught the interest of scientific inquiry for many decades now. Yet there has been more emphasis on the personalities or characteristics of the parents and parenting styles as they impact children, and seldom the reverse (Cohen, 2015). This is probably based on the assumption that both nature and nurture play greater roles than in any other field to conclude that it is by, of and for the parents that children become who they do. The literature on adulthood parenting has focused on intergenerational dynamics and more recently, intergenerational ambivalence, and not on parental roles like those of early parenting.

In the last four decades of the 20th century, radical changes took place in the social and economic conditions, demographic patterns and cultural perceptions affecting the generational cohorts differentially (Parker & Aldwin, 1997). The institution of family and practices of parenting have therefore been through changes as well, for reasons as yet not completely understood, although some have observed that change has always been the norm in family systems (Furstenberg, 2010). Parenting practices have been influenced by ideological shifts in areas such as women's education, greater involvement in the labour force, demands for equality at work and therefore greater demands on time outside home, time of marriage, fertility, age of childbearing, parental responsibility sharing, age and patterns of co-residency with offspring. Thus the changing climate of the times has given rise to the postmodern family. Six decades ago, people became "adults" early. The completion of schooling, leaving the nest, starting to work and marriage happened in their early twenties (Furstenberg, 2010). Consequently, midlife parents back then were relatively less duty-bound toward their "adult" children. The understanding and perception of adulthood have undergone major revisions since then. Eighteen years of age, is no longer a social benchmark for adulthood, albeit a legal one in many jurisdictions. In the recent days, the couple has married late, conceived later, shared parental responsibilities, been actively involved with and "invested in" their children, supporting their children longer until they become suitably prepared for skill-based professions.

The silent generation who were middle-aged during the period 1960–1980, the baby boomers who were in middle age during 1980–2000, generation X, who were middle-aged during 2000–2020 and millennials, who are approaching middle age currently, will all have experienced parenthood differently. Issues of co-residence with adult children, frowned upon by Western culture and held in esteem in the East, have now gradually gained ground.

Step-parenthood, single parenting, LGBTQ couple parenting and non-human parenting of today are a reflection of the changed socio-relational context.

Midlife Today

Approaches to Studying Midlife

Let us now ponder how midlife looks today. The theoretical approaches in understanding midlife have been about the silent generation who witnessed the Second World War as adults and were middle-aged in the 1960s. Earlier theorists viewing this generation spoke in terms of increasing maturity of the ego with advanced development, a renewed look at life or what was left of it, with "reality" setting in and the "illusion" of a fantastic life fading away, seeking fulfilment in more meaningful pursuits, resolving the conflict of "generativity and stagnation" through "care" (Erikson, 1950). While cross-sectional research (Levinson, 1978) spoke of a midlife crisis, longitudinal studies found no significant evidence of the same (Vaillant, 1977).

The 1980s were hailed as the postmodern period, and the approaches to studying midlife differed markedly. For one thing, the generational cohorts changed. The characteristics of the baby boomer generation were different from their earlier counterparts in midlife, at least partially attributable to having been exposed to significant social changes. The experience of midlife parenthood, too, was different and distinctly more personalized, less publicly defined, and hence more liberated. Longitudinal studies like MIDMAC (Foundation Research Network on Successful Midlife Development), a landmark in midlife study, were launched at the end of the same decade. The biopsychosocial angles of health came together with demography, epidemiology and health policymaking. It has strongly impacted the way midlife is understood today.

Midlife Lifestyle Demands and Fulfilment

Midlife has received the status of being a pivotal period in life today. That merely translates into saying that it is more of a walk on the tight rope than ever. With the evolution of family and society, there is an increasing need for parents to juggle demands of the workplace, maintain a home, look after own ageing parents, work out social relationships and look out for their own health and wellbeing all at the same time. Financial strains and shrinking safety nets are most notable in individuals above age 45 in countries like the USA (Thorne et al., 2018). There are more debts pertaining to the expensive charges for healthcare, housing and being co-signatories of student loans. The policies have yet to catch up with middle-aged carers. Individuals are either at the mercy of stagnant wages in ecession hit-times or in fear of loss of employment and bankruptcy altogether. It is only to be expected that their own health and wellbeing will be compromised when juggling responsibilities and battling the times all at once.

Children

The earlier half of midlife (forties–fifties) is when crucial changes in health and family begin. The effects on parental mental health are found to be related to the children they are parenting. Parenting minor children makes more demands on time, energy and resources, especially for mothers (Pollmann-Schult, 2014). It can also be rewarding and contribute to greater psychological wellbeing (Nomaguchi, 2012), but in varying degrees and depending on the age of the children. For instance, interpersonal conflict experienced with school-age or adolescent children can have adverse effects on the psychological wellbeing of parents. Understandably, marital status, marital quality and socioeconomic factors play strong roles in mediating the experiences with children. The fact that involvement in children's daily lives can be fulfilling and strenuous at the same time is generally agreed.

With adult children of middle-aged parents, it is not the degree of support but appraisal of it that determines life satisfaction for caregiving parents. Fingerman et. al. points out a bidirectionality in parental support and outcome whereby adult children set up for a successful launch draw on support from their parents as a future investment of sorts or because it is gratifying for parents to help well-set up adult children (Fingerman et al., 2009).

Ageing Parents

Those in midlife who are caring for their ageing parents in addition to their children are understandably under the most strain financially, emotionally and physically. It has been shown that financial insecurity has adverse effects on both physical and mental health (Feinberg, 2018), and in countries with inadequate paid leave policies for family care, it ultimately affects work life as well. Financial minorities like coloured and Hispanic communities can understandably access less formal support for caregiving than their white counterparts. In fact, research has established that multiple caregiving roles take a toll on life in general on factors from sleep to family relationships (DePasquale et al., 2016). Caregiving, however, can have many dimensions. For parents who suffer from gradually deteriorating conditions like dementia, the burden of care and the exhaustion experienced is bound to higher. Parents who remain more emotionally available lend a sense of support.

Health

In terms of the competing responsibilities that demand attention, that which is not prioritized takes a hit and takes it fast in midlife. A fast-paced life beset with cutting-edge responsibilities often comes with the cost of dietary compromises like reliance on processed food, sedentary lifestyle and obesity, which are risk factors for chronic conditions like metabolic syndromes (Infurna et al., 2020). Longitudinal studies have shown that lifestyle trends and unhealthy coping in youth affect midlife, and in turn have adverse implications for later life (Lachman, 2004). Compromises in physical health additionally have psychological impacts of helplessness, uncontrollability and vulnerability, which, combined with other psychosocial stressors, result in depression, associated mental health conditions and initial phases of well-compensated cognitive decline (Soederberg Miller & Lachman, 2000).

Selfhood

As a mediating factor between the stresses experienced and physical changes, the role of self is crucial for maintaining a sense of control and agency for effective psychological functioning. It could be reasonably assumed that the assumption of multiple responsible roles affects and is affected by a deepening sense of identity, better emotion regulation skills, coping skills, wisdom and insight. Experiences of overwhelming stress, especially associated with finance and children, are dealt through bringing about changes in the environment ("assimilative changes") or making adjustments and accepting them as a part of the necessary cost of living ("accommodative changes") (Lachman, 2004).

Contexts of Parenthood in Midlife

Normative Parenthood

Raising children awakens one's own relationship with one's parents. All relationships are complex and layered and can stir difficult emotions of self-criticism, fear, contempt, anger or rejection. This is especially true when it comes to parent–child relationships. Awareness of that ambivalence makes one reflect on whether to be like one's own parents, unlike them, or someone else altogether. Sometimes being a good mother can entail being a bad daughter if we are to go against the values taught to us. The task doesn't get simpler with age or maturity of the children. This task has close correspondence with the sense of identity and capacity for self-reflection of the individual.

i) Maturity of and relationships with children: As observed in the previous sections, there has been a gradual change in the normative relationships between midlife parents and their adult children in the past few decades. For one thing, contact between midlife parents and their children has grown significantly. This may partly be attributable to the rapid development and easy availability of communication devices during this period (Fingerman et al., 2012). Also, support of midlife parents for adult children has grown, ranging from instrumental, financial support as in earlier decades to emotional support, though the quantity and frequency of support is yet to be established. Co-residence with grown children, previously frowned upon, is a more frequent phenomenon (Fry, 2015). Unsurprisingly, middle-aged parents maintain closer contact with and are more supportive toward struggling adult children (Huo et al., 2019). It has been a consistent observation that the stress and wellbeing of midlife parents can be compromised even if a single offspring struggles or does not do well. Also, this adversely affects their perceived competence in having fulfilled the parental role (Fingerman et al., 2012).

ii) Co-residence with adult children: Research has established that adult children living with their middle-aged parents do so because they need the support of their parents, and seldom the other way round. This, however, needs to be seen in perspective. The nature of "investment" of parents in children, and for that matter parenting itself, has changed. With fewer of children, more investment in their extracurricular activities and college funds, the nature of parentchild involvement borders on close monitoring, anticipation of the children's needs and overprotection ("helicopter parenting"). It also often amounts to removing all obstacles from the child's life ("bulldozer parenting") or ensuring that they are on "the path to success" ("'tiger parenting") (Ebbert et al., 2019). The economic recession has made the path to the attainment of educational goals strew with as many loans as accolades. The parent–child relationship is affected by the changes in the socio-economic climate of the times. Having to share or shoulder these loans with children is an integral part of being a midlife parent. High financial liability is likely to invoke a stronger need to control and protect. It is more of a developmental task which the family goes through as a social unit, an acknowledgement that the markers of financial independence and social maturity have changed (Furstenberg, 2010).

Non-normative Parenthood

i) Postponement of parenthood: It is not surprising for individuals to be first-time parents in midlife today. The shift has been ongoing since the 1970s in industrialized nations owing to social perspective changes and pursuit of economic and relationship stability. Life stages including longer years of education, occupational transitions and lifestyle goals, more than age, have become the deciding factor for readiness for parenthood (Datta et al., 2023). This has understandably come closer to midlife than an earlier life stage. Ironically, the times which have revolutionized effective contraception and brought greater freedom of choice have also seen rising infertility and technological advancements in assisted reproduction and the consequences thereof for the offspring (Zacchini et al., 2022). The impact of delayed childbearing has other consequences in the form of increased risks for maternal health and the emotional complexities of navigating through hard choices like prenatal testing or selective abortion and the like which medical interventions bring into the mix. Yet the intentionality and the experience this life stage brings help approach parenthood with deeper understanding of self and appreciation of the role of a parent as a caregiver (Vance & Brandon, 2017).

ii) Children with developmental/mental health conditions: Parenting a child with special health needs has far-reaching consequences. Parent–child systems subject to chronic stressors like developmental or mental health conditions eat away at the normative age-related wellbeing associated with midlife parenting. Higher negative affect and poor physical and psychological wellbeing characterize such parents (Sloan et al., 2020). Previous longitudinal studies have warned that such conditions lead to prolonged restriction in activities of daily living and significant depressive features a decade later irrespective of parental gender (Smith & Grzywacz, 2014). However, it has been observed that "perceived control" serves as a protective factor for mothers rather than fathers. Sloan found that the negative affect of midlife fathers deteriorated more as a result of caregiving blues than that of mothers, probably attributable to lack of finding adequate social buffers (Sloan et al., 2020). Notably, the number of hours of social support offered were not found to be associated with physical or mental health status. However, the kinds of support or their desirability have yet to be explored (Resch et al., 2012).

iii) Step-parenthood: The changing picture of midlife parenthood has close associations with, among other factors, changing relationship paradigms. Remarriage is no longer non-normative, but is none the less stressful, contingent on individual characteristics, previous experiences and attitudes toward non-biological or grown-up children. While research into midlife step-parenthood has found greater stress associated with raising step-children, Pudrovska found that the association was mitigated by structural characteristics of the family, intergenerational ties and the quality of the marital relationship (Pudrovska, 2009). Gradual adaptive changes occur in a family with a crisis of remarriage and the associated ambiguity introduced to the family structure and dynamics (Pudrovska, 2008).

iv) Single parenthood: Single parenthood at midlife in the current times entails nearly all the stresses experienced by a couple and more. Research on single mothers shows that single parenthood is particularly stressful for mothers. However, the quality of life is significantly affected by the financial competence of the single mother. In a Korean study, the role of provider, if suitably fulfilled, together with a profession which brings a sense of accomplishment and meaningfulness, was found to be associated with greater life satisfaction for single mothers (Kim & Kim, 2020).

The postmodern family has brought about more involved and engaged fathers. The same era has also seen the rise of single parenthood or co-parenting. It is not fatherhood itself or living with the children per se, but the engagement and interaction with them that are associated with the broader connectedness of single fathers to society and altruistic acts (Eggebeen et al., 2010).

The assumption that single parents could be worse off than partnered parents at midlife is merely an assumption, and there are mediating factors like culture, norms and expectations and resourcefulness which affect the wellbeing of single parents (Stavrova & Fetchenhauer, 2015).

v) LGBTQ+ couple parenting: Midlife lesbian, gay, bisexual, transgender, and queer couples deciding to become parents is a phenomenon which brings together social, legal, political and economic factors. Midlife is a time of more independence and more clarity on what is wanted of life. Literature shows that marriage agrees with LGBTQ+ couples; recognition of their status by law and society strengthens the impact of wellbeing (Herek, 2006). "Mothering", for one thing, has been reported to be immensely fulfilling and more "mainstream" by women who identify as lesbian, with less need than their younger counterparts to seek validation from children (Donaldson, 2000). Some dedicated research has helped debunk myths associated with same-sex parenting and upheld the quality of family relationships as an important determinant of wellbeing (Patterson & Wainright, 2011). The one-of-its-kind "Work Love Play" longitudinal study on the LGBTQ community observed the changes in family dynamics and social support of families with same-sex parents (Power et al., 2010). Stepping down from a heteronormative standpoint and looking again, the wellbeing parameters of sexual minorities are hardly different from their more visible majority counterparts.

vi) Parenting non-human children: Although a controversial issue considering the animal rights movement, the rise in the number of families entering parent–pet relationships has been one of the outcomes of the major shift in the ways families and relationships are conceptualized and lived. Some research has associated the strong need for pet ownership with higher mental health burdens, mediated by the difficulty in dependence and anxiety in human relationships (Lass-Hennemann et al., 2022). Yet, from a sociological vantage point, the social construction of an inter-species family is fairly fluid if parenting, like family, is understood as a co-construction with a goal (Owens & Grauerholz, 2018). A qualitative enquiry revealed that older adults with human and pet children were different in their narrative compared to pet parents with no children or younger children. Their experience was less hurried, they were less preoccupied with training, reported less guilt regarding time spent, and some hinted at the process being more rewarding than raising human children (Owens & Grauerholz, 2018)! Although the sample size was small, the presence and effect of non-human children, given this prevalence, warrant more research attention.

Human life is myriad and complex. Yet the longing for it to continue beyond the designated years is reflected in human desires. In having children, some can envision a future where they will no longer belong, but experience a sense of continuity nonetheless. In a manner of speaking, it is similar to the sense of belongingness and identity which history lends humans. What of those parents who have had children and lost them? Parents who have been childless? How does a midlife parent imagine parenthood having once been one or having missed the opportunity to be one?

Bereavement, an off-time event, leaves parents with anger, resentment and inconsolable sadness, and adversely affects their mental health. However, the effects on psychological health differ depending on the age of the lost child (Pudrovska, 2009).

The literature speaks of parents who try to imagine what parenthood would be like and becomes "practice" parents through taking care of pet animals. There is cultural pressure to parent "intensively", and without any significant improvement in resources to aid the process. On the contrary, juggling responsibilities and managing everything that comes their way is considered the hallmark of success at midlife. It is understandable why individuals would want to defer taking on the additional responsibility of parenthood until other critical aspects of living has been adequately worked out, although this may eventually lead to having young children during midlife, which is a roller-coaster ride.

Relationship between Midlife, Wellbeing and Parenthood: A Multifaceted Lens

Traversing across the lifespan brings with it the dawning of the perception of an "end-point": the limitedness of life. While it is anxiety-provoking to some, it can generate increased acceptance and subsequent prioritization of the interpersonal, familial and other emotion-related goals (socioemotional selectivity theory) (Carstensen et al., 2003). With age, the ability to regulate emotions and experience positive emotions improves (Strengths and Vulnerability Integration Model) (Charles, 2010). The normative advantage of age, however, is compromised in the face of chronic stressors like developmental or mental health conditions in children, financial vulnerabilities, social discrimination (non-normative parents) or onset of chronic illnesses (like metabolic syndromes).

Involvement and intensive parenting and multiple caregiving roles in these postmodern times leads to similar psychological effects for both fathers and mothers. The differences that do exist are attributable to the structure of the parental role mediated by the quality of close interpersonal relationships.

The expected parental roles vary greatly based on individualist versus collectivist outlooks. Ssatisfaction in a particular role is contextual and is strongly associated with the expected standards of society. The European Values Study and the European Social Survey, a large-scale international survey of 43 countries revealed that collectivist nations and existing social norms that are biased toward two-parent families adversely affect the life satisfaction and wellbeing of non-normative (single-parent) parents (*European Values Study*, n.d.).

Gender-culture bias is another lens through which parenthood can be viewed. In countries like India, the attention on women's reproductive health far surpasses the attention devoted to menopause or midlife. The role of a woman as a caregiver overshadows every other role – especially that of being an individual with needs warranting attention and nurturing. A recent multimorbidity study on midlife women showed an association with an inferior quality of life and a need to debunk age-related stereotypes with action plan (Puri et al., 2022).

Conclusion

Time enters the midlife perceptual matrix of a parent, sometimes stealthily and sometimes like an epiphany. The experience of the limitedness of existence deepens the understanding of one's ageing parents, and a renewal of emotional connection with one's own childhood enhances the continuity of self (Erikson, 1950). With more life led than left, the future looks different than before. The capacity to genuinely care for people, things and ideas around oneself is the badge of adulthood, according to Erikson & Erikson (1998). Renowned psychoanalyst and novelist Sudhir Kakar says that adults fulfil their tasks by practising restraint, charity and compassion – qualities that practically define the desirable attributes of a parent. Midlife parenthood can look different for married couples versus those co-parenting, those with grown children versus those with younger ones, those with a stable and fulfilling profession, those in a non-normative relationship trajectory, and those who were midlife parents a few decades back versus now. In sum, societal, economic, family, policy and perspective changes are reflected in midlife parenthood today. Perhaps a singular identifiable factor that binds midlife parenthood and wellbeing is the quality of involvement with their children; it is not so much the intensity of support that determines satisfaction as the appraisal and meaningfulness of it.

References

Carstensen, L. L., Fung, H. H., & Charles, S. T. (2003). Socioemotional selectivity theory and the regulation of emotion in the second half of life. *Motivation and Emotion*, 27(2), 103–123. https://doi.org/10.1023/A:1024569803230

Charles, S. T. (2010). Strength and Vulnerability Integration (SAVI): A model of emotional well-being across adulthood. *Psychological Bulletin*, *136*(6), 1068–1091. https://doi.org/10.1037/a0021232

Cohen, S. T. (2015). Parenthood in midlife: Perceived parental roles, intergenerational ambivalence and well-being among parents of adult children. *Procedia - Social and Behavioral Sciences*, *209*, 137–144. https://doi.org/10.1016/j.sbspro.2015.11.269

Datta, J., Maxwell, K. J., Mitchell, K. R., Lewis, R., & Wellings, K. (2023). Factors shaping the timing of later entry into parenthood: Narratives of choice and constraint. *Social Sciences & Humanities Open*, *8*(1), 100700. https://doi.org/10.1016/j.ssaho.2023.100700
DePasquale, N., Davis, K. D., Zarit, S. H., Moen, P., Hammer, L. B., & Almeida, D. M. (2016). Combining formal and informal caregiving roles: The psychosocial implications of double- and triple-duty care. *The Journals of Gerontology Series B: Psychological Sciences and Social Sciences*, *71*(2), 201–211. https://doi.org/10.1093/geronb/gbu139
Donaldson, C. (2000). Midlife Lesbian parenting. *Journal of Gay & Lesbian Social Services*, *11*(2–3), 119–138. https://doi.org/10.1300/J041v11n02_06
Ebbert, A. M., Kumar, N. L., & Luthar, S. S. (2019). Complexities in adjustment patterns among the "best and the brightest": Risk and resilience in the context of high achieving schools. *Research in Human Development*, *16*(1), 21–34. https://doi.org/10.1080/15427609.2018.1541376
Eggebeen, D. J., Dew, J., & Knoester, C. (2010). Fatherhood and men's lives at middle age. *Journal of Family Issues*, *31*(1), 113–130. https://doi.org/10.1177/0192513X09341446
Erikson, E. H. (1950). *Childhood and society* (p. 397). W W Norton & Co.
Erikson, E. H., & Erikson, J. M. (1998). *The life cycle completed: Extended version* (Extended version). W.W. Norton & Company.
European Values Study. (n.d.). Retrieved April 29, 2024, from https://europeanvaluesstudy.eu/
Feinberg, L. F. (2018, September 4). *Breaking new ground: Supporting employed family caregivers with workplace leave policies*. https://www.aarp.org/ppi/info-2018/breaking-new-ground-supporting-employed-family-caregivers-with-workplace-leave-policies.html
Fingerman, K. L., Cheng, Y.-P., Tighe, L., Birditt, K. S., & Zarit, S. (2012). Relationships between young adults and their parents. In A. Booth, S. L. Brown, N. S. Landale, W. D. Manning, & S. M. McHale (Eds.), *Early adulthood in a family context* (pp. 59–85). Springer New York. https://doi.org/10.1007/978-1-4614-1436-0_5
Fingerman, K., Miller, L., Birditt, K., & Zarit, S. (2009). Giving to the good and the needy: Parental support of grown children. *Journal of Marriage and Family*, *71*(5), 1220–1233. https://doi.org/10.1111/j.1741-3737.2009.00665.x
Fry, R. (2015, July 29). More millennials living with family despite improved job market. *Pew Research Center*. https://www.pewresearch.org/social-trends/2015/07/29/more-millennials-living-with-family-despite-improved-job-market/
Furstenberg, F. F. (2010). On a new schedule: Transitions to adulthood and family change. *The Future of Children*, *20*(1), 67–87. https://doi.org/10.1353/foc.0.0038
Herek, G. M. (2006). Legal recognition of same-sex relationships in the United States: A social science perspective. *American Psychologist*, *61*(6), 607–621. https://doi.org/10.1037/0003-066X.61.6.607
Huo, M., Graham, J. L., Kim, K., Birditt, K. S., & Fingerman, K. L. (2019). Aging parents' daily support exchanges with adult children suffering problems. *The Journals of Gerontology Series B: Psychological Sciences and Social Sciences*, *74*(3), 449–459. https://doi.org/10.1093/geronb/gbx079
Infurna, F. J., Gerstorf, D., & Lachman, M. E. (2020). Midlife in the 2020s: Opportunities and challenges. *American Psychologist*, *75*(4), 470–485. https://doi.org/10.1037/amp0000591
Kim, G. E., & Kim, E.-J. (2020). Factors affecting the quality of life of single mothers compared to married mothers. *BMC Psychiatry*, *20*(1), 169. https://doi.org/10.1186/s12888-020-02586-0

Lachman, M. E. (2004). Development in midlife. *Annual Review of Psychology*, *55*(1), 305–331. https://doi.org/10.1146/annurev.psych.55.090902.141521
Lass-Hennemann, J., Schäfer, S. K., Sopp, M. R., & Michael, T. (2022). The relationship between attachment to pets and mental health: The shared link via attachment to humans. *BMC Psychiatry*, *22*(1), 586. https://doi.org/10.1186/s12888-022-04199-1
Levinson, D. J. (1978). *The seasons of a man's life* (1st ed, 1–1 online resource (xiv, 363 pages)). Knopf; WorldCat. http://books.google.com/books?id=b_RGAAAAMAAJ
Livingston, G. (2014, November 14). Chapter 2: The Demographics of Remarriage. *Pew Research Center*. https://www.pewresearch.org/social-trends/2014/11/14/chapter-2-the-demographics-of-remarriage/
Nomaguchi, K. M. (2012). Parenthood and psychological well-being: Clarifying the role of child age and parent-child relationship quality. *Social Science Research*, *41*(2), 489–498. https://doi.org/10.1016/j.ssresearch.2011.08.001
Nomaguchi, K. M., & Milkie, M. A. (2003). Costs and rewards of children: The effects of becoming a parent on adults' lives. *Journal of Marriage and Family*, *65*(2), 356–374. https://doi.org/10.1111/j.1741-3737.2003.00356.x
Owens, N., & Grauerholz, L. (2018). Interspecies parenting: How pet parents construct their roles. *Humanity & Society*, *43*, 016059761774816. https://doi.org/10.1177/0160597617748166
Parker, R. A., & Aldwin, C. M. (1997). Do aspects of gender identity change from early to middle adulthood? Disentangling age, cohort and period effects. In M. E. Lachman & J. B. James (Eds.), *Multiple paths of midlife development* (pp. 67–107). The University of Chicago Press.
Patterson, J. C., & Wainright, J. L. (2011). Adolescents with same-sex parents: Findings from the National longitudinal study of adolescent health. In D. M. Brodzinsky & A. Pertman (Ed.), *Adoption by lesbians and gay men: A new dimension in family diversity*. Oxford University Press. https://doi.org/10.1093/acprof:oso/9780195322606.001.0001
Pollmann-Schult, M. (2014). Parenthood and life satisfaction: Why don't children make people happy? *Journal of Marriage and Family*, *76*(2), 319–336. https://doi.org/10.1111/jomf.12095
Power, J. J., Perlesz, A., Schofield, M. J., Pitts, M. K., Brown, R., McNair, R., Barrett, A., & Bickerdike, A. (2010). Understanding resilience in same-sex parented families: The work, love, play study. *BMC Public Health*, *10*(1), 115. https://doi.org/10.1186/1471-2458-10-115
Pudrovska, T. (2008). Psychological implications of motherhood and fatherhood in midlife: Evidence from sibling models. *Journal of Marriage and Family*, *70*(1), 168–181. https://doi.org/10.1111/j.1741-3737.2007.00469.x
Pudrovska, T. (2009). Parenthood, stress, and mental health in late midlife and early old age. *International Journal of Aging & Human Development*, *68*(2), 127–147.
Puri, P., Sinha, A., Mahapatra, P., & Pati, S. (2022). Multimorbidity among midlife women in India: Well-being beyond reproductive age. *BMC Women's Health*, *22*(1), 117. https://doi.org/10.1186/s12905-022-01693-2
Resch, J. A., Elliott, T. R., & Benz, M. R. (2012). Depression among parents of children with disabilities. *Families, Systems, & Health*, *30*(4), 291–301. https://doi.org/10.1037/a0030366
Scott, J., & Alwin, D. F. (1989). Gender differences in parental strain: Parental role or gender role? *Journal of Family Issues*, *10*(4), 482–503. https://doi.org/10.1177/019251389010004004
Sloan, C. J., Mailick, M. R., Hong, J., Ha, J.-H., Greenberg, J. S., & Almeida, D. M. (2020). Longitudinal changes in well-being of parents of individuals with

developmental or mental health problems. *Social Science & Medicine*, *264*, 113309. https://doi.org/10.1016/j.socscimed.2020.113309
Smith, A. M., & Grzywacz, J. G. (2014). Health and well-being in midlife parents of children with special health needs. *Families, Systems, & Health*, *32*(3), 303–312. https://doi.org/10.1037/fsh0000049
Soederberg Miller, L. M., & Lachman, M. E. (2000). Cognitive performance and the role of control beliefs in midlife. *Aging, Neuropsychology, and Cognition*, *7*(2), 69–85. https://doi.org/10.1076/1382-5585(200006)7:2;1-U;FT069
Stavrova, O., & Fetchenhauer, D. (2015). Single parents, unhappy parents? Parenthood, partnership, and the cultural normative context. *Journal of Cross-Cultural Psychology*, *46*(1), 134–149. https://doi.org/10.1177/0022022114551160
Thorne, D., Foohey, P., Lawless, R. M., & Porter, K. M. (2018). Graying of U.S. Bankruptcy: Fallout from Life in a risk society. *SSRN Electronic Journal*. https://doi.org/10.2139/ssrn.3226574
Umberson, D., Chen, M. D., House, J. S., Hopkins, K., & Slaten, E. (1996). The effect of social relationships on psychological well-being: Are men and women really so different? *American Sociological Review*, *61*(5), 837. https://doi.org/10.2307/2096456
Vaillant, G. E. (1977). *Adaptation to life*. https://www.amazon.in/Adaptation-to-Life/dp/0316895202
Vance, A. J., & Brandon, D. H. (2017). Delineating among parenting confidence, parenting self-efficacy, and competence. *ANS. Advances in Nursing Science*, *40*(4), E18–E37. https://doi.org/10.1097/ANS.0000000000000179
Zacchini, F., Sampino, S., Ziętek, M., & Chan, A. (2022). Delayed parenthood and its influence on offspring health: What have we learned from the mouse model. *Biology of Reproduction*, *106*(1), 58–65. https://doi.org/10.1093/biolre/ioab202

9 Spirituality and Midlife Transition

Deepshikha Ray and Sanjukta Das

Spirituality as a concept is difficult to define, partly because of multiple perspectives related to it and partly because spirituality encompasses a highly personal and subjective experience, indescribable in words. William James (1902) construed spirituality as a real experience, indescribable by words, the faith in an "unseen order" and the active belief that "supreme good lies in harmoniously adjusting ourselves …", i.e., social adaptation. On the other hand, Fromm (1950) understands spirituality as an essential and distinctive aspect of human development, and considers it to be characterized by self-awareness, authenticity and self-transcendence. According to Fromm, human beings have this innate tendency to strive toward what is good in life, and such a striving itself is an indication of self-transcendence.

Allport and& Ross (1967) distinguished between intrinsic and extrinsic "religious orientation", where intrinsic orientation alludes to a sophisticated understanding of religion with an underlying motive to use the knowledge as a guiding force in life, in contrast to extrinsic religious orientation, which refers to an immature understanding of the sacred through which one tries to satisfy self-serving goals. Allport's conceptualization of "intrinsic religious orientation" is congruous with the concept of "spirituality". However, religiosity and spirituality share the common basis of a process of searching for something abstract; identifying something worthy of devotion/commitment – be it a god or a goal in life. Such an overlap between the psychological processes underlying religiosity and spirituality is also reflected in some of the definitions of spirituality. For example, Jankowski and Vaughn (2009) opined that "spirituality involves finding meaning in adherence to a set of larger beliefs, the exercise of faith as a way of knowing, and an experience of connection with [a higher power] and others". Similarly, Groen (2018) said that "Spirituality is about being aware and honoring the wholeness and interconnectedness of all things through the mystery of a higher power. It is about seeking a sense of purpose and ultimately making meaning in our lives." Sinnott (2002) proposed that spirituality is about individual pursuit and acquisition of self-awareness, and Groen (2018) reiterated that spiritual practices are personal exercises directed to connect with "a power and purpose greater than oneself" – e.g., contemplation, reflection, meditation etc. Spirituality has also been linked with "authenticity", which means living in a

DOI: 10.4324/9781003568360-11

way in which "word and deed, word and word, deed and deed are consistent with a personally owned value structure" (Chickering et al., 2015) and self-knowledge and authentic self-determination are considered as keys to leading a fulfilled life (Baumister, 1987).

Based on the myriad of understandings of spirituality, Knapik et al. (2010) have proposed five characteristics of spirituality:

- Connectedness: A sense of connection with something greater outside of oneself or outside of our usual experience;
- Aliveness/vitality: An energy and alertness not present before the experience;
- Wholeness/integrity: A sense of wholeness that may be with the world and with ourselves, including our present life and past life experiences;
- Peacefulness/serenity/joy/awe: An emotional response that may include peace or serenity, but may also include joy or awe or other strong emotions, depending on the situation;
- Meaning or purpose: From the experience, a new sense of meaning or purpose for life is derived.

Middle adulthood is a stage which is characterized by distinctive physical and psychosocial concerns that distinguish this stage from younger and older adult populations. Jung may be considered as the pioneer in highlighting the importance of psychosocial development in the second half of life. According to Jung (1954), personality processes expand in unique ways in middle adulthood, when individuals develop this tendency to understand the self in favour of focusing on external goals of life like consolidating identity, pursuing a career and relationship. Such a tendency to "look inwards", according to Jung (1957), not only complements the outer directed orientation of youth, but also leads to an increase in the subjective sense of spirituality in midlife and self-realization. However, Jung also forewarned that spiritual insights in middle adulthood can emerge through personal transformations mediated by intense critical appraisal of one's life's journey and the capacity to acquire new awareness and understanding of life.

Feldmeier (2004) has expanded this concept by stating that midlife is a stage when people reassess their values and satisfaction with life and try to take on a greater understanding of their life. It is in this phase of life that individuals start appreciating for the first time the transience of life in terms of developing mild age-related physical incapacities as well as confronting the impending death of elderly and fragile parents. Similar postulates have been put forward by Atchley (1997) – i.e., the inevitable physical constraints of growing older and the awareness of further degeneration make individuals opt for disengagement and narrowing down life's choices, which in turn provides opportunities for contemplation and spiritual development. The psychological changes in midlife (characterized by a spiritual bent) have also been conceptualized as a process of adapting to maturational demands (Sargent &

Schlossberg, 1988). In fact, cognitive developmental psychologists have also tried to explain midlife focus on spirituality in terms of enhanced intellectual potential whereby an individual embraces the paradoxical and circular reasoning characteristic of spiritual quest.

Spirituality in Midlife and Its Relation to Psychosocial Adjustment

Ageing is not merely a biological change, but is also marked by social and psychological transformations such as changes in family structure, personal and social roles as well as personal expectations. Hence, transition to middle adulthood may also encompass a distancing from activities characterizing initial phases of adulthood like searching for a partner, the quest for financial stability, childbearing, child-rearing etc. to a re-definition of life's priorities skewed in the direction of assimilation and savouring of experiences. In midlife, individuals have not only been found to show more interest toward religion and spirituality (Beit-Hallahmi & Argyle, 2014), but their religious interests of earlier ages are often transformed into a less moralistic and more personalized notion of spirituality (Bianchi, 2011). Thus, spiritual inclination in midlife may expand and reshape one's sense of self (Wink, 1999) and also help one cope with inevitable age-related developmental challenges.

Grof (1972) coined the term "spiritual emergency" to denote midlife psychosocial challenges such as divorce, bereavement due to loss of parents, and other traumatic emotional experiences that call for a need to undergo self-transformation through deep involvement in spirituality. Various researchers have explained that spirituality can act as a buffer to stressful experiences as it offers opportunities for alternative interpretations and tolerance of ambiguity, thereby ameliorating distress (Pargament & Brant, 1998; Sorajjakool, 1998). Lancaster and Palframan (2009) conducted qualitative research on the use of spiritual coping in middle-aged individuals who had undergone "a major life transformation (i.e., in terms of ideals, behaviour, concerns, spirituality) as a result of one or more life event(s)" such as "life-threatening illness to self", "major injury to close family members", "major disagreements with family in-laws", "domestic abuse", "alcoholism" etc. They found that spirituality functions as a subtle and insidious coping process characterized by self-transformation and the emergence of the ability to "let go" for these middle-aged individuals in their pathway to coping. Such a finding is in line with the conceptualizations of Park and Folkman (1997) that spirituality facilitates cognitive reappraisal of a negative life event, thereby ushering in a newer meaning of the crisis experience. Hirsch et al. (2014) provided evidence in favour of the association of spirituality with low levels of depression, hopelessness and suicidal ideation. Similarly, Nsamenang et al. (2013) reported that high spirituality is linked with lower perception of a thwarted need for belongingness and perception of self as a burden. Spirituality in midlife not only promotes mental health, but has also been found to improve adaptation to life-limiting physical illnesses as indexed by greater health-related quality of life (Hosseini et al., 2013).

A significant developmental task in midlife is the emergence of "generativity", a concept proposed by Erikson (1963) which represents a selfless concern for the welfare of future generations and/or the world at large. In this connection, the findings of Reischer et al. (2021) may be cited, who found out that increase in "ego integrity" (an index of generativity) is greater between young and middle adulthood in comparison to middle and late adulthood. Similar findings were also reported by McCarthy et al. (2013) and Upchurch (1999), who found subjective measures of ego integrity/self-transcendence to be greater enhanced in individuals in their midlife.

Ego integrity in middle adulthood also represents an ability to achieve a meaningful and coherent sense of self which fosters a sense of competence in understanding and managing life (Eriksson, 2017), and citizenship behaviour (Ravikumar & Jeyaprabha, 2022), and is also positively associated with a sense of satisfaction with life (del-Pino-Casado et al., 2019; McGee et al., 2018).

Generativity may be construed as an expression of beneficence, altruism and compassion, which are also common to spiritual needs (Bellah 1991). Spirituality and generativity may thus be considered to be conceptually analogous, as both psychological processes focus on resolving regrets and reconciling with the present (Kleijn et al., 2016). Irrespective of the definition, spirituality and/or ego integrity have been found to show a strong correlation with personality dimensions of "openness to experience" (Saroglou & Fiasse, 2003), emotional intelligence (Ravikumar & Jeyaprabha, 2022) and improved mental health (Smith et al., 2013).

Women and Spirituality in Midlife

Because of biological and social factors, the psychological antecedents and sequels of midlife transition are different for women in comparison to men (Gilligan, 1997; Levinson, 1996; Wong & Dillon, 2014). Midlife poses a different set of problems for women as middle adulthood also coincides with menopause in women, and it is only women that are effected by ageing constraints on reproductive and sexual functions with associated psychosocial consequences. Menopause/transition to menopause is marked by fluctuations in sex steroid hormones (Gyllstrom et al., 2007) and associated psychological and psychosomatic problems (Dennerstein et al., 2007), and even increased susceptibility to develop depression (Schmidt et al., 2004).

In midlife, women also go through a redefinition of their roles because of changes in family and professional roles and new roles as caregivers for elderly and ailing parents/spouses (Soares, 2014), adult-to-adult interaction with grown-up children, adjusting to new family members (by virtue of their children's marriage or birth of grandchildren) and even reassessment of their marital relationship (Khurram, 2017). In many traditional cultures, women share the primary responsibility of caring for elderly relatives, which may act as an additional stressor. Such experiences may increase the vulnerability of middle-aged women to developing depression. Spirituality in this context may help to find a meaning in suffering and coming to terms with the constraints of their life and thereby transcend suffering (Egnew, 2005).

At the same time, spiritual growth accompanying transition to midlife in women may also be empowering in the sense that women are ultimately able to integrate multiple and apparently incompatible aspects of self to become "what one is meant to be" (Smithson, 2012). Culture has also been found to play a critical role in shaping perspectives on middle adulthood in women. For example, Wong et al. (2012) reported that in cultures which viewed menopause less negatively, women reported fewer problems associated with menopause.

Another interesting observation is that in the new millennium, women often achieve milestones such as marriage and/or parenthood at the same time as the onset of middle adulthood (Degges-White & Myers, 2006). Such postponement of critical developmental tasks may be attributed to increased participation of women in higher education and employment as well as availability of modern medical technologies to buffer against the detrimental effect of ageing on pregnancy. But these experiences are not on a par with conventional norms, which might give rise to increased ambivalence regarding midlife in this cohort of women, and ensuing confusion regarding meaning in life.

However, recent studies have brought forth the idea that advanced maternal age should be viewed and analysed from a complex and multifactorial perspective. For example, delayed attainment of motherhood may bring psychosocial advantages for both the mother and the child because older mothers generally have a comparatively higher education, better financial stability and a longer married life in comparison to their younger counterparts. These factors often facilitate the development of subjective feelings of competence regarding taking care of a newborn, and a more balanced, nuanced readiness to face pregnancy and its sequelae (Ahmad et al., 2024).

Spirituality and Mental Health

It is reasonable to say that spirituality is relevant even today in the context of social and emotional adaptation (Plante 2007). The mediating role of spirituality in enhancing cognitive functions has been explored through neuroimaging techniques (Phillips et al., 2020; van Elk and Aleman, 2017). Also, spiritual practices like meditation and yoga have been examined in the context of biological parameters (Newberg & d'Aquili 2000). The various definitions of spirituality commonly focus on a personal quest to understand uncertain and uncontrollable aspects of life as well as an attempt to seek connectedness with transcendental experiences with nature and the sacred (Puchalsku et al., 2009; Koenig et al., 2001; Giacalone & Jurkiewicz, 2003). Such conceptualizations of spirituality inevitably link a spiritual bent of mind with wellbeing (Moberg, 1971; van Dierendonck, 2012). There is research literature showing positive correlations between measures of spirituality and measures of wellbeing, resilience and coping (Bai & Lazenby, 2015; Schwalm et al., 2022).

The contemporary understanding of "health" does not singularly focus on the absence of physical disease, but on a balanced ability to view oneself as a member of a social group, obligated to be concerned about others, to understand oneself and one's emotions, to be able to adjust to one's vocation, and finally the ability to trust, to accept others, to have a higher purpose in life, and to relate to concepts which are intangible and transcendental (spirituality) (Eberst, 1984). Hence, spirituality can be said to equip individuals with the ability to reappraise their relationships with others and the environment in an adaptive manner and thereby foster resilience (Hawley, 1993; Kearney et al., 2017).

The concept of "spiritual wellbeing" emerges in this context (Ellison, 1983), and consists of the following components:

- Relation with self;
- Relation with others;
- Relation with the environment;
- Relation with a transcendent Other.

It has been found that spiritual wellbeing is associated with increased hope and positive mood states. Thus, spiritual health can be envisaged as a "dynamic state of being" and measured in terms of the extent to which individuals can lead a life in harmony with self, others and nature.

Conclusion

With the growth of generative concern, midlifers gain access to heightened capacity for social care and connection. Their transcending selves allow them to utilize their resources for the upliftment of their work and living contexts. Such resource utilization, again, reinforces community wellbeing. The different personalized concepts of spirituality at midlife create a more meaningful milieu, ultimately culminating in an effective dynamic social network and paving a pathway to positive plasticity.

References

Ahmed, F. S., McMillan, T. M., Guenther, B. A., & Dearborn, P. (2024). Cognitive performance following single-or multi-session exercise intervention in middle age: A systematic review. *Experimental Aging Research*, *50*(1), 28–64.

Allport, G. W., & Ross, J. M. (1967). Personal religious orientation and prejudice. *Journal of Personality and Social Psychology*, *5*(4), 432.

Atchley, R. C. (1997). Everyday mysticism: Spiritual development in later adulthood. *Journal of Adult Development*, *4*, 123–134.

Bai, M., & Lazenby, M. (2015). A systematic review of associations between spiritual well-being and quality of life at the scale and factor levels in studies among patients with cancer. *Journal of Palliative Medicine*, *18*(3), 286–298.
Baumeister, R. F. (1987). How the self became a problem: A psychological review of historical research. *Journal of Personality and Social Psychology*, *52*(1), 163.
Beit-Hallahmi, B., & Argyle, M. (2014). The psychology of religious behaviour, belief and experience. Routledge.
Bellah, R. N. (1991). *Beyond belief: Essays on religion in a post-traditionalist world*. University of California Press.
Bianchi, E. C. (2011). *Aging as a spiritual journey*. Wipf and Stock Publishers.
Chickering, A. W., Dalton, J. C., & Stamm, L. (2015). *Encouraging authenticity and spirituality in higher education*. John Wiley & Sons.
Degges-White, S., & Myers, J. E. (2006). Women at midlife: An exploration of chronological age, subjective age, wellness, and life satisfaction. *Adultspan Journal*, *5*(2), 67–80.
del-Pino-Casado, R., Serrano-Ortega, N., López-Martínez, C., & Orgeta, V. (2019). Coping strategies and psychological distress in family carers of frail older people: A longitudinal study. *Journal of Affective Disorders*, *256*, 517–523.
Dennerstein, L., Lehert, P., Guthrie, J. R., & Burger, H. G. (2007). Modeling women's health during the menopausal transition: A longitudinal analysis. *Menopause*, *14*(1), 53–62.
Eberst, R. M. (1984). Defining health: A multidimensional model. *Journal of School Health*, *54*(3), 99–104.
Egnew, T. R. (2005). The meaning of healing: Transcending suffering. *The Annals of Family Medicine*, *3*(3), 255–262.
Ellison, C. W. (1983). Spiritual well-being: Conceptualization and measurement. *Journal of Psychology and Theology*, *11*(4), 330–338.
Erikson, E. H. (1963). *Childhood and society* (Vol. 2). Norton.
Eriksson, M. (2017). The sense of coherence in the salutogenic model of health. In *The handbook of salutogenesis* (pp. 91–96). Springer. https://doi.org/10.1093/heapro/dal016
Feldmeier, P. (2004). Spirituality in adulthood: Development and fruition. *Way-London-Society of Jesus Then the Way Publications*, *43*(1), 51–64.
Fromm, E. (1950). *Psychoanalysis and religion* (Vol. 12). Yale University Press.
Giacalone, R. A., & Jurkiewicz, C. L. (2003). Right from wrong: The influence of spirituality on perceptions of unethical business activities. *Journal of business Ethics*, *46*, 85–97.
Gilligan, S. (1997). *The courage to love: Principles and practices of self-relations psychotherapy*. WW Norton & Company.
Groen, J. E. (2018). Inner and outer congruence: An academic's quest to find spiritual wellness and health. *Journal for the Study of Spirituality*, *8*(2), 120–129.
Grof, S. (1972). Varieties of transpersonal experiences: Observations from LSD psychotherapy. *The Journal of Transpersonal Psychology*, *4*(1), 45.
Gyllstrom, M. E., Schreiner, P. J., & Harlow, B. L. (2007). Perimenopause and depression: Strength of association, causal mechanisms and treatment recommendations. *Best Practice & Research Clinical Obstetrics & Gynaecology*, *21*(2), 275–292.
Hawley, J. (1993). *Reawakening the spirit in work: The power of dharmic management*. Berrett-Koehler Publishers.
Hirsch, J. K., Nsamenang, S. A., Chang, E. C., & Kaslow, N. J. (2014). Spiritual well-being and depressive symptoms in female African American suicide attempters: Mediating effects of optimism and pessimism. *Psychology of Religion and Spirituality*, *6*(4), 276.

Hosseini, M., Davidson, P. M., Fallahi, K. M., & Green, A. (2013). Spiritual and religious interventions in health care: An integrative review (Reviews/Short Communication).

James, W. (1902). The reality of the unseen. In G. R. Hall (Ed.), *The* varieties *of* religious experience. Longmans, Green and Co.

Jankowski, P. J., & Vaughn, M. (2009). Differentiation of self and spirituality: Empirical explorations. *Counseling and Values*, *53*(2), 82–96.

Jung, C. G. (1954). *The development of personality* (Bollingen Ser No. XX). Pantheon Books.

Jung, C. G. (1957). The transcendent function. *The Journal of Analytical Psychology*, 2(2), 83.

Kearney, G., Fischer, L., & Groninger, H. (2017). Integrating spiritual care into palliative consultation: A case study in expanded practice. *Journal of Religion and Health*, *56*, 2308–2316.

Khurram, U. (2017). *Existential and spiritual support group for women of color in midlife transition*. Saint Mary's College of California.

Kleijn, G., Post, L., Witte, B. I., Bohlmeijer, E. T., Westerhof, G. J., Cuijpers, P., & Verdonck-de Leeuw, I. M. (2016). Psychometric characteristics of a patient reported outcome measures on ego-integrity and despair among cancer patients. *PLoS One*, *11*(5), e0156003.

Knapik, G. P., Martsolf, D. S., Draucker, C. B., & Strickland, K. D. (2010). Attributes of spirituality described by survivors of sexual violence. *Qualitative Report (Online)*, *15*(3), 644.

Koenig, H. G., & Larson, D. B. (2001). Religion and mental health: Evidence for an association. *International Review of Psychiatry*, *13*(2), 67–78.

Lancaster, B. L., & Palframan, J. T. (2009). Coping with major life events: The role of spirituality and self-transformation. *Mental Health, Religion and Culture*, *12*(3), 257–276.

Levinson, J. (1996). *The pleasures of aesthetics: Philosophical essays*. Cornell University Press.

McCarthy, V. L., Ling, J., & Carini, R. M. (2013). The role of self-transcendence: A missing variable in the pursuit of successful aging? *Research in Gerontological Nursing*, *6*(3), 178–186.

McGee, J. S., Zhao, H. C., Myers, D. R., & Seela Eaton, H. (2018). Spiritual diversity and living with early-stage dementia. *Clinical Gerontologist*, *41*(3), 261–267.

Moberg, D. O. (1971). *Spiritual well-being: Background*. White House Conference on Aging.

Newberg, A. B., & d'Aquili, E. G. (2000). The neuropsychology of religious and spiritual experience. *Journal of Consciousness Studies*, *7*(11–12), 251–266.

Nsamenang, S. A., Webb, J. R., Cukrowicz, K. C., & Hirsch, J. K. (2013). Depressive symptoms and interpersonal needs as mediators of forgiveness and suicidal behavior among rural primary care patients. *Journal of Affective Disorders*, *149*(1–3), 282–290.

Pargament, K. I., & Brant, C. R. (1998). Religion and coping. In *The handbook of religion and mental health* (pp. 111–128). Academic Press.

Park, C. L., & Folkman, S. (1997). Meaning in the context of stress and coping. *Review of General Psychology*, *1*(2), 115–144.

Phillips, J., El-Gabalawi, F., Fallon, B. A., Majeed, S., Merlino, J. P., Nields, J. A., & Norko, M. A. (2020). Religion and psychiatry in the age of neuroscience. *The Journal of Nervous and Mental Disease*, *208*(7), 517–523.

Plante, T. G. (2007). Integrating spirituality and psychotherapy: Ethical issues and principles to consider. *Journal of Clinical Psychology*, *63*(9), 891–902.

Puchalski, C., Ferrell, B., Virani, R., Otis-Green, S., Baird, P., Bull, J., & Sulmasy, D. (2009). Improving the quality of spiritual care as a dimension of palliative care: The report of the Consensus Conference. *Journal of Palliative Medicine*, *12*(10), 885–904.

Ravikumar, K., & Jeyaprabha, M. (2022). Social welfare schemes for downtrodden sections of Tamil Nadu an analytical study. *Neuro Quantology*, *20*(10), 30–44.

Reischer, H. N., Roth, L. J., Villarreal, J. A., & McAdams, D. P. (2021). Self-transcendence and life stories of humanistic growth among late-midlife adults. *Journal of Personality*, *89*(2), 305–324.

Sargent, A. G., & Schlossberg, N. K. (1988). Managing adult transitions. *Training & Development Journal*, *42*(12), 58–61.

Saroglou, V., & Fiasse, L. (2003). Birth order, personality, and religion: A study among young adults from a three-sibling family. *Personality and Individual Differences*, *35*(1), 19–29.

Schmidt, P. J., Murphy, J. H., Haq, N., Rubinow, D. R., & Danaceau, M. A. (2004). Stressful life events, personal losses, and perimenopause-related depression. *Archives of Women's Mental Health*, *7*, 19–26.

Schwalm, F. D., Zandavalli, R. B., de Castro Filho, E. D., & Lucchetti, G. (2022). Is there a relationship between spirituality/religiosity and resilience? A systematic review and meta-analysis of observational studies. *Journal of Health Psychology*, *27*(5), 1218–1232.

Sinnott, J. D. (2002). Introduction: Special issue on spirituality and adult development, part II. *Journal of Adult Development*, *9*, 1–2.

Smith, L., Webber, R., & DeFrain, J. (2013). Spiritual well-being and its relationship to resilience in young people: A mixed methods case study. *Sage Open*, *3*(2), 2158244013485582.

Smithson, M. (2012). *Ignorance and uncertainty: Emerging paradigms*. Springer Science & Business Media.

Soares, C. N. (2014). Mood disorders in midlife women: Understanding the critical window and its clinical implications. *Menopause*, *21*(2), 198–206.

Sorajjakool, S. (1998). Gerontology, spirituality, and religion. *Journal of Pastoral Care*, *52*(2), 147–156.

Upchurch, S. (1999). Self-transcendence and activities of daily living: The woman with the pink slippers. *Journal of Holistic Nursing*, *17*(3), 251–266.

Van Dierendonck, D. (2012). Spirituality as an essential determinant for the good life, its importance relative to self-determinant psychological needs. *Journal of Happiness Studies*, *13*, 685–700.

Van Elk, M., & Aleman, A. (2017). Brain mechanisms in religion and spirituality: An integrative predictive processing framework. *Neuroscience & Biobehavioral Reviews*, *73*, 359–378.

Wink, P. (1999). Addressing end-of-life issues: Spirituality and inner life. *Generations: Journal of the American Society on Aging*, *23*(1), 75–80.

Wong, C. M., & Dillon, D. (2014). Meaning making model: Inner purpose, goals, and religiosity/spirituality partially predict acceptance strategies and volunteerism behaviors. *International Journal of Existential Psychology and Psychotherapy*, *5*, 105–123.

PART III

Challenges, Community and Midlife

10 Crises and Challenges in Midlife

Papri Das and Sanjukta Das

Human development is a progressive lifelong process (Baltes, 1987) where midlife covers a large portion of adulthood and is a significant phase of transition. Research trends suggest that we are only at the initial phase of understanding midlife and how it is different from the other phases of adulthood (Lachman, 2004). Generally, major research in the area of midlife has revolved around midlife crisis, but the narratives surrounding midlife need to evolve and move beyond the misconceptions assigned to midlife crisis. The recent trends and current contextual changes emphasize considering midlife as rather a high-spirited phase of life with unparalleled opportunities and challenges (Infurna et al., 2020).

The term "midlife crisis" was first coined by Elliott Jaques (1965) through observing his midlife clients who were experiencing sudden changes in their lifestyle, functioning and productivity. Jaques (1965) also identified this phase as facing or recognizing one's limitations, along with increased importance for morality. The stereotypes often associated with the midlife crisis are buying fancy sports cars, marrying a younger partner, or seeking treatment and interventions to appear younger (Infurna et al., 2020). The incidence of midlife crises is questionable, and research reports that only 10–20% of individuals may experience them (Lachman, 2004). Research has also shown that the midlife crisis has also been considered a topic for humor, movies and entertainment shows. However, such usage of the concept of midlife crisis has often excluded psychological and physical concerns while attributing these features to midlife crisis (Lachman, 2015), and thus ignoring the basic understanding of such an important developmental phase.

Another much-researched phenomenon surrounding midlife crisis is empty nest syndrome. The initial conceptualization of empty nest syndrome was that, after caring for children for decades, women who primarily played the role of homemaker as well as mother experienced loneliness and depression after their children left home (Glenn, 1975; Harkness, 2008). This phase is also marked by the renegotiation of relationships with partners. Research reports that this phase is marked by different changes in relational patterns, ranging from women finding new roles and identities, and marital conflicts for some people to a positive and productive time for others (Mitchell, 2006). Moreover, challenges and crises may occur that require adjustment, which

DOI: 10.4324/9781003568360-13

may arise when sociocultural and personal norms, along with educational paths are dissimilar between parents and their grown-up children (Mitchell, 2006; Settersten & Hagestad, 1996).

It can be well understood that grown-up offspring leaving home is a real-life separation that is emotionally and psychologically overwhelming for the entire family structure (Kins et al., 2013). However, Lillian Rubin (1979) found that mothers who were homemakers felt relieved and relaxed when their grown-up offspring left home. Recent studies also confirmed that the majority of midlife parents might not experience long-standing emotional dysregulation with their grown-up offspring leaving home (Mitchell & Lovegreen, 2009; Mitchell & Wister, 2015). This research also found that it is not only the mothers who may experience emotional turmoil, but the fathers also equally experience similar emotional consequences (Mitchell, 2019).

However, with increasing longevity and reduced fertility rates, the concept of empty nest syndrome has changed and its timing has become delayed (Mitchell et al., 2009). Research has also reported a trend of grown-up offspring returning home after their initial departure to refill the empty nest as "incompletely launched adults" (Clemens & Axelson, 1985; Schnaiberg & Goldenberg, 1989), which has been attributed to socioeconomic and demographic changes, along with unstable partnerships and seeking higher education (Mitchell, 2019). This paradoxical pattern of grown-up offspring returning home is termed boomerang kids" (Mitchell, 2006).

Consequently, it can be well understood that midlife can be conceptualized as a pivotal period in the life course (Lachman et al., 2015), and middle-aged adults play a vital role in caring for and nurturing family members both financially and emotionally, which results in experiences of different opportunities and challenges during this remarkable life phase. The following sections discuss different dimensions, and trajectories that create challenges, crises as well as opportunities during middle adulthood.

Challenges and Crises Due to Physiological Changes

Midlife is a distinct phase from the other life stages like young adulthood or old age because it is not separated by any explicit legal or biological demarcation (Lachman et al., 2015). The transition from adolescence to adulthood is marked by a clear age boundary of 18 years as the legal age of majority in many countries across the world. Similarly, in the majority of wealthy countries across the world, ages from 60 onwards are marked as the eligibility criteria for age-related pension programmes. Biological factors also demarcate and distinguish some critical life stages, such as menarche among females, which signifies the transition from childhood to adolescence. However, the demarcations of middle adulthood are less definitive and rather are structured by various biopsychosocial and cultural factors (Cohen, 2012). The biological processes of menopause and andropause are considered to be significant markers during midlife transitions for women and men respectively. However, these biological processes lack clear-cut initiation and termination dates.

Menopause and Andropause among Middle-aged Adults

Menopause and andropause-related issues have been often associated with physiological changes during midlife. However, these biological concerns and the perceived experiences related to them are not common for every individual in this phase. The menopause usually begins between the late forties and early fifties and lasts about seven to ten years. The absence of menstruation about 12 months from the last menstrual period defines the menopause. Similarly, the andropause results from the lack of testosterone production among men, which usually starts around age 40, although the onset and progression of andropause vary widely (Sternbach, 1998). These age-related hormonal changes among men and women are associated with various physical symptoms like fatigue, sleep disorders, diminished libido, and obesity, which further contribute to hampering mental wellbeing and result in symptoms like depression (Martelli et al., 2021). Depression among women has been linked to reduced production of ovarian hormones, although most women successfully pass through the phase of transition without serious depressive episodes or symptoms (Maki et al., 2010). However, the risk of depression remains constant during perimenopausal and menopausal phases among women with a past psychiatric history of depression, high stress exposure and strained relationships (Sandilyan & Dening, 2011).

Other Related Biological Concerns among Middle-aged Adults

Age-related reduction in hypothalamic-pituitary-gonadal function in men can influence their mental health. Men experience a decline of testosterone from around 40 years onwards, which causes a range of symptoms in middle-aged and older men, including depression. However, research suggests that testosterone deficiency has only a moderate influence on mood disorders (Seidman, 2006).

Biological changes in midlife not only include hormonal changes, but some people during midlife also experience an initial onset of and gradual increase in chronic health conditions and functional limitations. The Health and Retirement Study in 2005 found increased levels of depressive symptoms triggered due to pharmacotherapy for different physical conditions, such as beta blockers, corticosteroids, anti-Parkinson's drugs and cancer treatment among middle-aged adults (Staff, 2017).

Challenges and Opportunities in Marital Relationships in Midlife

Recent sociocultural and contextual development has been discussing commitment-based models of marriage and expressive individualistic models of marriage as divorce rates during midlife have become alarming (Uhlenberg et al., 1990; Wu & Schimmele, 2007). During the 20th century, the rise in romantic love became the significant foundation upon which most marriages were built and maintained, which implied mutual responsibilities toward each other as partners. The relationship was maintained through commitment, and only in extreme conditions, where there was reciprocal strain on the relationship, would divorce ever be considered (Crowley, 2018).

However, in the middle of the 20th century, new philosophies regarding marriage evolved with a growing era of consumerism and significant sociopolitical changes, where the focus on expressive individualism was the priority (Russell, 2013). Expressive individualism means that everyone needs to prioritize their personal development. This change in perspective changed the concept of marriage, which became a site facilitating personal growth (Crowley, 2018). Furthermore, the success of the marriage was measured in terms of reciprocal abilities to facilitate each other's personal goals, failing which divorce would be easily considered, and separation and divorce became socially acceptable practices (Hackstaff, 1999; Wu & Schimmele, 2007). Moreover, research on middle-aged adults (aged 46–59) reported that there were significant etiological factors contributing to grey divorces, such as lack of emotional reciprocity and communication, presence of other long-term relationships, love affairs external to marriages, and physical and emotional abuse in marriages (Rokach et al., 2004).

Midlife divorces and widowhood often lead to depression and perceived loneliness. Re-partnering in the later phases of life (Brown & Lin, 2013) has eventually developed with the increase in life expectancy and other socio-contextual changes with modernization. This brings about a new opportunity and sense of belongingness and partnerhood during the later phase in the life course. Older adults generally enter into such relationships when both of the partners are physically and cognitively well-functioning. However, as the process of ageing continues, their health and functioning decrease (Devi, 2018) and they need assistance from others. Research has shown that middle-aged adults prefer their late-life partners rather than their children while seeking help and support during the process of ageing (Koren et al., 2016).

Challenges Faced in Family and Relationships

The structural and functional changes in the family influence the relationships of middle-aged adults with their ageing parents and grown-up children. Middle-aged adults need to adapt to the role of caregivers. Further, helping grown-up children to adapt to their adulthood issues is another critical role to develop for middle-aged adults. Middle adulthood also brings about challenges and opportunities offered by grandparenting. Among various underlying contemporary factors, middle-aged adults are supposed to deal with changing norms for single parenthood, separation and divorce, step-parenting due to re-marriage, blended families, and cohabiting families (Antonucci et al., 2011; Bengtson, 2001; Silverstein & Giarrusso, 2010). Therefore, changes in family structure and dynamics have resulted in changes in relationships, which significantly challenge middle-aged adults (Connidis, 2015).

The Crisis of Caring for Baby Boomers

Careing for ageing parents is stressful for middle-aged adults, and accepting the anxiety related to losing their parents adds to their vulnerabilities. Ageing parents act as a source of support for middle-aged adults, especially when their grown-up offspring encounter life problems. Supportive exchanges with ageing parents are positively associated with the daily health and wellness of middle-aged adults (Huo et al., 2019; Ryff et al., 1994). But despite this, the needs of ageing parents are increasing the strain on middle-aged adults as more baby boomers will live longer and the number of dementia cases will increase over time (Feinberg, 2018; Hebert et al., 2013). Research conducted in 2015 in the United States, Germany and Italy has found that middle-aged adults feel a need and an obligation to help their ageing parents (Fry, 2015), which is leading them to juggle caregiving responsibilities and full-time work (Gordon et al., 2012).

Along with informal caregiving for ageing parents, taking care of dependent grown-up offspring at the same time and working full-time are termed as double- and triple-duty caregiving. Double- and triple-duty caregiving among middle-aged adults has negative effects on health and work–life balance, affecting efforts to provide love and care as well as reducing work productivity as middle-aged adults have to coordinate these different types of roles (Aneshenshel et al., 1995). Middle-aged adults have reported significant work–family conflicts, psychological distress, poor sleep quality, marital issues and more acute health problems due to double- and triple-duty caregiving than non-caregivers (DePasquale et al., 2016, 2017; Polenick et al., 2018). They have found it difficult to manage double- and triple-duty caregiving roles and may have changed to less demanding jobs, resulting in a delay in career development or early voluntary retirement; they may also quit their jobs and move to being full-time caregivers due to excessive strain (Eifert et al., 2016; Feinberg, 2018).

Challenges of and Coping with Childlessness during Midlife

Infertility and childlessness during midlife may lead to mental health difficulties due to societal norms and expectations. Erikson (1963) in his theory of personality development spoke about the attainment of generativity as the major concern during midlife. It has been defined as the ability to influence or contribute to future generations (Erikson, 1963). This developmental phase has been associated with parenthood as one of the prime factors for the attainment of generativity (Hansen et al., 2009; Rothrauff & Cooney, 2008), and Erikson (1978) has mentioned parenthood as one of the many ways to achieve generativity during midlife (An & Cooney, 2006; McAdams

& de St. Aubin, 1992). Major sociocultural themes have often placed a significant focus on parenthood concerning generativity through the parent–child relationship, nurturing the children and leaving a genetic legacy (Bures, 2009; Connidis, 2001; Morgan & King, 2001). Achievement of generativity is not only limited to parenting, teaching, mentoring and caregiving, it may occur through other routes (Cox et al., 2010; McAdams et al., 1997; Wojciechowska, 2011).

Research has indicated that there remains no significant difference in psychological wellbeing and generativity among childless middle-aged adults and middle-aged adults with children (Rothrauff & Cooney, 2008), which further indicates that parenthood is not the only route to generativity. It is often observed that childless middle-aged couples engage in parenting or nurturing their nephews or nieces, taking care of their older parents, or mentoring younger generations in their workspace (Milardo, 2005). Childless middle-aged adults have also been observed to adopt pets, which fulfils their parental aspirations (Albert & Bulcroft, 1988; Hansen, 2012).

Studies on involuntarily childless middle-aged couples have reported resilience as one of the significant factors that helps couples overcome the psychosocial pain and difficulties concerning infertility and childlessness (Peters et al., 2011). Although infertility and childlessness in the initial years of marriage have been often found to be difficult factors to adapt to, with increasing years several benefits to childlessness, like less stress, lower financial responsibilities and more freedom, have been observed (Hansen et al., 2009; Mirowsky & Ross, 2002).

Challenges of Caring for Children during Midlife

With changes in sociocultural norms and increasing financial competition, women may take time out from their careers to get married and eventually procreate. Reports have suggested that early childbearing leads to reduced wages among women due to negative effects on their careers (Taniguchi, 1999), whereas women who decide to delay childbearing have a higher tendency to remain stable in their careers throughout their working years (Pienta, 1999). These concerns are leading to greater instances of childbearing and child-rearing during midlife.

Childbearing during midlife or around the late thirties often leads to difficulties with conception due to compromised fertility, which can apply equally to men and women. However, it is not always problematic for couples to bear children during their middle adulthood even though there can be social and psychological effects of child-rearing during midlife.

Reports have suggested that late child-rearing is related to more emotional preparedness for the stresses of parenthood among older parents (Reece 1993). Studies have suggested that with increasing age of motherhood and delayed parenthood, child–mother interactions are increased, with positive maternal affect and less negative emotions (Ragozin et al., 1982; Conger et al., 1984, Walter 1986). Contrastingly other studies have shown that children of older mothers experience a sense of separation and lack of intimacy (Daniels & Weingarten, 1982, Yarrow, 1991). Delayed child-rearing has also been found to have positive effects on father–child relationships and a lower depression rate among fathers (Cooney et al., 1993). Late fatherhood is associated with increased interactions with their children and more nurturing behaviour toward them (Heath, 1994). Older fathers engage in less physical play but may establish stronger emotional bonds with their children (Neville & Parke, 1997).

Challenges Arising from Relationships With Grown-up Offspring

Changes in relationship dynamics and structure among middle-aged adults and their grown-up children have taken place due to frequent intergenerational contact, continuous support from the middle-aged parents, and cohabitation and reciprocal emotional needs (Fingerman, 2017). The frequency of contact between middle-aged parents and their grown-up offspring has grown over the past 30 years due to technological developments and usage (Fingerman et al., 2012). The contact between middle-aged parents and their grown-up offspring is also increasing due to the problems of children and middle-aged adults providing more support to them (Huo et al., 2019), which may stress the middle-aged adults and make them believe that they have failed as parents (Byers et al., 2008; Fingerman et al., 2012). The nature and style of parenting have evolved gradually in middle adulthood with the increasing demands, engagement and financial resources needed for raising grown-up offspring. Protecting grown-up offspring from any hardships or disappointment, and financial pressures for their higher education have led to growing attention to "helicopter" or "bulldozer" parents or "tiger moms" (Ebbert et al., 2019). Grown-up offspring are more reliant on their middle-aged parents because of greater engagement with them anddependence due to the costs of higher education attainments (Settersten & Ray, 2010). Research has shown that compared to recent decades, more grown-up offspring are now cohabitating with their middle-aged parents (Fry, 2015). Research in the United States also shows that middle-aged parents are involved with their grown-up offspring's higher education where they act as the cosigner of the financial debt required for the education. This engagement increases the financial risk added to other challenges like future savings for retirement, mortgage payments, and liability for paying the debt for education if the grown-up offspring are unable to (Walsemann & Ailshire, 2017).

Challenges and Opportunities of Grandparenting

Research has found variations in the type of grandparenting and ways of getting involved with grandchildren, ranging from rare interactions with them to grandchildren taking care of them, along with custodial grandparenting (Meyer & Kandic, 2017). Among of the many positives of grandparenting, it offers an opportunity to get involved in fulfilling family roles and demands, and this helping behaviour in turn offers meaningfulness and purpose during middle adulthood, promoting wellbeing and quality of life (Bengtson, 2001; Hilbrand et al., 2017). Grandparenting has positive outcomes which can be beneficial for their significant others. Retired grandparents get involved with careing for their grandchildren or helping their adult divorced offspring by babysitting the grandchildren, which reduces the burden on their grown-up offspring (Coall & Hertwig, 2010). Research has shown that a proper balance in the frequency and intensity of caregiving and helping behaviour in middle-aged adults fosters cognitive functioning, quality of life, physical health and mental wellbeing and also promotes long life (Arpino & Bordone, 2014).

On the other hand, divorce and separation in families result in tension and ambivalence which negatively influences intergenerational cargiving or grandparenting (Connidis, 2015). Added responsibilities of grandparenting may arise due to the re-marriage of their offspring and an increase in the number of family members. Further, disconnection with grandchildren due to custodial parenting (Antonucci et al., 2011) may generate feelings of isolation and emotional dysregulation, but may also provide an opportunity to explore new roles and interests.

Other downsides of grandparenting include middle-aged adults becoming full-time caregivers or taking primary custody of the grandchildren. However, custodial grandparenting makes a positive contribution to the community, where providing full-time caregiving to the grandchildren leads to handling stressful situations with care (Meyer & Kandic, 2017). Custodial grandparents also face significant financial strain, lowered social support, disturbances in lifestyle and ignorance in the workspace (Meyer & Kandic, 2017). Furthermore, multiple studies have found that middle-aged adults raising their grandchildren report lower mental wellbeing and physical health than non-caregivers (Hayslip et al., 2017).

Crises and Challenges in Work–family Balance

Work provides a sense of independence and freedom and boosts the ego in individuals regardless of their developmental phase. But work in middle adulthood not only provides a sense of entitlement, it also encroaches, with challenges due to technological advancements, consumerism and excessive engagement in social media. As discussed in an earlier section, midlife is a phase of double- and triple-duty responsibility, where balancing work with the family burden of caring for ageing parents and financially supporting grown-up offspring create a disparity in attitudes toward their social roles. Therefore, maintenance of work–family balance is a critical task in middle adulthood, which provides a scaffolding for existential wellbeing.

Work–family balance has been defined as a comprehensive appraisal of the extent of efficacy and satisfaction of the individual in work and family roles to be consistent with their values in life at a particular point in time (Greenhaus & Allen, 2011). Work–family conflict has also been widely attended to and investigated in terms of work-family balance. Work–family conflict has been defined as a type of inter-role conflict that consists of role pressures both from the work and family domains that are mutually conflictual in one apect or other (Greenhaus & Beutell, 1985). A Japanese study by Tomida et al. (2022) considered familial factors among middle-aged adults (e.g., participation in household chores, caring for older parents and child-rearing), and various lifestyle factors including health-promoting and health-damaging habits (e.g., sleep cycle, diet and nutrition, and substance intake) to be the influencing factors of workk–family roles. The study also reported that middle-aged adults with high work–life balance and low work–family facilitation were the ones who were working for long hours with regular employment and living with family members. These individuals experienced the heavy burden of household responsibilities (e.g. child-rearing, and assisting others in the family) and problematic lifestyles, leading to difficult work–family balance (Tomida et al., 2022). The importance of social support and relationships has also been highlighted as an essential factor for a healthy work–family balance among middle-aged adults. Middle-aged adults receiving social support from family and non-family members have been found to have better mental health, lower depressive symptoms, high life satisfaction and better work–family balance (Tomida et al., 2022). Social support can act as a mediator or a buffer in the relationship between work–family balance and mental wellbeing (Greenhaus & Beutell, 1985). Moreover, receiving social support regardless of work, family or leisure domain positively influences an employee's mental health (Viswesvaran et al., 1999).

Social Media and Middle-aged Adults

Social media plays a recreational role and helps people strengthen ties with family and friends among middle-aged adults (Sleek, 2014). Middle-aged adults have work and family lives where remaining connected to family and frequent communication at work becomes extremely pivotal, and social media plays a significant role in this context. Various research studies have found that smartphones play a necessary role for middle-aged adults in managing their workload, but they also create pressure on middle-aged adults to remain virtually connected to their friends and family.

However, spending too much time on social media has rather negative results, leading to perceived loneliness, isolation and aggravated mental health concerns like anxiety and depression. Excessive and addictive use of social media often leads to significant mental health issues. Studies have found that problematic use of social media is significantly associated with perceived social isolation among middle-aged adults (Meshi et al., 2020). On the other hand, a few studies have confirmed that using social media has resulted in a reduced sense of loneliness and improved mental health by remaining connected to their loved ones (Coto et al., 2017).

Financial Challenges and Related Concerns during Middle Adulthood

Employment with career growth and financial stability are the prime aspects of midlife. Employment's significance has been highlighted in various research programmes on work-related factors like work hazards, complexity and occupation status that influence physical and mental health, cognitive functioning and longevity in middle and older adulthood (Fisher et al., 2014; Hülür et al., 2019; Super, 1990).

The aftermath of the economic recession of 2008 in the US showed that middle-aged adults are more vulnerable to failure in the economy and labour market volatility than adults in other age groups. Factors resulting in the recession included various hardships (like soaring unemployment rates, falls in housing and financial conditions, and depletion in retirement accounts) rather than a single cause (Burgard & Kalousova, 2015). This recession further led to financial crises, job insecurity, lack of wage rises, frequent phases of unemployment, and increased loans (Burgard & Kalousova, 2015). The long-term effects of job insecurity, financial crises and other related financial losses can lead to anxiety, depression, substance and behavioural addiction and suicidal behaviour (Haw et al., 2015; Phillips & Nugent, 2014). Cyclical economic hardships also lead to cognitive problems from midlife to the old age phase (Leist et al., 2014). Research has also shown that the economic crisis and the status of grown-up offspring of middle-aged adults negatively contributed to their physical and mental health. Middle-aged parents remain under stress and pressure about their grown-up offspring's economic crises and future, which leads to higher levels of anxiety and depression among middle-aged adults (Stein et al., 2011). This was reinforced by the lack of employment opportunities during middle adulthood, further leading to financial instability and difficulty in managing health needs (Rajmil et al., 2014). Research during the 2008 recession showed that particular sections of people were hit harder than others: the middle adults with low–middle socio-economic status who lost their jobs, and middle-aged parents with children experiencing disabilities (Lam et al., 2014; Riumallo-Herl et al., 2014; Song et al., 2018). Also, women of colour were found to be most vulnerable to low psychological wellbeing and physical health with financial vulnerabilities due to labour market volatility (Castro Baker et al., 2019; Kirsch & Ryff, 2016; Wang et al., 2018). The labour market volatility in the US has contributed to reduced social and healthcare safety nets among middle-aged adults. It has been most striking for middle-aged adults who play caregiver roles for their aged parents with limited access to increasingly high-cost healthcare services. Healthcare services are becoming increasingly costly and growing out of control for daily consumers (Paez et al., 2009; Woolhandler & Himmelstein, 2019). Healthcare insurance with less comprehensive benefits may result in heightened anxiety, financial debts and restriction in access to and availability of proper medical care and management (Grande et al., 2013), further disrupting household budgets and access to social activities (Salamon et al., 2009).

COVID-19 and Challenges during Midlife

Several recent studies on the impact of COVID-19 on middle-aged adults have been conducted across the globe. COVID-19 was an unprecedented public health issue that not only affected physical health across all sections of society but also had significant psychological impacts. Moreover, individuals falling in the age group of 40 years and above who had one or more health complications were at a higher risk of developing serious complications after contracting the disease (Ranjan et al., 2020; Williamson et al., 2020). Due to this, preventive measures of social distancing and isolation at home were the identified strategies for mitigating and controlling the spread of the disease. These preventive measures created an adverse effect on middle-aged adults due to sudden limitations in their social life (Amritage & Nellums, 2020).

COVID-19 created a significant psychological impact among middle-aged adults. Being in the vulnerable age group instilled a significant sense of fear and anxiety about contamination. These also affected the lifestyle-related behaviour of middle-aged adults. Increased dietary awareness was found to be one of the significant changes among middle-aged adults, wherein they started consuming a healthy diet and balanced food (FAO, 2020). Giustino et al. (2020) also found that home confinement had negatively affected the overall physical health of middle-aged adults due to reduced physical activity. Lack of physical activity led to disturbed circadian rhythms and disturbed sleeping hours and patterns (Emerson, 2020), which have been associated with depression, reduced life satisfaction and negative effects on overall wellbeing. Additionally, the preventive measures for COVID-19 led to significant behavioural changes in middle-aged adults, which included frequent hand-washing, social distancing and avoidance of social gatherings as well as frequent disinfecting behaviour (Brooke & Clark, 2020). Apart from that, there have been some mixed behavioural changes among middle-aged adults in activities like spending time with family members as well as frequent engagement in social media and attending online wellness programmes (Brooke & Clark, 2020).

COVID-19, Mental Health and Financial Vulnerabilities

Moulton et al. (2023) have discussed the fact that economic inequalities and unemployability during the pre-pandemic phase among individuals with psychological distress across the life course seem to have been exacerbated by the economic shock of COVID-19. Middle-aged adults with prior mental health issues were more vulnerable to the economic shock. Moulton et al. (2023) have also pointed out that during the pandemic, vulnerable groups were more likely to seek financial help from the economic response packages of the UK government. However, after subsequent cuts in financial support from the government during the post-pandemic phase, economic challenges were likely to put further mental and financial strain on the vulnerable groups. Moreover, to cope with the financial strain during the COVID-19 pandemic, the vulnerable groups may have indefinitely relied on their savings or reduced consumption during the period of increasing inflation; which may in turn have led to an increase in psychological distress and reduction in the chances of improvements in mental health concerns (Moulton et al., 2023; Douglas et al., 2020; Di Gessa et al., 2022).

Crises among Middle-aged Adults belonging to the LGBTQ+ Community

Old age comes with various mental health concerns, especially cognitive impairment, Alzheimer's disease and other forms of dementia (Alzheimer's Association, 2016). Various research has also shown that older adults belonging to the LGBTQ+ community are more prone to experiencing fragile mental health as they face extreme discrimination, social isolation (Fredriksen-Goldsen et al., 2013, Cornwell & Waite, 2009) and an increased death rate (Steptoe et al., 2013). Reports also have found that middle-aged people belonging to the LGBTQ+ community face identity concealment, unique family composition and dynamics that result in barriers to receiving and providing caregiving activities (Fredriksen-Goldsen et al., 2018). Due to their already fragile mental health and experience of sociocultural traumas, older adults belonging to the LGBTQ+ community are vulnerable to impairment and decline in cognitive functioning as well as diagnosis of Alzheimer's disease and other types of dementias (Fredriksen-Goldsen et al., 2018, Cacioppo & Hawkley, 2009). Other than neurocognitive concerns, older adults from the LGBTQ+ community are also vulnerable to HIV/AIDS, which may further complicate their other health conditions and is also associated with significant cognitive decline, resulting in HIV-associated dementia (Huang, 2015). Fredriksen-Goldsen, Kim, et al. (2013) have also reported that lesbian and bisexual women have higher rates of cardiovascular diseases and obesity, and one-third of them experience depression.

Challenges in Recent Contextual Changes

Changing sociocultural structure, gender and relationship fluidity, and same-sex relationships have led to changes in normative sociocultural phenomena in many societies around the globe. These changes are not easily accommodated by a varied spectrum of members of the community due to stereotypical ideologies. Middle-aged adults may face challenges and dilemmas in accommodating the changes in sociocultural structures. Cramer and Roach (1988) witnessed that relationships between parents and their gay sons were usually strained immediately after the sons came out, and the families experienced extensive periods of turmoil. It was also found that parents of gay children who had not come out had strong traits associated with homophobia. As the majority of the middle-aged adult mothers had more traditional sex-role attitudes and the fathers were highly orthodox, the stereotypical ideologies imprinted inflexible perspectives and attitudes among the middle-aged adults about the current sociocultural and contextual changes. Moreover, this resulted in conflicting relationship dynamics and affected overall psychological wellbeing among middle-aged adults.

Wellbeing and Opportunities in Middle Adulthood

The earlier sections have delineated the challenges and crises faced by middle-aged adults, but it is untrue to say that midlife is only about challenges and crises. This phase of life is extremely critical and significant at the same time, as it also brings opportunities that fuel the overall wellbeing of middle-aged adults. There are various areas like job positions, earnings, leadership, family relationships, self-efficacy, decision-making capacities, and contributing toward the community and the next generation (Infurna et al., 2020) which bring various opportunities for middle-adults. Studies have shown that individuals with fewer years of education move up the ladder of earnings during their late forties, whereas individuals with more years of education move up their ladder of earnings in their early fifties (Bhuller et al., 2017). Those in midlife has been significantly observed to gain in emotional experiences (Carstensen et al., 1999), abilities to acquire new knowledge and skills, and control of their values and beliefs (Lachman, 2006). Middle adulthood brings about the major opportunity of grandparenting, which acts as a road map to generativity and multi-generational relationships, like day-to-day caregiving for their grandchildren (Bengtson, 2001).

Research has suggested that the opportunities of middle adulthood are socially structured. Individuals from higher socioeconomic strata have more opportunities to experience better-quality and more consistent medical care, better leisure activities, and less exposure to negative and stressful life events with significant access to financial, social and psychological resources (Kirsch & Ryff, 2016). In contrast, individuals with lower socioeconomic status have reduced gains in episodic memory and executive function in comparison to individuals with higher socioeconomic status (Zahodne et al., 2017). Research has also suggested that in terms of psychological wellbeing, socioeconomic status plays a very vital role in experiencing gains in life among middle-aged adults. Chen et al. (2019) found that white middle-aged adults experienced higher rates of depression and anxiety in comparison to other racial or ethnic groups.

Conclusion

Middle adulthood can be identified as the phase of life that strives for balance amidst multiple co-occurring crises and challenges while coping with transitions of self, work, family and relationships. Gradually, the narratives of midlife are shifting and also changing in other ways, including changes in the lives of younger adults and the health status of older adults. Biological, social, cultural and economic changes over time bring about distress as well as fulfilment in the lives of middle adults.

It is well understood that middle adulthood is a phase for a multitude of challenges as well as opportunities to adjust to changes and transition which impact mental wellbeing. These issues make it important to focus on holistic intervention and policy-making for middle-aged adults to promote resilience among them, improving their overall health and financial strength, reducing caregiving stresses or burdens, and enhancing mental wellbeing through support groups and community engagements. Policies that involve the shrinking of the social and healthcare safety nets need to be considered carefully along with policies involving flexible working hours for middle adults who have to fulfil multiple social and familial responsibilities. This will further help and empower middle-aged adults. The focus on and optimization of the wellbeing of middle-aged adults may also be helpful for younger adults and older adults who remain dependent on middle-aged adults for considerable periods.

References

Albert, A., & Bulcroft, K. (1988). Pets, families, and the life course. *Journal of Marriage and the Family, 50*, 543–552. http://doi.org/10.2307/ 352019

Alzheimer's Association. (2016). 2016 Alzheimer's disease facts and figures. Alzheimer's & Dementia, 12(4), 459-509.

An, J. S., & Cooney, T. (2006). Psychological well-being in mid to late life: The role of generativity development and parent-child relationships across the lifespan. *International Journal of Behavioral Development, 30*, 20–31. http://doi.org/10.1177/0165025406071489

Aneshensel, C. S., Pearlin, L. I., Mullan, J. T., Zarit, S. H., & Whitlatch, C. J. (1995). Profiles in caregiving: The unexpected career. Elsevier.

Antonucci, T. C., Birditt, K. S., Sherman, C. W., & Trinh, S. (2011). Stability and change in the intergenerational family: A convoy approach. *Ageing & Society*, 31, 1084–1106. http://dx.doi.org/10.1017/ S0144686X1000098X

Armitage, R., & Nellums, L. B. (2020). COVID-19 and the consequences of isolating the elderly. *The Lancet Public Health*, *5*(5), e256.

Arpino, B., & Bordone, V. (2014). Does grandparenting pay off? The effect of child care on grandparents' cognitive functioning. *Journal of Marriage Family, 76*, 337–351.

Baltes, P. B. (1987). Theoretical propositions of life-span developmental psychology: On the dynamics between growth and decline. *Developmental Psychology, 23*(5), 611–626.

Bengtson, V. L. (2001). Beyond the nuclear family: The increasing importance of multigenerational bonds. *Journal of Marriage and Family, 63*, 1–16. http://dx.doi.org/10.1111/j.1741-3737.2001.00001.x

Bhuller, M., Mogstad, M., & Salvanes, K. G. (2017). Life-cycle earnings, education premiums, and internal rates of return. *Journal of Labor Economics, 35*, 993–1030.

Brooke, J., & Clark, M. (2020). Older people's early experience of household isolation and social distancing during COVID-19. *Journal of Clinical Nursing*, *29*(21–22), 4387–4402.

Brown, S. L., & Lin, I. F. (2013). *Age variation in the remarriage rate, 1990–2011.* National Center for Family & Marriage Research. http://www.firelands.bgsu.edu/content/dam/BGSU/college-of-arts-and-sciences/NCFMR/documents/FP/FP-13-17.pdf
Bures, R. M. (2009). Childlessness, parenthood, and depressive symptoms among middle-aged and older adults. *Journal of Family Issues, 30*, 670–687. http://doi.org/10.1177/0192513X08331114
Burgard, S. A., & Kalousova, L. (2015). Effects of the great recession. *Applied Psychology Health and Well-Being, 41*, 181–203.
Byers, A. L., Levy, B. R., Allore, H. G., Bruce, M. L., & Kasl, S. V. (2008). When parents matter to their grown-up offsprings: Filial reliance associated with parents' depressive symptoms. *Journals of Gerontology: Series B, Psychological Sciences and Social Sciences, 63*, P33–P40. http://dx.doi.org/10.1093/geronb/63.1.P33
Cacioppo, J. T., & Hawkley, L. C. (2009). She perceived social isolation and cognition. *Trends in Cognitive Sciences, 13*(10), 447–454.
Carstensen, L. L., Isaacowitz, D. M., & Charles, S. T. (1999). Taking time seriously. *American Psychologist, 54*(3), 165–181.
Castro Baker, A., West, S., & Wood, A. (2019). Asset depletion, chronic financial stress, and mortgage trouble among older female homeowners. *Gerontologist, 59*, 230–241. http://dx.doi.org/10.1093/geront/gnx137
Chen, R., Kessler, R. C., Sadikova, E., Nemoyer, A., Sampson, N. A., Alvarez, K., & Williams, D. R. (2019). Racial and ethnic differences in individual-level and area-based socioeconomic status and 12-month DSM-IV mental disorders. *Journal of Psychiatric Research, 119*, 48–59.
Clemens, A. W., & Axelson, L. J. (1985). The not-so-empty-nest: The return of the fledgling adult. *Family Relations, 34*, 259–264.
Coall, D. A., & Hertwig, R. (2010). Grandparental investment: Past, present, and future. *Behavioral and Brain Sciences, 33*, 1–19. http://dx.doi.org/10.1017/S0140525X09991105
Cohen, P. (2012). *In our prime: The invention of middle age.* Simon and Schuster.
Conger, R. D., McCarty, J. A., Yang, R. K., Lahey, B. B., & Burgess, R. L. (1984). Mother's age as a predictor of observed maternal behavior in three independent samples of families. *Journal of Marriage and the Family, 46*, 411–424.
Connidis, I. A. (2001). *Family ties and aging.* Sage.
Connidis, I. A. (2015). Exploring ambivalence in family ties: Progress and prospects. *Journal of Marriage and Family, 77*, 77–95.
Crimmins, E. M., & Zhang, Y. S. (2019). Aging populations, mortality, and life expectancy. *Annual Review of Sociology, 45*, 69–89.
Cooney, T. M., Pedersen, F. A., Indelicato, S., & Palkovitz, R. (1993). Timing of fatherhood: Is "on-time" optimal? *Journal of Marriage and the Family, 174*, 205–215.
Cornwell, E. Y., & Waite, L. J. (2009). Social disconnectedness, perceived isolation, and health among older adults. *Journal of Health and Social Behavior, 50*(1), 31–48.
Coto, M., Lizano, F., Mora, S., & Fuentes, J. (2017). Social media and elderly people: research trends. In *Social computing and social media. applications and analytics: 9th International Conference, SCSM 2017, held as part of HCI International 2017, Vancouver, BC, Canada, July 9–14, 2017, Proceedings, Part II 9* (pp. 65–81). Springer International Publishing.
Cox, K. S., Wilt, J., Olson, B., & McAdams, D. P. (2010). Generativity, the big five, and psychosocial adaptation in midlife adults. *Journal of Personality, 78*, 1185–1208. http://doi.org/10.1111/j.1467-6494. 2010.00647.x

Cramer, D. W., & Roach, A. J. (1988). Coming out to mom and dad: A study of gay males and their relationships with their parents. *Journal of Homosexuality, 15*(3–4), 79–92.

Crowley, J. (2018). *Gray divorce: What we lose and gain from mid-life splits.* University of California Press.

Daniels, P., & Weingarten, K. (1982). Sooner or later: The timing of parenthood in adult lives. *(No Title).*

DePasquale, N., Davis, K. D., Zarit, S. H., Moen, P., Hammer, L. B., & Almeida, D. M. (2016). Combining formal and informal caregiving roles: The psychosocial implications of double- and triple-duty care. *Journals of Gerontology: Series B, Psychological Sciences and Social Sciences, 71*, 201–211. http://dx.doi.org/10.1093/geronb/gbu139

DePasquale, N., Polenick, C. A., Davis, K. D., Moen, P., Hammer, L. B., & Almeida, D. M. (2017). The psychosocial implications of managing work and family caregiving roles: Gender differences among information technology professionals. *Journal of Family Issues, 38*, 1495–1519. http://dx.doi.org/10.1177/0192513X15584680

Devi, J. (2018). The scales of functional assessment of activities of daily living in geriatrics. *Age and Ageing, 47*(4), 500–502. https://doi.org/10.1093/ageing/afy050

Di Gessa, G., Maddock, J., Green, M. J., Thompson, E. J., McElroy, E., Davies, H. L., & Patalay, P. (2022). Pre-pandemic mental health and disruptions to healthcare, economic and housing outcomes during the COVID-19 pandemic: Evidence from 12 UK longitudinal studies. *The British Journal of Psychiatry, 220*(1), 21–30.

Douglas, M., Katikireddi, S. V., Taulbut, M., McKee, M., & McCartney, G. (2020). Mitigating the wider health effects of covid-19 pandemic response. *Bmj, 369*, m1557.

Ebbert, A. M., Kumar, N. L., & Luthar, S. S. (2019). Complexities in adjustment patterns among the "best and the brightest": Risk and resilience in the context of high achieving schools. *Research in Human Development, 16*, 21–34. http://dx.doi.org/10.1080/15427609.2018.1541376

Eifert, E. K., Adams, R., Morrison, S., & Strack, R. (2016). Emerging trends in family caregiving using the life course perspective: Preparing health educators for an aging society. *American Journal of Health Education, 47*, 176–197. http://dx.doi.org/10.1080/19325037.2016.1158674

Emerson, K. G. (2020). Coping with being cooped up: Social distancing during COVID-19 among 60+ in the United States. *Revista Panamericana de Salud Pública, 44*, e81.

Erikson, E. H. (1963). *Childhood and society* (2nd ed.). Norton.

Erikson, E. H. (1978). *Adulthood.* Norton.

FAO. (2020). *Maintaining a healthy diet during the COVID-19 pandemic.* FAO.

Feinberg, L. F. (2018). Breaking new ground: Supporting employed family caregivers with workplace leave policies. https://www.aarp.org/content/dam/aarp/ppi/2018/08/breaking-new-ground-supportingemployed-family-caregivers-with-workplace-leave-policies.pdf

Fingerman, K. L. (2017). Millennials and their parents: Implications of the new young adulthood for midlife adults. *Innovation in Aging, 1*(3), igx026. http://dx.doi.org/10.1093/geroni/igx026

Fingerman, K. L., Pillemer, K. A., Silverstein, M., & Suitor, J. J. (2012). The baby Boomers' intergenerational relationships. *Gerontologist, 52*, 199–209. http://dx.doi.org/10.1093/geront/gnr139

Fisher, G. G., Stachowski, A., Infurna, F. J., Faul, J. D., Grosch, J., & Tetrick, L. E. (2014). Mental work demands, retirement, and longitudinal trajectories of cognitive functioning. *Journal of Occupational Health Psychology, 19*, 231–242. http://dx.doi.org/10.1037/a0035724

Fredriksen-Goldsen, K. I., Emlet, C. A., Kim, H. J., Muraco, A., Erosheva, E. A., Goldsen, J., & Hoy-Ellis, C. P. (2013). The physical and mental health of Lesbian, Gay Male, and Bisexual (LGB) older adults: The role of key health indicators and risk and protective factors. *The Gerontologist, 53*(4), 664–675.

Fredriksen-Goldsen, K. I., Jen, S., Bryan, A. E., & Goldsen, J. (2018). Cognitive impairment, Alzheimer's disease, and other dementias in the lives of Lesbian, Gay, Bisexual and Transgender (LGBT) older adults and their caregivers: Needs and competencies. *Journal of Applied Gerontology, 37*(5), 545–569.

Fry, R. (2015). *More millennials living with family despite improved job market.* Pew Research Center.

Giustino, V., Parroco, A. M., Gennaro, A., Musumeci, G., Palma, A., & Battaglia, G. (2020). Physical activity levels and related energy expenditure during COVID-19 quarantine among the Sicilian active population: A cross-sectional online survey study. *Sustainability, 12*(11), 4356.

Glenn, N. D. (1975). Psychological well-being in the postparental stage: Some evidence from national surveys. *Journal of Marriage and the Family, 37*, 105–110.

Gordon, J. R., Pruchno, R. A., Wilson-Genderson, M., Murphy, W. M., & Rose, M. (2012). Balancing caregiving and work: Role conflict and role strain dynamics. *Journal of Family Issues, 33*, 662–689. http://dx.doi.org/10.1177/0192513X11425322

Grande, D., Barg, F. K., Johnson, S., & Cannuscio, C. C. (2013). Life disruptions for midlife and older adults with high out-of-pocket health expenditures. *Annals of Family Medicine, 11*, 37–42. http://dx.doi.org/10.1370/afm.1444

Greenhaus, J. H., & Allen, T. D. (2011). Work-family balance: A review and extension of the literature. In J. C. Quick & L. E. Tetrick (Eds.), *Handbook of occupational health psychology* (pp. 165–183). American Psychological Association.

Greenhaus, J. H., & Beutell, N. J. (1985). Sources of conflict between work and family roles. *Academy of Management Review, 10*, 76–88. http://doi.org/10.5465/amr.1985.427 7352

Hackstaff, K. (1999). *Marriage in a culture of divorce* (Vol. 105). Temple University Press.

Hansen, T. (2012). Parenthood and happiness: A review of folk theories versus empirical evidence. *Social Indicators Research, 108*, 29–64. http://doi.org/10.1007/s11205-011-9865-y

Hansen, T., Slagsvold, B., & Moum, T. (2009). Childlessness and psychological well-being in midlife and old age: An examination of parental status effects across a range of outcomes. *Social Indicators Research, 94*, 343–362.

Harkness, S. (2008). Empty nest syndrome. In S. J. Loue & M. Sajatovic (Eds), *Encyclopedia of aging and public health* (pp. 318–319). Springer US.

Haw, C., Hawton, K., Gunnell, D., & Platt, S. (2015). Economic recession and suicidal behaviour: Possible mechanisms and ameliorating factors. *International Journal of Social Psychiatry, 61*, 73– 81. http://dx.doi.org/10.1177/0020764014536545

Hayslip, B., Jr., Fruhauf, C. A., & Dolbin-MacNab, M. L. (2017). Grandparents raising grandchildren: What have we learned over the past decade? *Gerontologist, 57*, 1196. http://dx.doi.org/10.1093/geront/ gnx124

Heath, D. T. (1994). The impact of delayed fatherhood on the father-child relationship. *The Journal of Genetic Psychology, 155*(4), 511–530.

Hebert, L. E., Weuve, J., Scherr, P. A., & Evans, D. A. (2013). Alzheimer disease in the United States (2010–2050) estimated using the 2010 census. *Neurology, 80*, 1778–1783. http://dx.doi.org/10.1212/WNL.0b013e31828726f5

Hilbrand, S., Coall, D. A., Gerstorf, D., & Hertwig, R. (2017). Caregiving within and beyond the family is associated with lower mortality for the caregiver. *Evolution*

and Human Behavior, 38, 397– 403. http://dx.doi.org/10.1016/j.evolhumbehav.2016.11.010
Huang, J. (2015). *HIV-associated dementia* (Merck Manual Professional Version). http://www.merckmanuals.com/professional/neurologic-disorders/delirium-and-dementia/hiv-associated-dementia
Hülür, G., Ram, N., Willis, S. L., Schaie, K. W., & Gerstorf, D. (2019). Cohort differences in cognitive aging: The role of perceived work environment. *Psychology and Aging, 34*, 1040–1054. http://dx.doi.org/10.1037/pag0000355
Huo, M., Graham, J. L., Kim, K., Birditt, K. S., & Fingerman, K. L. (2019). Aging parents' daily support exchanges with grown-up offspring suffering problems. *Journals of Gerontology: Series B, Psychological Sciences and Social Sciences, 74*, 449–459. http://dx.doi.org/10.1093/geronb/gbx079
Infurna, F. J., Gerstorf, D., & Lachman, M. E. (2020). Midlife in the 2020s: Opportunities and challenges. *American Psychologist, 75*(4), 470.
Jaques, E. (1965). Death and the midlife crisis. *International Journal of Psychoanalysis, 46*, 502–514.
Kins, E., Soenens, B., & Beyers, W. (2013). Separation anxiety in families with emerging adults. *Journal of Family Psychology, 27*(3), 495.
Kirsch, J. A., & Ryff, C. D. (2016). Hardships of the great recession and health: Understanding varieties of vulnerability. *Health Psychology Open, 3*(1). https://doi.org/10.1177/2055102916652390
Koren, C., Simhi, S., Lipman-Schiby, S., & Fogel, S. (2016). The partner in late-life repartnering: Caregiving expectations from an intergenerational perspective. *International Psychogeriatrics, 28*(9), 1555–1565. https://doi.org/10.1017/s1041610216000181
Lachman, M. E. (2004). Development in midlife. *Annual Review of Psychology, 55*(1), 305–331.
Lachman, M. E. (2006). Perceived control over aging-related declines: Adaptive beliefs and behaviors. *Current Directions in Psychological Science, 15*, 282–286.
Lachman, M. E. (2015). Mind the gap in the middle: A call to study midlife. *RHD, 12*, 327–334.
Lachman, M. E., Teshale, S., & Agrigoroaei, S. (2015). Midlife as a pivotal period in the life course: Balancing growth and decline at the crossroads of youth and old age. *International Journal of Behavioral Development, 39*(1), 20–31.
Lam, J., Fan, W., & Moen, P. (2014). Is insecurity worse for well-being in turbulent times? Mental health in context. *Society and Mental Health, 4*, 55–73.
Leist, A. K., Hessel, P., & Avendano, M. (2014). Do economic recessions during early and mid-adulthood influence cognitive function in older age? *Journal of Epidemiology and Community Health, 68*, 151–158. http://dx.doi.org/10.1136/jech-2013-202843
Maki, P. M., Freeman, E. W., Greendale, G. A., Henderson, V. W., Newhouse, P. A., Schmidt, P. J., & Soares, C. N. (2010). Summary of the NIA-sponsored conference on depressive symptoms and cognitive complaints in the menopausal transition. *Menopause (New York, NY), 17*(4), 815.
Martelli, M., Zingaretti, L., Salvio, G., Bracci, M., & Santarelli, L. (2021). Influence of work on andropause and menopause: A systematic review. *International Journal of Environmental Research and Public Health, 18*(19), 10074.
McAdams, D. P., & de St. Aubin, E. (1992). A theory of generativity and its assessment through self-report, behavioral acts, and narrative themes in autobiography. *Journal of Personality and Social Psychology, 62*, 1003–1015. http://doi.org/10.1037/0022-3514.62.6.1003
McAdams, D. P., Diamond, A., de St.Aubin, E., & Mansfield, E. (1997). Stories of commitment: The psychosocial construction of generative lives. *Journal of*

Personality and Social Psychology, 72, 678–694. http://doi.org/10.1037/0022-3514.72.3.678

Meshi, D., Cotten, S. R., & Bender, A. R. (2020). Problematic social media use and perceived social isolation in older adults: A cross-sectional study. *Gerontology, 66*(2), 160–168.

Meyer, M. H., & Kandic, A. (2017). Grandparenting in the United States. *Innovation in Aging, 1*(2), igx023. http://dx.doi.org/10.1093/geroni/igx023

Milardo, R. (2005). Generative uncle and nephew relationships. *Journal of Marriage and Family, 67*, 1226–1236. http://doi.org/10.1111/j.1741-3737.2005.00212.x

Mirowsky, J., & Ross, C. E. (2002). Depression, parenthood, and age at first birth. *Social Science & Medicine, 54*(8), 1281–1298.

Mitchell, B. A. (2006). The boomerang age from childhood to adulthood: Emergent trends and issues for aging families. *Canadian Studies in Population [ARCHIVES], 33*(2), 155-178.

Mitchell, B. A. (2019). Empty nest. In D. Gu, & M. Dupre (Eds.), *Encyclopedia of gerontology and population aging*. Springer. https://doi.org/10.1007/978-3-319-69892-2_317-1

Mitchell, B. A., & Lovegreen, L. D. (2009). The empty nest syndrome in midlife families: A multimethod exploration of parental gender differences and cultural dynamics. *Journal of Family Issues, 30*(12), 1651–1670.

Mitchell, B. A., & Wister, A. V. (2015). Midlife challenge or welcome departure? Cultural and family-related expectations of empty nest transitions. *The International Journal of Aging and Human Development, 81*(4), 260–280.

Morgan, S. P., & King, R. B. (2001). Why have children in the 21st century? Biological predisposition, social coercion, rational choice. *European Journal of Population/Revue européenne de démographie, 17*, 3-20.

Moulton, V., Sullivan, A., Goodman, A., Parsons, S., & Ploubidis, G. B. (2023). Adult life-course trajectories of psychological distress and economic outcomes in midlife during the COVID-19 pandemic: Evidence from the 1958 and 1970 British birth cohorts. *Social Psychiatry and Psychiatric Epidemiology*, 1–16. https://doi.org/10.1007/s00127-022-02377-w

Neville, B., & Parke, R. D. (1997). Waiting for paternity: Interpersonal and contextual implications of the timing of fatherhood. *Sex Roles, 37*, 45–59.

Paez, K. A., Zhao, L., & Hwang, W. (2009). Rising out-of-pocket spending for chronic conditions: A ten-year trend. *Health Affairs, 28*, 15–25. http://dx.doi.org/10.1377/hlthaff.28.1.15

Peters, K., Jackson, D., & Rudge, T. (2011). Surviving the adversity of childlessness: Fostering resilience in couples. *Contemporary Nurse, 40*(1), 130–140.

Phillips, J. A., & Nugent, C. N. (2014). Suicide and the great recession of 2007–2009: The role of economic factors in the 50 U.S. states. *Social Science & Medicine, 116*, 22–31. http://dx.doi.org/10.1016/j.socscimed.2014.06.015

Pienta, A. (1999). Early childbearing patterns and women's labor force behavior in later life. *Journal of Women & Aging, 11*(1), 69–84.

Polenick, C. A., DePasquale, N., Eggebeen, D. J., Zarit, S. H., & Fingerman, K. L. (2018). Relationship quality between older fathers and middle-aged children: Associations with both parties' subjective wellbeing. *Journals of Gerontology: Series B, Psychological Sciences and Social Sciences, 73*, 1203–1213. http://dx.doi.org/10.1093/geronb/gbw094

Ragozin, A. S., Basham, R. B., Crnic, K. A., Greenberg, M. T., & Robinson, N. M. (1982). Effects of maternal age on parenting role. *Developmental Psychology, 18*(4), 627.

Rajmil, L., Fernandez de Sanmamed, M. J., Choonara, I., Faresjö, T., Hjern, A., Kozyrskyj, A. L., & Taylor-Robinson, D. (2014). Impact of the 2008 economic

and financial crisis on child health: A systematic review. *International Journal of Environmental Research and Public Health, 11*, 6528–6546. http://dx.doi.org/10.3390/ijerph110606528
Ranjan, P., Kumar, A., Chowdhury, S., Pandey, S., Choudhary, A., Bhattacharya, A., & Vikram, N. K. (2020). Is excess weight a risk factor for the development of COVID 19 infection? A preliminary report from India. *Diabetes & Metabolic Syndrome: Clinical Research & Reviews, 14*(6), 1805–1807.
Reece, S. M. (1993). Social support and the early maternal experience of primiparas over 35. *Maternal-Child Nursing Journal, 21*(3), 91–98.
Riumallo-Herl, C., Basu, S., Stuckler, D., Courtin, E., & Avendano, M. (2014). Job loss, wealth and depression during the Great Recession in the USA and Europe. *International Journal of Epidemiology, 43*, 1508–1517. http://dx.doi.org/10.1093/ije/dyu048
Rokach, R., Cohen, O., & Dreman, S. (2004). Triggers and fuses in late divorce: The role of short term crises vs. ongoing frustration on marital break-up. *Journal of Divorce & Remarriage, 40*(3–4), 41–60.
Rothrauff, T., & Cooney, T. M. (2008). The role of generativity in psychological well-being: Does it differ for childless adults and parents? *Journal of Adult Development, 15*, 148–159. http://doi.org/10.1007/ s10804-008-9046-7
Rubin, L. B. (1979). Women of a certain age: The midlife search for self. *(No Title)*.
Ryff, C. D., Lee, Y. H., Essex, M. J., & Schmutte, P. S. (1994). My children and me: Midlife evaluations of grown children and of self. *Psychology and Aging, 9*, 195–205. http://dx.doi.org/10.1037/0882-7974.9.2.195
Salamon, L. M., Geller, S. L., & Spence, K. L. (2009). Impact of the 2007–09 economic recession on nonprofit organizations (Communique No. 14). Johns Hopkins Listening Post Project website: http://ccss.jhu.edu/wp content/uploads/downloads/2011/09/LP_Communique14_2009.pdf
Sandilyan, M. B., & Dening, T. (2011). Mental health around and after the menopause. *Menopause International, 17*(4), 142–147.
Schnaiberg, A., & Goldenberg, S. (1989). From empty nest to crowded nest: The dynamics of incompletely-launched young adults. *Social Problems, 36*(3), 251–269.
Seidman, S. N. (2006). Normative hypogonadism and depression: Does 'andropause'exist. *International Journal of Impotence Research, 18*(5), 415–422.
Settersten, R. A., & Hagestad, G. O. (1996). What's the latest? Cultural age deadlines for family transitions. *The Gerontologist, 36*, 178–189.
Settersten, R. A., & Ray, B. (2010). What's going on with young people today? The long and twisting path to adulthood. *Future of Children, 20*, 19–41. http://dx.doi.org/10.1353/foc.0.0044
Silverstein, M., & Giarrusso, R. (2010). Aging and family life: A decade review. *Journal of Marriage and Family, 72*, 1039–1058. http://dx.doi.org/10.1111/j.1741-3737.2010.00749.x
Sleek, S. (2014). The psychological toll of the smartphone. *APS Observer, 27*, 347–366.
Song, J., Mailick, M. R., & Greenberg, J. S. (2018). The impact of the great recession on midlife and older parents of individuals with a mental health problem or a developmental disability. *Gerontologist, 58*, 448–455. http://dx.doi.org/10.1093/geront/gnw269
Staff, H. R. S. (2017). *Sample sizes and response rates*. Survey Research Center, Institute for Social Research, University of Michigan.
Stein, C. H., Abraham, K. M., Bonar, E. E., Leith, J. E., Kraus, S. W., Hamill, A. C., & Fogo, W. R. (2011). Family ties in tough times: How young adults and their parents view the U.S. economic crisis. *Journal of Family Psychology, 25*, 449–454. http://dx.doi.org/10.1037/a0023697

Steptoe, A., Shankar, A., Demakakos, P., & Wardle, J. (2013). Social isolation, loneliness, and all-cause mortality in older men and women. *Proceedings of the National Academy of Sciences*, *110*(15), 5797–5801.
Sternbach, H. (1998). Age-associated testosterone decline in men: Clinical issues for psychiatry. *American Journal of Psychiatry*, *155*(10), 1310–1318.
Super, D. E. (1980). A life-span, life-space approach to career development. *Journal of vocational behavior*, *16*(3), 282-298.
Taniguchi, H. (1999). The timing of childbearing and women's wages. *Journal of Marriage and the Family*, *61*, 1008–1019.
Tomida, M., Nishita, Y., Tange, C., Nakagawa, T., Otsuka, R., Ando, F., & Shimokata, H. (2022). Typology of work–family balance among middle–aged and older Japanese adults. *Frontiers in Psychology*, *13*, 751879.
Uhlenberg, P., Cooney, T., & Boyd, R. (1990). Divorce for women after midlife. *Journal of Gerontology*, *45*(1), S3–S11.
Viswesvaran, C., Sanchez, J. I., & Fisher, J. (1999). The role of social support in the process of work stress: A meta-analysis. *Journal of Vocational Behavior, 54*, 314–334. http://doi.org/10.1006/jvbe.1998.1661
Walsemann, K. M., & Ailshire, J. A. (2017). Student debt spans generations: Characteristics of parents who borrow to pay for their children's college education. *Journals of Gerontology: Series B, Psychological Sciences and Social Sciences, 72*, 1084–1089. http://dx.doi.org/10.1093/geronb/gbw150
Walter, C. A. (1986). *The timing of motherhood*. Free Press.
Wang, H., Wang, C., & Halliday, T. J. (2018). Health and health inequality during the great recession: Evidence from the PSID. *Economics and Human Biology, 29*, 17–30. http://dx.doi.org/10.1016/j.ehb.2018.01.001
Williamson, E. J., Walker, A. J., Bhaskaran, K., Bacon, S., Bates, C., Morton, C. E., & Goldacre, B. (2020). OpenSAFELY: Factors associated with COVID-19 death in 17 million patients. *Nature*, *584*(7821), 430.
Wojciechowska, L. (2011). Basic hope and generativity in middle adulthood. *Polish Psychological Bulletin, 42*, 188–197. http://doi.org/10.2478/v10059-011-0025-7
Woolhandler, S., & Himmelstein, D. U. (2019). Single-payer reform—"Medicare for All". *JAMA*, *321*(24), 2399–2400.
Wu, Z., & Schimmele, C. (2007). Uncoupling in late life. *Generations*, *31*(3), 41–46.
Yarrow, A. L. (1991). Latecomers: Children of parents over 35. *(No Title)*.
Zahodne, L. B., Manly, J. J., Smith, J., Seeman, T., & Lachman, M. E. (2017). Socioeconomic, health, and psychosocial mediators of racial disparities in cognition in early, middle, and late adulthood. *Psychology and aging*, *32*(2), 118.

11 COVID-19 and Midlife

Masroor Jahan, Amool R. Singh and Rahul Sharma

Ageing is a continuous and complex process, and people still tend to expect and assess important events in their lives according to a "social clock". There are certain common challenges that are experienced by individuals belonging to a certain age group. Middle age typically comprises of individuals aged 40–65 years. According to Carl Jung, both men and women express previously suppressed aspects of their personalities at midlife. Acknowledging mortality and letting go of the idea of youth are two essential steps. Humanistic theorists such as Maslow and Rogers see middle age as an opportunity for positive change. Erikson, in his theory of psychosocial development, held that individuals experience a stage of generativity versus stagnation. Generativity can be expressed through parenting and grandparenting, teaching or mentorship, productivity or creativity, self-development, and positively impacting the world. On the other hand, "stagnation" represents feeling stuck, unproductive and lacking purpose. Those who experience stagnation may feel a sense of emptiness, lack of growth or a lack of fulfilment in their lives, and eventually a lack of meaning or purpose in life.

During middle age, many key psychosocial issues and themes may emerge, including the midlife crisis, identity development and psychological wellbeing. Every parent wants their children to grow up and lead independent lives, but letting go is bittersweet and emotionally challenging. This can be liberating for the majority, but may be stressful for couples whose identity is dependent on the parental role or couples who will have to face previously submerged marital problems. It is relatively uncommon to see divorce, at midlife although it is becoming more common these days. For some couples, this phase of life can be followed by an improved relationship after the children leave home. As lifespans lengthen, more and more ageing parents become dependent for care on their middle-aged children. The role of caregiving responsibility increases, especially for women. This and other responsibilities had increase severalfold for all age groups in general, and the middle-aged in particular, when the world witnessed one of the major threats in the first half of the 21st century.

The world has witnessed several pandemics in the past, like the Spanish flu, the HIV/AIDS pandemic, swine flu, avian flu, ebola and zika. Epidemics have become more common as urban areas have grown, even though

DOI: 10.4324/9781003568360-14

communicable diseases existed long before humans relied solely on hunting and gathering for food (History.com Editors, 2020). The World Health Organization (WHO) designated severe acute respiratory syndrome-coronavirus (SARS-CoV-2) as a global health emergency on January 30, 2020. The disease is the most contagious respiratory illness, with a high rate of human-to-human transmission, commonly known as coronavirus disease 2019 (COVID-19). On March 11, 2020, the World Health Organization formally declared the virus to be a pandemic as it continued to spread, affecting 114 countries and killing over 4,000 people (Sohrabi et al., 2020). The most common symptoms were fever, cough and shortness of breath, as well as normal or decreased leukocyte counts and fatigue.

As COVID-19 continued to spread around the world, numerous national and local governments implemented drastic health measures, such as isolation, quarantine, lockdowns, physical distancing, closure of unnecessary services, and travel restrictions (Government of Canada, 2021). In a large PHOSP-COVID study, it was found that 7 in 10 patients admitted to hospital with COVID-19 reported "long COVID" symptoms an average of five months after discharge, and symptoms were more prevalent in women aged 40–60 (Evans et al., 2021).

A wide range of adversities, such as difficulties meeting basic needs, increased caregiving responsibilities, difficulties accessing healthcare unrelated to COVID-19, employment and financial loss, and disruption of social networks have been experienced by many people during and after previous outbreaks, such as the ebola and SARS outbreaks. These events may increase the risk of mental illness during and after the outbreaks. The rapidly expanding mass hysteria and panic of COVID-19 may have long-term psychological implications, which could be more detrimental than the virus itself. Preventive measures like social distancing and self-isolation were found to be effective in mitigating and controlling the spread of the disease (Ranjan et al., 2020). These measures may have a negative impact on middle-aged and senior citizens whose major social contact is outside the home, such as meeting friends, attending family functions, religious ceremonies and places of worship, and being involved in some kinds of recreational activities and other group activities.

Contrary to the dire circumstances seen in Italy, the US and Spain, early lockdown deployment in several countries, including India, helped buy more time to upgrade the current healthcare infrastructure despite the hardships people endured (Golechha, 2020). However, the worldwide shutdown also helped the telecommunications sector and decreased pollution levels. Information and communication technology advancements have somewhat lessened the impact of COVID-19.

The impact it has had is complex to understand. Research on lifespan development and COVID has so far concentrated on the study of childhood, adolescence, young adulthood and old age; relatively few studies have concentrated on the years in between – the two decades from 40 to 60 years, what is commonly called the phase of midlife (Dörner, 2005). There is a need to address the psychosocial and behavioural impact that COVID-19 may have on the lives of people of this age group.

Who Is Affected?

General Public

Mass fear of COVID-19, rightly termed "coronaphobia" (Asmundson et al., 2020), mainly due to the unpredictable and uncertain nature of the course of the disease, intolerance of uncertainty, perceived risk of acquiring the infection etc., can lead to a host of psychological problems, including maladaptive behaviours, emotional distress and avoidance reactions among common people (Taha et al., 2014). Middle-aged people who had to go out to buy essential groceries or to work were at a heightened risk of acquiring the infection. They were also worried about transmitting the virus to their children or elderly parents. Non-realistic panic among the public regarding scarcity of emergency and essential services due to the lockdowns led to the stockpiling of daily essentials or resources like hand sanitizer, medications, protective masks or even toilet paper. This "herd behaviour" (Banerjee, 1992; Singh & Mishra, 2020) can have a detrimental effect on communities that is actually in need and can promote black marketing of such products, leading to social disruption and injustice (Sen, 2009; Mahase, 2020). The abundance of information available at our fingertips via social media, the cost and availability of basic and medical resources, and the efficiency of the regional public health systems have all had an impact on psychological distress levels (Wang et al., 2020). The majority of the carers were worried about financial restraints during lockdown, getting infected and difficulty in adjusting to the new normal. Lockdown also had an impact on emergency medical services because there were not enough options for transportation. People felt an inability to take their ailing parents for treatment. Also, the inability to find closure and bury loved ones who died as a result of COVID-19 could leave bereaved families with long-term psychiatric consequences as well as psychological trauma, anger and resentment (Ho, 2020; *New York Times*, 2020). There was a rise in the cases of xenophobia related to infection, and also reports of verbal and physical attacks against Chinese people (Chung, 2020). Such preconceived opinions can impact access to services and can also lead to stress and altered health behaviours.

Health Professionals and Other Frontline Workers

The outbreak of COVID-19 lead to unavoidable stress, fear and anxiety among the higher-risk groups such as healthcare professionals (HCPs) and other frontline workers, including bankers, police, the armed forces etc. Health workers' mental health suffered from exposure to COVID-19 cases in hospitals, isolation, the illness or death of a relative or friend from the virus, and increased self-perception of danger due to the virus's lethality (Wu et al., 2009; Liu et al., 2012; Greenberg et al., 2020). Inadequate hospital supply of required hygiene tools (Biswas & Chatterjee, 2014) and personal protective equipment) for healthcare practitioners who were at the highest risk of transmission (Chen et al., 2020) again compounded the problem. Addressing the psychological aspects of patients requires a specific set of skills, and if these skills are missing, it can be difficult to manage the patients in a holistic manner, further leading to a sense of insufficiency.

Middle-aged HCPs also had to bear the brunt of remaining separated from family members for an extended periods of time. Anxiety regarding the fear of transmitting the disease to their own family members was suspected to have increased in those who were performing hospital duties on a daycare basis and returned home (Chen et al., 2020). Amidst the pandemic, there was news of assaults on doctors after the death of COVID-19 patients, and some of the doctors were asked to vacate their rented house (Giordano, 2020). Such inhuman behaviour can have long-term psychological implications and can lead to decreased interest in social service and an increase in being self-centred.

Informal Sector

It has been extensively documented in the literature that the pandemic's effects have mostly followed the path of pre-existing vulnerabilities in a number of economies (Couch et al., 2020; Desphande & Ramachandran, 2020). These studies emphasize how some racial, gender, caste, religious, social, demographic and economic groups – who were already marginalized before the pandemic – were disproportionately impacted. The informal sector is hardly covered by any social security or insurance schemes, thereby making its members vulnerable to exploitation. Low pay, unstable working conditions, a lack of social protection, and, at its worst, a reliance on daily earnings for subsistence are characteristics of informal employment (International Labour Organisation, 2018). Any interruption in economic activity immediately eliminates or destroys jobs and wages for that labour force. Issues of precarity and informality are exacerbated by decades of underfunding public services without a meaningful extension of the social safety net (SWI, 2019). It has also been observed that those returning to employment are earning less. This could be due to the financial crunch or the notion that workers have few work opportunities and will accept whatever they are offered. Also, there is a further shift toward informality and self-employment. Middle-aged people, who generally are thought to be financially stable, lack this stability when it comes to those working in the informal sector. Notably, recovery has taken many different forms for different social groups, with women recovering at a significantly slower rate (Bertrand et al., 2020).

Service Sector

Many workers, especially those in middle age, in a variety of industries were afraid of losing their jobs as the "new normal" necessitated learning new coping mechanisms for an uncertain future. There is a consensus among the specialized financial literature that in spite of the devastation caused by COVID-19, at least two groups of the formal sector have been thriving: home delivery, and grocery stores and supermarkets (Times, 2020; Financial, 2020). Hospitality value chains were affected, with the cancellation of events and shutdown of leisure parks, restaurants, hotels and accommodation. The tourism sector was disrupted due to global as well as domestic travel restrictions. Due to the lack of proper social security for citizens, COVID-19 saw lay-offs and bankruptcies. It becomes very difficult for a person who is in their forties or fifties to start afresh when there are a multitude of responsibilities on their shoulders at a time when there is a dearth of opportunities. This is also usually a time when the person starts to feel a loss of control over their children as they have grown up to be adults, there is also a slow but progressive deterioration of their physical health, and COVID-19 added to this loss of control over their environment.

Marginalized Community (Migrants, Those on Daily Wages and Slum Dwellers)

The majority of international migrants and refugees live in areas severely affected by the pandemic, and also experience significant accessibility problems with the public health system, making them disproportionately susceptible to stigma, discrimination and exclusion (WHO, 2020). The risk of contracting and spreading the disease increased for migrants, refugees and slum dwellers because of the lethal communicability of this disease (UN News, 2020). These people were not able to maintain basic hand hygiene measures (which have been of utmost importance in control of the COVID-19 outbreak) because of the scarcity of sufficient, safe and affordable water supplies, thereby making them vulnerable to feelings of deprivation, neglect and segregation. Furthermore, the communities where home quarantine was implemented stigmatized and were suspicious of immigrants and refugees as speculated sources of the outbreak. The lockdowns and the rapid increase in the number of cases led to misery for these migrant workers, those on daily wages and billions of slum dwellers worldwide. During the lockdowns, lack of work and financial means to survive in urban areas resulted in anxiety and pushed migrants and daily wage earners to travel kilometres on foot to reach their native places. In India, incidences of death while migrating (*Washington Post*, 2020), mass chemical spraying of migrants (Coronavirus BBC, 2020) and quarantine on trees or boats (TRT world, 2020) were reported. Also, the continuous reverse migration of millions of migrant workers to their native villages could be detrimental for mental health, and the rural population may be particularly susceptible to suicide in the near future due to the heavy economic load of jobless migrant workers (Nelson, 2020). The vulnerability of middle-aged male migrant workers to mental health issues, including depression, is exacerbated by the absence of family. Stress levels also increased due to feelings of helplessness to attend to family members and the loss of loved ones. The marginalised, slum dwellers, the poor andpeople living in rural areas neither had access to technology nor were equipped (age being one of the factors) to get any benefit from it, including online health services. This excluded middle-aged people belonging to marginalized communities even further. Those who remained in urban areas had to work extra shifts to boost production. The absence of protective welfare laws led to longer working hours, reduced rest time and increased psychological stress, which can result in occupational mental illnesses.

People Living with HIV

A vast majority of people living with HIV (PLWH) worldwide are living in countries with poor health infrastructure and are over 50 years of age. This is probably due to the effectiveness of treatment with HIV medicine (called antiretroviral therapy, or ART); people with HIV who are diagnosed early and who get and stay on ART can keep the virus suppressed and live long and healthy lives. According to the Center for Systems Science and Engineering (2020), South Africa and India, which have the highest COVID-19 burden, are also among the nations with the highest rates of HIV infections. It has been noted in several studies that COVID-19 mortality among PLWH does not differ from the general population. According to Lee et al. (2020), there was no difference in mortality based on HIV status. In fact, those who had

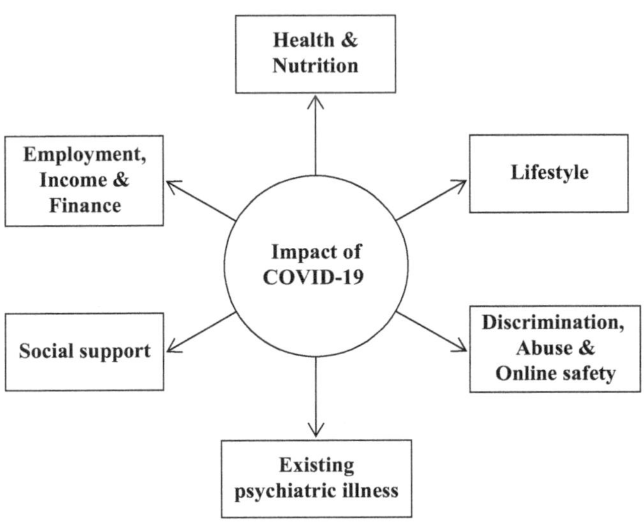

Figure 11.1 Impact of COVID-19

HIV were more likely to exhibit clinical improvement or be released from the hospital within 28 days of admission. But it has been found in several countries that the fear of COVID-19 has pushed PLWH to practise poor health care (Kowalska et al., 2020). People who have faced stigma for a long time due to their HIV status are hesitant to engage in care when the prospect of getting infected with COVID-19 is high. Some of them even avoid going to pharmacies to collect ART for fear of getting infected. Due to the lockdowns, existing care was hampered significantly. Many people faced accessibility problems owing to suspension of nationwide public and private transportation. Migrant workers who had to relocate to rural areas also lostaccess to HIV care in the cities where they lived (Lodge & Kuchukhidze, 2020). After substance abuse, depression is the second most prevalent mental health illness among PLWH and presents another obstacle to receiving treatment (Rabkin, 2008). Financial crunches due to the loss of livelihood also contributed to it. Due to the discontinuation of ongoing treatment or failure to detect new HIV cases, the number of PLWH is going to increase further and this may lead to poorer prognoses.

Impact on Health and Nutrition

Middle-aged people may experience health issues related to ageing. When the pandemic hit the world, these vulnerabilities got multiplied manyfold. Psychological distress, depression, anxiety and stress can be due to food insecurity (Malek Rivan et al., 2021). With food being such a basic need, its unavailability can be an alarming situation for an individual. During the COVID-19 pandemic, many scheduled procedures and outpatient visits were cancelled or postponed by patients and healthcare providers (Wright et al., 2020). There was also a rise in seriously uncontrolled chronic diseases, including diabetes, which was noted to be linked with the pandemic's delays in care and poor access to specialized care and treatment, especially in vulnerable populations. Telemedicine health services became essential given the restrictions caused by the pandemic. These services acted as a buffer during the pandemic as ailing patients were able to connect with health professionals. Although the satisfaction of being treated in person could not be achieved, it was a silver lining.

Infection with COVID-19

The majority of infected individuals experienced mild to moderate illness and recovered without the need for hospitalization, and they may or may not have experienced fever, diarrhoea, aches and pains, taste loss and sore throats, among other symptoms (World Health Organisation, 2020). Middle age is the time of life when degeneration of biological and psychological functioning can begin. Infection with COVID-19 may lead to respiratory failure, arrhythmias, shock, kidney failure, cardiovascular damage or liver failure, especially in patients with other underlying diseases. There is a high risk of mortality among middle-aged and elderly people owing to multi-morbidity in this age group. The pandemic was accompanied not just by physical illnesses but also psychological disturbances. While many studies have shown worse mental health outcomes during the early weeks of the pandemic, some sources have shown a steady reduction in symptoms of depression and anxiety during lockdown (Fancourt et al., 2021).

Impact on Food Behaviour and Nutrition

An increase in calory intake and a decrease in nutritional quality have been found to be associated with the COVID-19 pandemic (Bahl et al., 2021). This could be due to an increase in frequency of snacking, as reported among adults aged 18 years and older (Bahl et al., 2021). The probable reason behind increase in snacking may be people facing temptations at home, being bored, having more leisure time and stress, but there were also money shortages which inhibited individuals from buying vegetables and fruits.

From the beginning of the COVID-19 pandemic, there has been a rise in the popularity of online grocery shopping (Chang & Meyerhoefer, 2021). People in their middle years who live in cities now don't have to go to the marketplace to get groceries and other household items, thus reducing the risk of infection. Cooking at home has increased concurrently (Wong et al., 2023). This could be attributed to an increased availability of time and policies requiring a mandatory stay at home.

Impact on Employment, Income and Finances

There have been adverse economic consequences of the COVID-19 pandemic since the modern-day economy is interdependent. There was a twin threat from the impact on health and reduced labour demand and supply. Manufacturing, accommodation and food services, wholesale, the retail trade, real estate and business activities have been the hardest-hit sectors. Due to home delivery services being in operation during lockdown, the urban transport sector was still operational. Domestic workers faced serious challenges because people for whom they worked were fearful of getting infected by them. Also, due to low earnings and availability of time, people preferred doing household chores themselves.

Due to long-term absences of workers, production has been disrupted. The aggregate demands for commodities have gone down due interruptions in supply chains. Business owners who cannot conduct their businesses due to lockdown measures were concerned because their means of livelihood were affected, especially in countries where social welfare programmes are not very effective. Some middle-aged employees were pushed to seek early retirement to compensate for the loss of work. It was a trade-off between economic activities and restricting the spread of the infection. As proposed by Acemoglu et al. (2020), lockdowns of social groups are likely to create serious economic problems for some of the targeted groups. The vast majority of the poor, regardless of whether they have COVID-19 or are awaiting the results of testing for it, have little choice but to work (if they can) in the absence of government financial assistance. Additionally, compared to the wealthy, they are more likely to be in jobs where they cannot work from home, such as cleaning or driving taxies and buses in higher-income nations. For those who migrated to villages, the agriculture sector may serve as a refuge employer. There may be a host of factors limiting economic recovery, including supply and demand synchronization problems, travel restrictions and fear of contracting COVID-19. There may be an enhanced emphasis on automation to help comply with physical distancing measures. Many tasks in dining establishments and retail stores may be automated, and the use of robots may rise in an effort to encourage contactless activities and reduce reliance on human resources (Hess & Liu, 2020). This may adversely impact unskilled middle-aged employees because they will no longer be needed.

Impact on Lifestyle

The COVID-19 pandemic has brought about drastic changes, and with many people working from home, there has been a significant reduction in contact with people other than family members. These changes have brought about less physical activity, altered rhythms of daily life and led to unhealthier lifestyles specifically among the middle-aged. Additionally, they ma ybe more prone to circadian rhythm disorders owing to increased snacking during lockdown. Although COVID-19 is not always fatal for those who have it, lifestyle-related illnesses like obesity, diabetes and hypertension seem to make it more severe and increase the risk of death (Richardson et al., 2020). An international online survey identified unhealthier food consumption and meal patterns as well as decreased physical activity and increased sedentary time during quarantine (Ammar et al., 2020). The literature clearly showed that confinement led to a decrease in physical activity at all levels and an increase in daily sitting and screen time (Ammar et al., 2020). This may be due to restrictions on social gatherings and reduced access to parks and sports facilities. In a long-term population health study conducted in Singapore, data from wearable wrist sensors revealed significant shifts in the rest–activity rhythm, including later bedtimes and significantly lowers levels of physical activity (Ong et al., 2020). In particular, women have seemed more prone to psychological distress during the COVID-19 pandemic (Casagrande et al., 2020). It can be due to fear of getting infected, increased caregiving responsibilities etc. Some research has even pointed toward a positive impact on lifestyles (regular meal consumption, healthy eating) which was attributed to fear of coronavirus infection, preferring home-cooked food and less involvement in eating out and socializing (Chopra et al., 2020). A possible reason for the difference in consumption of Western food in India could be due to the high preference for home-cooked food there. There were some favourable changes observed during the pandemic, including that parents were better able to take care of their children by helping them with their homework and cooking meals for them in addition to managing their own online remote work tasks. This was also an opportunity for middle-aged people to renew their bonds with their children and spouse as they had more time to spend together, thus compensating for the negative impacts of COVID-19.

Sleep–wake Schedule

During the pandemic, people's sleep–wake schedules changed. They were going to bed later and taking frequent naps during the day. Based on the various roles women play in families, previous research on women in eight different African and Asian countries revealed that women reported more sleep problems than men, and more females than males were confirmed to be susceptible to insomnia and high levels of post-traumatic stress symptoms (Liu et al., 2020; Stranges et al., 2012; Zhang & Wing. 2006). This could be due to stresses of work and uncertainty about the future.

Working from Home

Working from home is a concept where individuals make use of technology to do their jobs in their own home. The concept of working from home was adopted to keep work going during lockdown and at the same time ensure the safety of employees. The work environment has completely changed since the pandemic, especially for workers in corporate settings. An Indian study by Kaushik and Guleria (2020) looked at how the COVID-19 pandemic affected the workplace. They noted that the major hurdle that came into play was how to connect with employers again after lockdown. There are technical challenges as well being faced, like poor connectivity, no separate space at home to work uninterrupted, lack of sophisticated technical devices, concerns about security of confidential data and poor skills in handling the devices required. There was also a decrease in community feeling among employees, leading to a decreased motivation to work. The responsibility for a working women to coordinate the dual responsibility of managing work and home is quite complex to understand, as some researchers found that women were better able to manage this dual responsibility as they no longer had to commute, whereas others found that their responsibilities increased as all the family members were staying at home. Although there were challenges associated with working from home, one good thing was that people no longer had to undergo long-distance commutes and were able to spend more time with their families and strike a better work–life balance. The benefits also included gains in productivity. An interesting finding from Adam Grant's Nick Bloom experiment was that an increase of 13%n productivity was noted for call centres when staff worked from home. This was attributed to the flexibility around where they were working, how they were working and when they were working, and most importantly they felt that they were not being micromanaged, which led to a boost up morale. It is also important to note that technology might be ready to serve during the "new normal", but people in their middle age are a bit reluctant to accept change. , the abrupt shift to working from home has caused the lines separating personal and work time to become hazier in novel and unusual ways. Days are blending with night, and weekdays are mixed with weekends.

Physical Activity

Middle age is often associated with a decline in physical activity, likely as a result of workload or household or caregiving responsibilities. Being physically active can help middle-aged and older adults improve their longevity. It can also protect them from various lifestyle diseases. Due to the imposition of lockdown, people, especially those in urban areas, were unable to engage in physical activities. Adults aged 55 years and older with lower levels of education exercised less during lockdown (Constandt et al., 2020).

Food Access and Affordability

The global lockdown affected how people accessed food and disrupted the production of certain food products. One of the primary causes of increased food insecurity was a decline in earnings and revenues, a shortage of food in markets and food outlets, and a reduction in travel. In India, 62% of the farm households Harris et al. (2020) interviewed talked about dietary disruptions. Specifically, nearly 50% of the households reported consuming significantly less fruit and foods derived from animals other than dairy. Those declines in different aspects of food security did not affect only populations in low-income countries. Niles et al. (2020) demonstrated that there has been a nearly one-third increase in household food insecurity since the COVID-19 pandemic in Vermont, USA using the six-item validated food security module. Of food insecure households, 35.5% were classified as newly food insecure. However, in developed countries, food insecurity is not a major concern as the major impact has been on food diversity, especially for imported food items. In line with other studies that made similar findings, middle-aged and older adults who experienced food insecurity reported feeling more stressed than those who did not (Ma et al., 2020; Wolfson et al., 2020).

Impact on Social Support

Human beings have always lived together to satisfy certain basic needs in order to survive. Social support involves emotional support, instrumental support and informational support etc. Social support may moderate genetic and environmental vulnerabilities and confer resilience to stress and other psychopathology. It can protect us or decrease the functional consequences of developing trauma-related psychopathology. Social isolation and low levels of social support have been shown to be associated with increased morbidity and mortality.

Socializing

During the pandemic, due to the high transmission rate of the virus, people were fearful of socializing. High perception of risk and lowered trust are related to feelings of anxiety and lack of control. The lack of control over one's environment gives rise to various psychological consequences. However, digital platforms replaced face-to-face socialization to a great extent.

Social Relationships and Social Networks

Social relationships can be of many types, including those with spouses, co-workers, friends and acquaintances. During lockdown, face-to-face interaction became restricted to very close networks, only and connections were lost with those who were not included in them. Individuals living in dysfunctional families had no choice but to live under the same roof in the absence of community support. Middle-aged individuals, although at a disadvantage due to poor skills in handling technology were more likely to adapt to such changes by shifting to new ways of engaging, probably because of their maturity in handling relationships. Social support is one of the the most significant resilience factors following stressful events. Opportunities for spontaneous social interactions have been disrupted. For instance, having chats with co-workers in the break room gives a chance to socialize with people outside your immediate social circle, and these side discussions can act as a kind of social support (Patulny, 2020). This has significantly reduced indirect support-seeking opportunities. However, alongside this disruption, new opportunities to interact and obtain social support have arisen. The initial lockdown triggered a surge in social support from the community, which is often observed in response to unfavourable events such as natural disasters (Kaniasty et al., 2020). Although since the pandemic online social support systems have grown significantly, disparities in social support still exist in society, which were exacerbated by COVID-19 For example, people with lower socioeconomic status and older adults are more likely to be socially disadvantaged. Large social gatherings like weddings, assemblies and athletic events also offer important chances for affirming and assimilating interactional norms, create a sense of community and shared identity, and promote cooperation between social groups (Watson-Jones & Legare, 2016). Social norms were drastically changed by COVID-19, especially those that were used to express trust, affinity, empathy and respect (e.g., hugging, physical comforting). Lockdown has resulted in weakening of the ties in society. The loss of intergroup contact may even lead to more prejudiced attitudes toward out-groups.

Intimacy

A fundamental human need is satisfied when there is emotional connection through romantic, friendship or family relationships (Pietromonaco & Collins, 2017). Emotional connection also has a positive impact on health, lowering blood pressure, improving mental health, reducing stress and lowering the risk of heart disease (Pietromonaco & Collins, 2017). Middle-aged individuals whose major contacts were outside the home were unable to share intimacy with colleagues or romantic partners if they didn't stay together during lockdown. COVID-19 also provided an opportunity for individuals to reconnect and strengthen bonds within the household due to the availability of quality time after lockdown. Physical touch is also regarded as an important component of intimacy. It is a basic human need that is essential for fostering and preserving intimacy in close relationships, but restrictions and fear of infection restricted the range of people with whom intimacy could be shared.

Impact on Existing Psychiatric Illness

Middle age is undoubtedly a testing ground during which the vulnerabilities of many individuals can come to the fore. Opportunities are restricted and individuals are compelled to take stock of where they have got to in life. The discrepancy between one's ambitions and achievements can trouble the vulnerable mind. The change in physical health and bodily appearance can be stressful for many. In women, the physical changes of menopause and associated symptoms can provide them with a reminder that they are moving into the declining half of their lifecycle. COVID-19 was another reminder for them.

Numerous areas, including America, Asia, the Middle East and Europe, have reported on the pandemic's effects on mental health, including high rates of anxiety, depression and post-traumatic stress disorder in the general population (Xiong et al., 2020). A range of factors have been found to be associated with the emergence of psychiatric symptoms in the COVID-19 crisis, such as demographic factors, economic challenges, contact with social media, coping styles, quality of life, social support, psychological resilience, history of chronic and medical/psychiatric diseases, and government support policies (Banerjee 2020; Wang et al., 2020). Loneliness and being away from family were found to be linked to increased risk of mood disorders and worsening of pre-existing mental health conditions during the pandemic (Holmes et al., 2020). Middle-aged people who were working away from their families or those who were demographically separated from their children were at particularly high risk.

Mentally challenged patients are substantially more prone to develop infectious diseases such as pneumonia (Seminog & Goldacre, 2013), and the risk of more negative physical as well as psychological outcomes increases manyfold. Due to cognitive decline, diminished awareness, distorted risk perception and decreased concern for personal hygiene, these individuals are more likely to contract an infection (Yao, 2020). Individuals with a history of mental illness were more likely to experience a recurrence or worsening of their current symptoms. People who suffer from obsessive compulsive disorder (OCD) may, for example, wash their hands more frequently after it became the new norm and check for infections more frequently. There are high chances of discontinuation of therapeutic counselling schedules and difficulty in accessing prescribed psychiatric medications due to the strict nationwide regulations regarding transport and quarantine (Xiao, 2020). Also, it was interesting to note that individuals with "high illness anxiety" (OCD, generalized anxiety disorder, somatization disorder) were more likely to misinterpret the benign symptoms of cough or pain as signs of being infected with COVID-19.

Alcoholism

When considering the social, psychological and biological experiences of milife accompanied with social isolation due to the pandemic, individuals sought maladaptive coping strategies like indulging in heavy alcohol use. The factors tidentified to be associated with increased intake of alcohol were loneliness, social isolation, anxiety, depression, disruption of one's regular schedule, less clear delineation between work and leisure time, drinking alcohol with meals at home and boredom (Statistics Canada, 2021; Nanos, 2020; Shield et al., 2020). There could be any motive behind the intake of alcohol. Whatever the drivers might be, of concern are the known associations between moderate and high levels of alcohol use and adverse health outcomes, aggression, violence and domestic abuse (Sontate et al., 2021), and impaired driving (Canadian Centre on Substance Use and Addiction, 2021). The prevalence of heavy alcohol consumption was found to be greater in higher-income groups, whereas individuals belonging to lower-income groups reported greater frequency and quantity consumed (Centers for Disease Control and Prevention, 2012). Anxiety may give rise to alcohol use, or alcohol use may give rise to anxiety, or both may be related to a common third factor (Anker, 2019). This leads to a deterioration in health in middle-aged people. On the other hand, a handful of studies reported that due to loss of income, reduced opportunity to socialize, adhering to COVID-19 public health measures and other factors, there was a decrease in the consumption of alcohol (Garnett et al., 2021).

Anxiety and Depression

Middle age can be a turning point when people with failed marriages, discrepancies between their achievements and ambitions, declining physical health and poor social support to slip into withdrawal and isolation. The COVID-19 pandemic was a period during which individuals felt a sense of stagnation, that they are not going anywhere in life nor were they able to contribute to the next generation. For some, it was a really tough time with no social and financial support. During the start of the pandemic, there was confusion surrounding the disease as many people didn't know what exactly needed to be done to protect themselves from it.

Prior research has shown a correlation between joblessness, uncertain employment, instability in finances, and food insecurity and anxiety, depression and stress (Wolfson et al., 2020; Xiong et al., 2020; Wilson et al., 2020). A lingering concern was also getting infected themselves and fear for family members' health. Middle-aged adults experienced higher levels of stress due to social isolation brought on by quarantine restrictions and orders to remain at home (Bahl et al., 2021), especially those with a lower socioeconomic status (Kantamneni, 2020). This can be explained by the fear of COVID-19 outbreak, vulnerability to being infected, social distancing requirements, exposure to or close contact with someone who had been infected, and changes to social and personal daily care routines (Park et al. 2020). In addition, some respondents who were not at retirement age may have had children at home, which may be a factor for increased stress. Research has indicated increased stress related to parenting, including routine adjustments for children, the demands of online learning, and COVID-19 (Adams et al. 2021). This can also be true for middle-aged grandparents who were involved with their grandchildren with little opportunity for respite during this time. Many people were unable to access a variety of healthcare services during the pandemic, such as basic healthcare, diagnostic procedures, surgical procedures and guidance. For those who were already living with a mental health condition, the inability to assess healthcare services, led to new or worsening depressive symptoms over time. Depressive symptoms which may result from delayed care can reduce motivation and limit achievement of goals, especially when they are complex and require multiple steps, such as making an appointment with a healthcare provider (Egede & Osborn, 2010). Additionally, it has been demonstrated that depression lowers interest in achieving favourable healthcare outcomes and delays the use of healthcare services (Kim et al., 2022). According to a Chinese study, during the pandemic, those without a job or with low incomes were much more likely to experience depression (Lei et al., 2020). It has been noted that low economic status is a potential risk factor for psychological distress even during outside the COVID-19 period.

Suicide

Compared to other age groups like adolescents or the elderly, the suicide rate among the middle-aged has been documented to be relatively lower. However, a rise in the suicide rate has also been noted during crisis situations. A reason for this may be that middle-aged adults have greater financial, familial and occupational responsibilities compared to their older counterparts, which can be affected severely during a crisis. As the COVID-19 pandemic spread, researchers observed an exceptionally high level of susceptibility to serious mental health repercussions, including both thoughts of suicide and attempts (Brown & Schuman, 2020). People were generally fearful of getting infected as well as burdened by the loss of employment and limited access to social and health-related services. This additional load increased their likelihood of acting on their desperation by committing deadly self-harm. Suspicion that this burden was not evenly distributed is warranted. People in high-risk groups, such as the elderly, the chronically ill, the socially and physically isolated, and those with high daily exposure to an increased health risk such as the virus (e.g., emergency responders and frontline healthcare workers), were more likely to consider and carry out suicide than people who did not fall into these categories (Elovaino et al., 2017; Holmes et al., 2020). However, a person's perceived level of mastery and control over their destiny (Pearlin et al., 1981) as well as their resources, such as their religious affiliation and religiosity (Lawrence et al., 2016), could act as a buffer.

Impact on Discrimination, Abuse and Online Safety

In both developing and developed countries, women are more likely to be poorer than their male counterparts. Living in such conditions can increase the vulnerability of middle-aged women to violence. Women are often expected to provide caregiving responsibilities, while some women are prevented from building any savings. A perpetrator may exploit a middle-aged worker's vulnerability in terms of physical ability, social skills and availability of financial resources. During the lockdown period, when people were isolated from friends, family and community along with having limited access to services or support in the event of violence, the vulnerability of middle-aged women increased severalfold.

Middle-aged adults who have lower technological literacy can be at high risk of privacy-related harms. They are also more likely to engage in risky password practices (e.g., using passwords that can be guessed easily, using the same password over multiple platforms). Also, people who are glued to their screen for a long time in one position can experience strain in their eyes or postural problems.

Regarding the use of social media and feeling connected, researchers disagree. People were unable to establish face-to-face contact as frequently as they had in the past during the COVID-19 lockdowns. During this period, social media remained one of the important means of socialization although they also had a negative impact in the form of loneliness and isolation for those who spent too much time on such platforms. Some adults also felt jealous and dissatisfied with their current life when they consumed content portraying others' lives tas "perfect".

People who were infected or suspected of being infected and those considered responsible for the spread of the virus were the victims of negative attitudinal reactions directed toward them.

Gender-based Violence

Gender-based violence has been prevalent in society before the COVID-19 pandemic, but it worsened unexpectedly during lockdown. Domestic violence is another stressful and common occurrence that contributes to mental health issues in women (Jungari, 2020). Domestic violence is defined by the Protection of Women from Domestic Violence Act (Government of India 2005) as "any act of commission or omission or conduct resulting in physical, verbal, emotional, sexual and economic abuse", and this can range from calling names, insulting, humiliating, controlling behaviour, physical violence to sexual violence). The increased level of frustration due to job loss, physical confinement, unavailability of alcohol and multitasking experienced by male partners and lack of social support to female partners led to an increase in domestic violence against women. Occupation and earning sources for females work as a cushion against violence since their income supports the family financially, but unemployed females lose this cushion and become more vulnerable to violence at the hands of partners. Females who do not have a paid occupation are also dependent on their male partners, and face the loss of social ties and being locked up with their abusers (Nigam, 2020). The National Commission for Women logged 58 reports of domestic violence in the first week following the nationwide lockdown in March, 2020, nearly twice as many as it usually received on a weekly basis (Roy & Bagchi, 2021). This data might be an under-representation of the actual situation due to lack of awareness and access to digital services and phone calls for women, especially those from rural backgrounds. The UN Deputy Secretary General also called on all governments, civil society organizations and individuals to address gender-based violence as a major issue in all domestic COVID-19 response plans.

Social Media and News

Social media can provide a real-time account of the happenings around the world. It worked as an important tool for tracking the pandemic and for taking necessary measures. However, the modern "info media ecosystems", also known as social media, can also have some terrible effects on the management and course of an infectious disease pandemic (Al-Garadi et al., 2016). Days after the COVID-19 outbreak in China began, the "social media panic", which was marked by an unrelenting abundance of false information and badly skewed misinformation, spread more quickly than the virus itself (Depoux et al.; Shimizu, 2020). The WHO director-general called this a "coronavirus infodemic" which spread fear and panic through sensationalism, flamboyant news propaganda and unrestrained, mind-boggling rumours (Zarocostas, 2020). The circulation of fake content without its authentication and verification can lead to anxiety in anyone who consumes it. Some users faked COVID-19 symptoms in order to gain instant popularity, deliberately sowing confusion and panic among the public because sensationally charged and appalling contents draw the most attention and garner the most traffic in social media (Sokolov, 2020). Even in those who were not infected, this resulted in feelings of fear, anxiety, irritability, obsession and delusion that they had COVID-like symptoms. On the other hand, some other netizens shared social media posts that portrayed the disease too lightly, leading to a casual attitude toward the pandemic and thereby leading to the violation of rules. Since the beginning of the COVID-19 pandemic, social media have been a major factor in the global rise of anti-Chinese sentiment (Chung, 2020). The detrimental effects of this careless behaviour by netizens and media outlets may include long-term sustained stigma, shame, stress and a wide range of mental health issues.

Stigma and Discrimination

Healthcare providers, particularly general practitioners, involved in COVID-19 patient care were found to be more prone to stigmatization (Verma et al., 2004). They were the ones who were dealing with affected persons one-to-one on a daily basis. Due to stigmatization, people may not seek care until an advanced stage of infection, and may even hide their travel history. This behaviour can in turn increase the community transmission of the virus. Stigmatization and societal rejection of quarantine measures, including discrimination, neighbourhood mistrust and avoidance, property insecurity, workplace discrimination and withdrawal from social events even after epidemics have been contained are other crucial aspects to consider (Robertson et al., 2004).

Conclusion

It remains difficult to quantify the exact impact the global pandemic had on people in general, and the middle-aged in particular. But it is clear that there has been a rapid decline in social interactions, a looming global economic depression, loss of lives and changes in social as well as personal dynamics. The impact has been long-term in the form of changes observed in lung capacity, decreased immunity, mild to moderate cognitive impairment and increased risk of stroke. A lot of COVID-19 survivors have suffered from poor sleep quality, fatigue, anxiety, depression, and post-traumatic stress disorder even in the longer term. The pandemic-related increase in weight brought about a burden of obesity and numerous other non-communicable diseases, including cancer, diabetes and cardiovascular disease. The COVID-19 outbreak will make it harder for non-retired adults to achieve their long-term financial goals. It may be even tougher for middle-aged marginalized adults working in the informal sector to become part of the mainstream.

A variety of approaches is needed to address the stressors and challenges caused by the COVID-19 pandemic. These approaches should include telemedicine as an option to avoid disrupting healthcare access, improving unemployment insurance, fostering supportive workplace environments and policies, ensuring adequate access to support for basic needs and resources, facilitating access to online and telephone support services, and expanding opportunities for safe social participation. Since stigma can result in under-reporting of symptoms and decreased use of medical facilities, preventing the spread of attitudes and behaviours linked to stigma can help slow the spread of such a pandemic. It is important for states to learn a lesson from this pandemic and recognize public mental health as an important priority area that needs to be integrated into public health preparedness and emergency response plans. There is also a dire need for monitoring and counselling for the public as well as dissemination of authentic information during a crisis like the COVID-19 pandemic. Putting culturally sensitive health-promoting interventions into practice is also crucial. Building strategies for utilizing both online and offline social support avenues in complementary, as opposed to antagonistic, ways should also be a goal. We also have to understand that middle age is characterized by multiple morbidities and that every sign and symptom should not be attributed to the effect of COVID-19.

References

Acemoglu, D., Chernozhukov, V., Werning, I., & Whinston, M. D. (2020). *Optimal targeted lockdowns in a multi-group SIR model.* Economic Fluctuations and Growth, Health Economics, Public Economics. National Bureau of Economic Research. https://www.nber.org/papers/w27102

Adams, E. L., Smith, D., Caccavale, L. J., & Bean, M. K. (2021). Parents are stressed! Patterns of parent stress across COVID-19. *Frontiers in Psychiatry*, *12*, 626456.

Al-Garadi, M. A., Khan, M. S., Varathan, K. D., Mujtaba, G., & Al-Kabsi, A. M. (2016). Using online social networks to track a pandemic: A systematic review. *Journal of Biomedical Informatics*, *62*, 1–11.

Ammar, A., Brach, M., Trabelsi, K., Chtourou, H., Boukhris, O., Masmoudi, L., et al. (2020). Effects of COVID-19 home confinement on eating behaviour and physical activity: Results of the ECLB-COVID19 international online survey. *Nutrients*, *12*(6). https://doi.org/10.3390/nu12061583

Anker, J. J., & Kushner, M. G. (2019). Co-occurring alcohol use disorder and anxiety: Bridging psychiatric, psychological, and neurobiological perspectives. *Alcohol Research: Current Reviews*, *40*(1). https://doi.org/10.35946/arcr.v40.1.03

Asmundson, G. J., & Taylor, S. (2020). Coronaphobia: Fear and the 2019-nCoV outbreak. *Journal of Anxiety Disorders*, *70*, 102196.

Bahl, M., Francis, S. L., Litchfeld, R., Coleman, S., & Naig, A. (2021). Assessing and responding to COVID-19 pandemic nutrition and wellness impacts on Iowans. *Journal of Extension*, *58*(6). Retrieved May 4, 2022, from https://tigerprints.clemson.edu/joe/vol58/iss6/12/

Banerjee, D. (2020). The impact of Covid-19 pandemic on elderly mental health. *International Journal of Geriatric Psychiatry*, *35*(12), 1466–1467. https://doi.org/10.1002/gps.5320

Banerjee, A. V. (1992). A simple model of herd behavior. *The Quarterly Journal of Economics*, *107*(3), 797–817.

Bertrand, M., Dizon-Ross, R., Krishnan, K., & Schofield, H. (2020). *Employment, income and consumption in india during and after the lockdown: A v-shape recovery?* Report. Rustandy Center for Social Sector Innovation Blog.

Biswas, P., & Chatterjee, S. (2014). Hand hygiene compliance among doctors in a tertiary care hospital of India. *The Indian Journal of Pediatrics*, *81*, 967–968.

Brown, S., & Schuman, D. L. (2020). Suicide in the time of COVID19: A perfect storm. *Journal of Rural Health, 0*, 1–4. https://doi.org/10.1111/jrh.12458

Canadian Centre on Substance Use and Addiction. (2021). Impaired driving in Canada. https://www.ccsa.ca/sites/default/files/2021-03/CCSA-Impaired-Driving-Canada-Summary2021-en.pdf

Casagrande, M., Favieri, F., Tambelli, R., & Forte, G. (2020). The enemy who sealed the world: effects quarantine due to the COVID-19 on sleep quality, anxiety, and psychological distress in the Italian population. *Sleep Medicine, 75*, 12–20. https://doi.org/10.1016/j.sleep.2020.05.011

Centers for Disease Control and Prevention (CDC). (2012). Vital signs: Binge drinking prevalence, frequency, and intensity among adults-United States, 2010. *MMWR. Morbidity and Mortality Weekly Report*, *61*(1), 14–19.

Chang, H. H., & Meyerhoefer, C. D. (2021). COVID-19 and the demand for online food shopping services: Empirical evidence from Taiwan. *American Journal of Agricultural Economics*, *103*(2), 448–465.

Chen, Q., Liang, M., Li, Y., Guo, J., Fei, D., Wang, L., He, L., Sheng, C., Cai, Y., Li, X., Wang, J., & Zhang, Z. (2020). Mental health care for medical staff in China during the COVID-19 outbreak. *The Lancet Psychiatry*, *7*(4), e15–e16.

Chopra, S., Ranjan, P., Singh, V., Kumar, S., Arora, M., Hasan, M. S., & Baitha, U. (2020). Impact of COVID-19 on lifestyle-related behaviours-a cross-sectional audit of responses from nine hundred and ninety-five participants from India. *Diabetes & Metabolic Syndrome: Clinical Research & Reviews*, *14*(6), 2021–2030.

Chung, R. Y., Li, M. M. (2020). Anti-Chinese sentiment during the 2019-nCoV outbreak. *The Lancet, 395*, 686e7.

Constandt, B., Thibaut, E., De Bosscher, V., Scheerder, J., Ricour, M., & Willem, A. (2020). Exercising in times of lockdown: An analysis of the impact of COVID-19 on levels and patterns of exercise among adults in Belgium. *International Journal of Environmental Research and Public Health, 17*(11), 4144. https://doi.org/10.3390/ijerph17114144

Coronavirus BBC. (2020). Anger as migrants sprayed with disinfectant in India. Retrieved April 1, 2020, from https://www.bbc.com/news/world-asia-india-52093220

Couch, K. A., Fairlie, R. W., and Xu, H. (2020). The impacts of COVID-19 on minority unemployment: First evidence from April 2020 CPS microdata. http://dx.doi.org/10.2139/ssrn.3604814

COVID-19 Dashboard by the Center for Systems Science and Engineering at Johns Hopkins University. (2020). https://coronavirus.jhu.edu/map.html

Deshpande, A., & Ramachandran, R. (2020). *Is COVID-19 "The great leveler?" The critical role of social identity in lockdown-induced job losses* (No. 622). GLO discussion paper.

Dörner, J., Mickler, C., & Staudinger, U. M. (2005). Self-development at midlife. In *Middle adulthood: A lifespan perspective* (pp. 277–317). Sage. https://doi.org/10.4135/9781452225999.n9

Egede, L. E., & Osborn, C. Y. (2010). Role of motivation in the relationship between depression, self-care, and glycemic control in adults with type 2 diabetes. *Diabetes Educator*, *36*, 276–283.

Elovaino, M., Hakulinen, C., Pulkki-Råback, L., Virtanen, M., Josefsson, K., Jokela, M., Vahtera, J., & Kivimäki, M. (2017). Contribution of risk factors to excess mortality in isolated and lonely individuals: An analysis of data from the UK Biobank cohort study. *The Lancet Public Health*. https://doi.org/10.1016/s2468-2667(17)30075-0

Evans, R. A., McAuley, H., Harrison, E. M., PHOSP-COVID Collaborative Group. (2021). Physical, cognitive and mental health impacts of COVID-19 following hospitalisation: A multi-centre prospective cohort study. *medRxiv* [preprint]. https://doi.org/10.1101/2021.03.22.21254057

Fancourt, D., Steptoe, A., & Bu, F. (2021). Trajectories of anxiety and depressive symptoms during enforced isolation due to COVID-19 in England: a longitudinal observational study. *The Lancet Psychiatry*, *8*(2), 141-149.

Financial, A. (2020). Grocery stores thriving amid the coronavirus outbreak. https://amtrustfinancial.com/blog/small-business/grocery-stores-thriving-coronavirus%20Last

Garnett, C., Jackson, S., Oldham, M., Brown, J., Steptoe, A., & Fancourt, D. (2021). Factors associated with drinking behaviour during COVID-19 social distancing and lockdown among adults in the UK. *Drug and Alcohol Dependence, 219*, 108461.

Golechha, M. (2020). COVID-19, India, lockdown and psychosocial challenges: What next?. *International Journal of Social Psychiatry*, *66*(8), 830–832.

Greenberg, N., Docherty, M., Gnanapragasam, S., & Wessely, S. (2020). Managing mental health challenges faced by healthcare workers during covid-19 pandemic. *bmj*, *368*, m1211.

Harris, J., Depenbusch, L., Pal, A. A., Nair, R. M., & Ramasamy, S. (2020). Food system disruption: Initial livelihood and dietary effects of COVID-19 on vegetable producers in India. *Food Security*, *12*(4), 841–851.

Hess, A., & Liu, J. (2020). 13 ways the coronavirus pandemic could forever change the way we work. Retrieved May 14, 2020, from https://www.cnbc.com/2020/04/29/how-the-coronaviruspandemic-will-impact-the-future-of-work.html

History.com. (2020). Pandemics that changed history. Retrieved August 17, 2020, from https://www.history.com/topics/middle-ages/pandemics-timeline

Ho, C. S., Chee, C. Y., & Ho, R. C. (2020). Mental health strategies to combat the psychological impact of COVID-19 beyond paranoia and panic. *Annals of the Academy of Medicine of Singapore*, *49*(1), 1–3.

Holmes, E. A., O'Connor, R. C., Perry, V. H., Tracey, I., Wessely, S., Arseneault, L., Ballard, C., Christensen, H., Cohen Silver, R., Everall, I., Ford, T., John, A., Kabir, T., King, K., Madan, I., Michie, S., Przybylski, A. K., Shafran, R., Sweeney, A., … Bullmore, E. (2020). Multidisciplinary research priorities for the COVID-19 pandemic: A call for action for mental health science. *Lancet Psychiatry*, *7*(6), 547–560. https://doi.org/10.1016/S2215-0366(20)30168-1

Giordano, C. (2020, March 25). *Doctor kicked out by landlord over coronavirus fears*. The Independent. https://www.independent.co.uk/news/health/coronavirus-latest-nhs-doctor-evicted-covid-19-oxford-a9425166.html

International Labour Organisation. (2018). *India wage report: Wage policies for decent work and inclusive growth*. International Labor Organization.

Jungari, S. (2020). Maternal mental health in India COVID-19. *Public Health, 185*, 97–898.

Kaniasty, K., de Terte, I., Guilaran, J., & Bennett, S. (2020). A scoping review of post-disaster social support investigations conducted after disasters that Struck the Australia and Oceania continent. *Disasters, 44,* 336–366.

Kantamneni, N. (2020). The impact of the COVID-19 pandemic on marginalized populations in the United States: A research agenda. *Journal of Vocational Behavior, 119,* 103439. https://doi.org/10.1016/j.jvb.2020.103439

Kaushik, M., & Guleria, N. (2020). The impact of pandemic COVID-19 in workplace. *European Journal of Business and Management*, *12*(15), 1–10.

Kim, K., Kim, H., Lee, J., Cho, I.-K., Ahn, M. H., Son, K. Y., Kim, J. E., Kim, H. J., Yoon, S. M., & Kim, S. H. (2022). Functional impairments in the mental health, depression and anxiety related to the viral epidemic, and disruption in healthcare service utilization among cancer patients in the COVID-19 pandemic era. *Cancer Research and Treatment Official Journal of Korean Cancer Association, 54*, 671–679.

Kowalska, J. D., Skrzat-Klapaczyńska, A., Bursa, D., Balayan, T., Begovac, J., Chkhartishvili, N., & ECEE Network Group. (2020). HIV care in times of the COVID-19 crisis—Where are we now in Central and Eastern Europe? *International Journal of Infectious Diseases, 96*, 311–314.

Lawrence, R. E., Oquendo, M. A., & Stanley, B. (2016). Religion and suicide risk: A systematic review. *Archives of Suicide Research, 20*, 2–121. https://doi.org/10.1080/13811118.2015.1004494

Lee, M., Smith, C., Snell, L., et al. (2020). Comparative outcomes in hospital admissions with COVID-19 in people living with HIV and people living without HIV: A retrospective study. *AIDS*. 2020. Virtual: 2020.

Lei, L., Huang, X., Zhang, S., Yang, J., Yang, L., & Xu, M. (2020). Comparison of prevalence and associated factors of anxiety and depression among people affected by versus people unaffected by quarantine during the COVID-19 epidemic in Southwestern China. *Medical Science Monitor: International Medical Journal of Experimental and Clinical Research, 26*, e924609-1.

Liu, N., Zhang, F., Wei, C., Jia, Y., Shang, Z., Sun, L., & Liu, W. (2020). Prevalence and predictors of PTSS during COVID-19 outbreak in China hardest-hit areas: Gender differences matter. *Psychiatry Research, 287*, 112921.

Liu, X., Kakade, M., Fuller, C. J., Fan, B., Fang, Y., Kong, J., et al. (2012). Depression after exposure to stressful events: Lessons learned from the severe acute respiratory syndrome epidemic. *Comprehensive Psychiatry, 53*, 15–23.

Lodge, W., & Kuchukhidze, S. (2020). COVID-19, HIV, and migrant workers: The double burden of the two viruses. *AIDS Patient Care STDS, 34*, 249–250. https://doi.org/10.1089/apc.2020.0092

Ma, Z. F., Zhang, Y., Luo, X., Li, X., Li, Y., Liu, S., & Zhang, Y. (2020). Increased stressful impact among general population in mainland China amid the COVID-19 pandemic: A nationwide cross-sectional study conducted after Wuhan city's travel ban was lifted. *International Journal of Social Psychiatry, 66*(8), 770–779. https://doi.org/10.1177/0020764020935489

Mahase, E. (2020). Covid-19: Hoarding and misuse of protective gear is jeopardising the response, WHO warns. *BMJ, 368*, m869.

Malek Rivan, N. F., Yahya, H. M., Shahar, S., Ajit Singh, D. K., Ibrahim, N., Mat Ludin, A. F., & Kamaruddin, M. Z. A. (2021). The impact of poor nutrient intakes and food insecurity on the psychological distress among community-dwelling middle-aged and older adults during the COVID-19 pandemic. *Nutrients, 13*(2), 353.

Nanos. (2020). *COVID-19 and increased alcohol consumption: NANOS poll summary report*. Commissioned for Canadian Centre on Substance Use and Addiction. https://www.ccsa.ca/sites/default/files/2020-04/CCSA-NANOS-AlcoholConsumption-During-COVID-19-Report-2020-en.pdf

Nelson, V. M. (2020). Suicide Prevention India Foundation. http://www.rfi.fr/en/international/20200514-mental-illness-suicides-on-the-rise-in-india-during-covid19-lockdown

Nigam, S. (2020). *COVID-19, lockdown and violence against women in homes*. Lockdown and Violence against Women in Homes (April 28, 2020).

Niles, M., Bertmann, F., Belarmino, E., Wentworth, T., Biehl, E., & Neff, R. (2020). The early food insecurity impacts of COVID-19. *Nutrients, 12*(7), 2096. https://doi.org/10.3390/nu12072096

Ong, J. L., Lau, T., Massar, S. A. A., Chong, Z. T., Ng, B. K. L., Koek, D., et al. (2020). COVID-19 related mobility reduction: Heterogenous effects on sleep and physical activity rhythms. *Sleep*. https://doi.org/10.1093/sleep/zsaa179

Park, C. L., Russell, B. S., Fendrich, M., Finkelstein-Fox, L., Hutchison, M., & Becker, J. (2020). Americans' COVID-19 stress, coping, and adherence to CDC Guidelines. *Journal of General Internal Medicine, 35*(8), 2296–2303. https://doi.org/10.1007/s11606-020-05898-9

Patulny, R. McKenzie, J. J., Bower, M. & Olson, R. E. (2020-, April 27). Reconnecting after coronavirus - 4 key ways cities can counter anxiety and loneliness. *The Conversation*, 1–4.

Pearlin, L. I., Menaghan, E. G., Lieberman, M. A., & Mullan, J. T. (1981). The stress process. *Journal of Health and Social Behavior, 22*, 337–356. https://doi.org/10.2307/2136676

Pietromonaco, P. R., & Collins, N. L. (2017). Interpersonal mechanisms linking close relationships to health. *American Psychologist*, *72*, 531–542.

Rabkin, J. G. (2008). HIV and depression: 2008 review and update. *Current HIV/AIDS Reports*, *5*, 163–171. https://doi.org/10.1007/s11904-008-0025-1

Ranjan, R. (2020). Predictions for COVID-19 outbreak in India using epidemiological models. MedRxiv, 2020-04

Richardson, S., Hirsch, J. S., Narasimhan, M., Crawford, J. M., McGinn, T., Davidson, K. W., et al. (2020). Presenting characteristics, comorbidities, and outcomes among 5700 patients hospitalized with COVID-19 in the New York City Area. *JAMA*. https://doi.org/10.1001/jama.2020.6775

Robertson, E., Hershenfield, K., Grace, S. L., & Stewart, D. E. (2044). The psychosocial effects of being quarantined following exposure to SARS: A qualitative study of Toronto health care workers. *The Canadian Journal of Psychiatry, 49*, 403e7.

Roy, A. S., Sen, N., & Bagchi, S. S. (2021). Gender-based violence in India in Covid-19 lockdown. *Journal of Comparative Literature and Aesthetics*, *44*(1), 41–55.

Seminog, O. O., & Goldacre, M. J. (2013). Risk of pneumonia and pneumococcal disease in people with severe mental illness: English record linkage studies. *Thorax*, *68*(2), 171–176.

Sen, A. (2009). *The idea of justice*. Belknap Press of Harvard University Press.

Shield, K., Young, M., & Agic, B. (2020). *Alcohol consumption and the COVID-19 pandemic: Synthesizing knowledge for policy action: Draft CIHR knowledge synthesis report*. CIHR.

Shimizu, K. (2020). 2019-nCoV, fake news, and racism. *Lancet, 395*, 685e6.

Singh, A. K., & Misra, A. (2020). Herd mentality, herds of migrants/people, and COVID-19 in India. *Diabetes & Metabolic Syndrome*, *14*(4), 497.

Sohrabi, C., Alsafi, Z., O'Neill, N., et al. (2020). World Health Organization declares global emergency: A review of the 2019 novel coronavirus (COVID-19). *International Journal of Surgery, 76*, 71–76. https://doi.org/10.1016/j.ijsu.2020.02.034

Sokolov, M. (2020). The pandemic infodemic: How social media helps [and hurts] during the coronavirus outbreak. *The Drum*.

Sontate, K. V., Kamaluddin, M. R., Mohamed, I. N., Mohamed, R. M. P., Shaikh, M. F., Kamal, H., & Kumar, J. (2021). Alcohol, aggression and violence: From public health to neuroscience. *Frontiers in Psychology*, *12*, 699726. https://doi.org/10.3389/fpsyg.2021.699726

Statistics Canada. (2021). Alcohol and cannabis use during the pandemic: Canadian Perspectives Survey Series 6. https://www150.statcan.gc.ca/n1/daily-quotidien/210304/dq210304a-eng.htm

Stranges, S., Tigbe, W., Gómez-Olivé, F. X., Thorogood, M., & Kandala, N. B. (2012). Sleep problems: an emerging global epidemic? Findings from the INDEPTH

WHO-SAGE study among more than 40,000 older adults from 8 countries across Africa and Asia. *Sleep, 35*(8), 1173–1181.
Taha, S., Matheson, K., Cronin, T., & Anisman, H. (2014). Intolerance of uncertainty, appraisals, coping, and anxiety: The case of the 2009 H 1 N 1 pandemic. *British Journal of Health Psychology, 19*(3), 592–605.
The New York Times. (2020). Coronavirus means funerals must Wait: 'We can't properly bury our dead'. Retrieved April 3, 2020, from https://www.nytimes.com/2020/03/25/us/coronavirus-funerals.html
The Washington Post. (2020). In India, the world's biggest lockdown has forced migrants to walk hundreds of miles home. Retrieved April 1, 2020, from https://www.washingtonpost.com/world/asia_pacific/india-coronavirus-lockdown-migrant-workers/2020/03/27/a62df166-6f7d-11ea-a156-0048b62cdb51_story.html
Times, F. (2020). Prospering in the pandemic: The top 100 companies. *Financial Times.*
TRT World. (2020). Indian workers self-quarantine in trees. Retrieved April 1, 2020, from https://www.youtube.com/watch?v¼f7I6zsqmQIE
UN News. (2020). Water access critical to beating back COVID-19 spread in slum areas. Retrieved April 1, 2020, from https://news.un.org/en/story/2020/03/1060042
Verma, S., Mythily, S., Chan, Y. H., Deslypere, J. P., Teo, E. K., & Chong, S. A. (2004). Post-SARS psychological morbidity and stigma among general practitioners and traditional Chinese medicine practitioners in Singapore. *Annals of the Academy of Medicine of Singapore, 33*, 743e8.
Wang, C., Pan, R., Wan, X., Tan, Y., Xu, L., Ho, C. S., et al. (2020). Immediate psychological responses and associated factors during the initial stage of the 2019 Coronavirus Disease (COVID-19) epidemic among the general population in China. *International Journal of Environmental Research and Public Health, 17*(5). https://doi.org/10.3390/ijerph17051729
Wang, Y., Di, Y., Ye, J., & Wei, W. (2020). Study on the public psychological states and its related factors during the outbreak of coronavirus disease 2019 (COVID-19) in some regions of China. *Psychology, Health & Medicine, 30,* 1e10.
Watson-Jones, R. E., & Legare, C. H. (2016). The social functions of group rituals. *Current Directions in Psychological Science, 25*, 42–46.
WHO. (2020). OHCHR. IOM, UNHCR and WHO joint press release: The rights and health of refugees, migrants and stateless must be protected in COVID-19 response. Retrieved April 1, 2020, from https://www.who.int/news-room/detail/31-03-2020-ohchr-iomunhcr-and-who-joint-press-release-the-rights-and-health-of-refugees-migrants-and-stateless-must-be-protected-in-covid-19-response
Wolfson, J. A., Leung, C. W., & Kullgren, J. T. (2020). Food as a critical social determinant of health among older adults during the coronavirus disease 2019 (COVID-19) pandemic. *JAMA Health Forum, 1*(7), e200925. https://doi.org/10.1001/jamahealthforum.2020.0925
Wong, L. Y., Francis, S. L., Genschel, U., Arthur, A., Xu, F., Weidauer, L., & Kendall, C. (2023). A cross-sectional assessment of food practices, physical activity levels, and stress levels in middle age and older adults' during the COVID-19 pandemic. *Journal of Public Health, 31*(10), 1567–1583.
World Health Organization (WHO). (2020). Weekly epidemiology update on corona virus disease (COVID-19). Retrieved March, 2020, from https://www.who.int/emergencies/diseases/novel-coronavirus-2019/situation-reports
Wright, A., Salazar, A., Mirica, M., Volk, L. A., & Schiff, G. D. (2020). The invisible epidemic: Neglected chronic disease management during COVID-19. *Journal of General Internal Medicine, 35*, 2816–2817.

Wu, P., Fang, Y., Guan, Z., Fan, B., Kong, J., Yao, Z., et al. (2009). The psychological impact of the SARS epidemic on hospital employees in China: Exposure, risk perception, and altruistic acceptance of risk. *The Canadian Journal of Psychiatry, 54*, 302–311.

Xiao, C. (2020). A novel approach of consultation on 2019 novel coronavirus (COVID-19)-related psychological and mental problems: Structured letter therapy. *Psychiatry Investigation*, *17*(2), 175.

Xiong, J., Lipsitz, O., Nasri, F., Lui, L. M. W., Gill, H., Phan, L., et al. (2020). Impact of COVID19 pandemic on mental health in the general population: A systematic review. *Journal of Affective Disorders, 277*, 55–64. https://doi.org/10.1016/j.jad.2020.08.001

Yao, H., Chen, J. H., & Xu, Y. F. (2020). Patients with mental health disorders in the COVID-19 epidemic. *The Lancet Psychiatry*, *7*(4), e21.

Zarocostas, J. (2020). How to fight an infodemic. *The Lancet*, *395*(10225), 676.

Zhang, B., & Wing, Y.-K. (2006). Sex differences in Insomnia: A meta-analysis. *Sleep, 29*(1), 85–93. https://doi.org/10.1093/sleep/29.1.85

12 Conversations on Marginalization

Dovetailing Lived Experiences of Marginal Urban Groups of India

Ritwik Saha, Jayeeta Naskar Das and Anindita Chaudhuri

Conceptualising Marginalisation and Self

The presence of stories from the margins is sometimes overlooked in the grand narrative of human lore. The minor voices in this story remain muffled, if not unheard. Those who are not taken into account within the dominant socioeconomic and cultural framework are considered marginalized. Thus, it is imperative that scholarly attention be given to the phenomenon of marginalization and its associated trajectory, as well as its exclusion from the mainstream psychosocial discourse. These factors posit a structural incomprehension of the cultural, social and existential ground of the various marginal groups in urban settings.

An attempt is made to comprehend lived experiences via the lens of postmodernism, setting aside the ubiquitous hegemonic rhetoric of marginalization, the subjective narratives of human life and the interpretative framework of the individual in a particular sociocultural setup. Since its introduction into sociological theory in 1928, the notion of marginalization has been used to describe a variety of situations. Later, as the traditional economic market and stable employment opportunities gradually declined, psychological perspectives on marginalization were added. An increasing number of communities are experiencing a wide range of mobility and marginality as a result of the decline of traditional industries, the acceleration of the Industrial Revolution and the expansion of global capitalism (Chomsky, 2000). A wide range of exclusions occurred due to the severe oppression of the labour market which prevents people from participating meaningfully in society (Young, 2000).

Social marginality and the subjective assessment of one's exposure to a specific society, culture and environment are the foundations of the psychological perspective on marginality. The lived experiences through encountering the lives of various urban marginal groups and adding meaning to them in the context of various sociocultural setups that aim to understand the multiplicity of identities and narratives are characteristic of postmodernism, which is defined by subjectivity, multiculturalism and social constructivism.

DOI: 10.4324/9781003568360-15

Furthermore, compared to the traditional nature of work, identity and relationships, the postmodern era is marked by globalization, insecurities and related experiences of precarious existence and the transient status of relationships with friends, family and co-workers (Standing, 2014). The change in emphasis is due to the evolving as well as shifting nature of personal relationship perspectives, the variety of subjective experiences, and the identity and power dynamics of the various marginalized groups (socioeconomic, religious, cultural, biological, demographic, ethnic etc.), which are all contributing factors to the change in focus.

Their daily lives are impacted by intersectional inequality and the power dynamics of many social groupings, and as a result, their self-evaluations may vary from others. The experiences of many marginalized groups and their voices are structurally devalued in the postmodern era by the dominant discourse of popular culture, but marginalization (in many forms) and its distinctiveness themselves triumph over the inclusive function of academia's gatekeeping role. As Fisk calls for centring and discusses the "failure of the politics of the uncentered differences", their experiences have largely diverged from the recognition of the dominant theoretical discourse, which means that knowledge cannot be shared to transform their lives (Fisk, 1992).

The deliberate endeavour to comprehend and empower culturally varied and socially excluded groups by exposing their layer of deprivation is the overall strategic process of centring for meaningful involvement in society that is exemplified by their self-representation. Furthermore, the subjective sensations of derecognition from the immaterial angle by the dominant narratives and the sense of loneliness or despair resulting from the unfavourable situation are radically different. This could convey a part of the central experience, wherein a sense of detachment allows for viewpoints not available from central locations (Kurtz et al., 2009). Therefore, the attempt to comprehend marginalization is sparked by the perspectives of those on the edges and their perception of reality.

Because of its multifaceted dynamic nature, marginality can be both global and local. In many literary works, marginality is regarded as social exclusion. Therefore, feeling like you don't belong, that you can't contribute much to your community, that you can't access the opportunities and services that others can and that you're not a valued member of the community, all of which contribute to your feeling of exclusion from society, are interchangeable with being marginalized (Frisen et al., 2012; Razer et al., 2013).

Nonetheless, marginalization has two unique aspects, according to Messiou (2012): the experiences of marginalization and the acknowledgement of it by an individual or by others (due to the subjective nature of the individual). As a result, it is clear that marginalization encompasses more than simply the subjective perceptions, feelings and moods themselves. Put another way, it is not a fixed state, but rather a series of intricate processes that deny people access to resources or involvement in a range of social activities. A group of people who carry and share a common range of emotions and experiences because they have been victimized (economically, socially, psychologically or in any other way) by the prevailing order in a specific culture is referred to as a "marginalized group or community". Furthermore, their identity, sense of belonging and social interactions are adversely correlated with their psychological wellbeing when their physical location shifts (Flynn, 2017). Thus, in order to adapt to or oppose the perceived threat of the new setup, a complex process of reconstructing selfhood or moulding identity becomes active in the urban marginal group's transitory period (Vasas, 2005).

Complexity is seen as the subjective experience of marginalization within the framework of mainstream culture and the reconstruction of group identity (such as ethnicity) as a strategy for adapting to a new setting. Migrants and ethnic minorities are marginalized groups that have lower social status and power, are more likely to face discrimination, and have less representation in the host society. They also hold different sociocultural values and are frequently caught between two opposing sets of cultural values, which strengthens their sense of commitment to and belonging to their group or culture (Phinney, 1990). In line with Phinney's theory of ethnic identity formation, young adults either advance with unquestioned beliefs or hold their ethnicity in high regard by investigating community or societal attitudes and immersing themselves in the history and culture of their group in order to develop a strong sense of their ethnic identity (Phinney, 1993).

Intersectional Vulnerability through the Lens of Marginalization

Marginalization is an experience (Kagan & Burton, 2005) that impacts negatively upon societies (Mowat, 2015) and affects millions of people worldwide. People belonging to certain marginalized communities termed as social, sexual or related to any stigmatized profession seem to possess some common criteria like exclusion, being subjected to negative public attitudes and having limited access to resources (Kagan & Burton, 2005).

Being a multi-layered concept, marginalization deals with several aspects which can be covered by the intersectionality approach. Vulnerability is such an aspect that became very prominent for these marginalized communities due to their social status which they achieved by being a part of the communities. In order to unravel the dynamics of vulnerability and resilience, intersectionality approaches are very helpful as this aim to understand intra-group differences and the existence of multiple axes of identity that govern an individual's or group's relationship to power (Osborne, 2015). This particular approach enables us to view marginalization in the form of vulnerability from a new angle. Rather than as the characteristic of some socio-demographic groups, intersectionality allows us to see it as the result of different and interdependent societal stratification processes that result in multiple dimensions of marginalization (Kuran et al., 2020). However, by origin, the concept of intersectionality is the work of a black feminist researcher to understand the position of African-American women in their respective social structures. The intersectional theory of Kimberle Crenshaw (1989) a leading scholar of critical race theory, is about the power structure, how the exercise of power affects individuals having social inequalities with multiple marginalizations through domination and oppression, and how people's social identities can overlap to magnify the experiences of discrimination (Crenshaw, 1989; Kuran et al., 2020). The intersectional perspective is not only concerned with showing how oppressive power is submerged in societal structure (Collins & Bilge, 2020) but also pays attention to expressing the differences in terms of individual lives, social practices, cultural ideologies and the results of this interaction with respect to power (Davis, 2008). It is quite evident to view the lived experiences of such marginalized (which refers to communities that experience discrimination and exclusion socially, politically and economically because of unequal power relationships across economic, political, social, and cultural dimensions) communities of India through the lens of the intersectionality approach as it will allow us to explore the struggle they face in their everyday life in order to fit themselves within the host culture despite having different cultural ideologies irrespective of particular gender, but as a community as a whole.

Feelings of rootlessness magnify the feelings of being alone and sometimes create a voidness that makes these communities more vulnerable in terms of their members' individual identities or their identity as a community. An intersectional approach toward vulnerability will provide us with a way through which we can examine and capture the processes, practices and policies and understand the dilemma and discrimination they face due to their overlapping identities. Growing feelings of "being alone have escalated the desperation that drove them toward their "own", which shows the vulnerable side of being a migrant population in a country like India which also exhibits feelings of insecurity, alienation and loss. Kuran et al. (2020) successfully exhibit how applying an intersectionality perspective in the study of vulnerable groups across Europe in times of hazards and crisis helps authorities and agencies to put together guidelines to meet the respective needs. The ability to uncover the social differences along with the interplay of multiple power structure and social inequalities in certain contexts make the intersectionality approach viable to study the concerned populations. Chaplin et al. (2019) not only demonstrate identifying vulnerability or exercise of power in a particular social structure, but the intersectional perspective also shines a light on vulnerability reduction and resilience-building with the aim of informing institutional policy and operational practice. IN order to understand a marginalized community from an intersectional perspective, it is necessary to recognize how inequality categories cross paths or intersections, and how that reflects people's everyday experiences and practices (Fylling & Melboe, 2019). Being a marginalized community, feelings of deprivation in accessing basic amenities most of the time make them question their existence, and an intersectional approach explores this uncertainty and the crises they face during their life course. Several studies show how the intersectional perspective seems to be effective in gaining a deep insight into the studies of marginal communities. The gendered implication of the migrant women population from South Rajasthan (Dutta et al., 2020), accessing welfare service by Sami people from the Northern Arctic region (Fylling & Melboe, 2019) or legal conditions of immigrant sex workers from Berlin (Altay et al., 2021), and many more.

Migration and Marginalization

In order to achieve psychological wellbeing, a marginalized group of migrants may go through a period of identity remodelling while they are transitioning into the destination society. This chapter will explore the subjective and experiential point of view, and the consequential factors that accompany migration, such as social exclusion, alienation and various disqualifying parameters in the host society, that lead to marginalization, despite the fact that migration is a highly discussed topic in contemporary trends of globalization and socioeconomic activities. Therefore, it is important to have a broad understanding of the idea of marginalization in the context of this chapter. By exploring the lived experiences of India's urban marginal migrant populations, the qualitative features of marginalization which can be either actively or passively linked to migration are uncovered.

Lack of Social Support

n connection with the conversation on marginalization, migration is the contemporary trend that leads to the experience of living on the edge. Migration is a phenomenon that involves integration, acculturation and assimilation into a new society (Sreedharan & Murale, 2018), but beyond that, in the transitional phase, the lack of social support and positive connection in the host society makes the urban migrant (socioeconomically poor) feel alone, and perceived inferiority reshapes their confidence and self-concept, which negatively affects their psychosocial life. Thus, the insignificant living experiences of marginal migrants in urban society probably compel them to work hard and fulfil the basic livelihood demands, but apart from that, the thirst to earn status in life is another urge to seek coherence in their transitioning existence.

Desire for a Future

Besides all the adversity, a strong desire for a future is another phenomenon that probably keeps urban migrants resilient while experiencing hardship in the host society. Contributing hard labour or compromising their social life to follow a better future for their family members is the reality with which they keep on moving. The physical world of hardship or adversity of the new destination is a less-valued phenomenon while futuristic desire overwhelms, leading to some persistence in their experiences in life.

Developing a Sense of Alienation

In relation to the marginal experiences of people and groups, sociocultural alienation or helplessness results from being rejected or disregarded by mainstream society (Giddens, 2001). This affects the exposed person as well as the family, neighbours and support systems in the community on a psychological level. The idea of social disintegration, which represents the individual condition of isolation and a sense of social alienation, is developed as a result of socioeconomic marginalization.

However, in addition to the disintegrative factors, the new normal period's health measures hasten the state of social detachment, leading to psychological anguish that disproportionately impacts the poor and marginalized. Additionally, social detachment has been found to hasten the experience of social isolation, which is adversely linked to psychological wellbeing (Cacioppo et al., 2011; Swader, 2019). Living in extreme poverty on the one hand and experiencing a sense of uprooting on the other, along with the lack of psychological and transcendental cues to establish emotional connections, can cause one to feel alone and unrelieved. In addition, long-term family separation, losing one's independence and autonomy, lack of leisure time and lack of face-to-face social interaction all likely contribute to mental distress, particularly in middle age (Bai et al., 2004). The subliminal emotional attachment and accompanying identification with one's natal location are frequently unreimbursed in the destination setup for the underprivileged migratory population. Strong ties to a location can provide significance, social status and support for the development of an individual's identity and sense of belonging (Benson & Jackson, 2013). Urban society's lack of traditional networks and cultural cues, combined with its relatively diverse and modern sociocultural practices, is thought to exacerbate negative psychological outcomes like social isolation, increased loneliness and micro-aggression, which are especially harmful to marginalized migrant populations. Furthermore, even when the original motivation for migrating is satisfied, the destination fails to provide the subjective sense of social detachment, freedom from concerns and lack of emotional support from loved ones, and finally, the solace that comes from comforting oneself. Therefore, more research is necessary to understand the subjective experiences of such discontent and how to make meaning of it for one's existence and resilience.

Making sense of life, as seen from an Indian perspective, is the contextual process of encountering and interpreting the experiences one has on a daily basis (Salagame, 2016). Indian society endeavours to incorporate sociocultural tools such as mutual trust, understanding, public relations and interaction with associates. These tools are considered to be social capital that may be lacking, particularly for the marginalized class. Furthermore, a degree of social distrust was sparked by pandemic measures, as noted by Aassve et al. (2021), which could have detrimental effects. Meanwhile, interacting with the environment for a living and having a physical link to society and its economic domain are two quite different experiences. The living element that creates a sense of connection and belonging is positive interaction with society and keeping oneself informed about events around one. Because of these buffering space limits, it is challenging for the marginalized population to integrate into a society that is very different from their own, which breeds micro-aggression and a sense of alienation.

Therefore, the other aspect to be revealed in the literature is the process of meaning-making and the subjective experiences of being marginalized or living on the edge, aside from its structural concept. The prevalent social recognition that was built up through family ties, sociopolitical involvement, sociocultural customs, and the everyday use of language and cultural capital in the native place is frequently rejected and disqualified in the host social contexts during the migration process. Furthermore, the dominant narratives, the sociocultural system and the social power structure all work together to create barriers to the integration of alternative identities. The socioeconomic status, education and living standards of urban migrants are all factors in their social exclusion. In addition, being away from friends and family and the unwelcome satisfaction of typical middle-aged psycho-physical requirements further marginalizes them. Furthermore, the migrant population with lower socioeconomic positions in urban settings are badly impacted by the current global socioeconomic trends, which are frequently at odds with the regional and sociocultural variety of various Indian states/people along with distinct ethnic identities. Middle-aged migrant groups experience a perceived devaluation of their sociocultural identity, isolation from family and friends, and related experiences in their host community, which leads to the shaping and reshaping of their identity to fit their new location. The absence of acknowledgement in the host society results in a lack of political representation, which means that the lived experiences of social exclusion and the hardships faced by marginalized migrant groups are not taken into account by the dominant discourse (Schlossberg, 2004). Additionally, because of the marginal population's precarious living conditions brought on by their informal settlement and means of subsistence, they have poor access to resources and are disproportionately exposed to environmental hazards (such as floods and landslides) (Banks et al., 2011; Chu & Michael, 2019). Ironically, the emerging state (in the COVID-19 period) and the ensuing circumstances necessitate substantial social and economic assistance, or means of subsistence, which is not provided at their place of employment. As a result, they have been forced to return home out of desperation in order to survive. The act of returning home, which they used to do on a regular basis, now becomes a survival instinct (Singh, 2020).

Furthermore, a number of social issues, like having small social networks and facing discrimination for risks of spreading the coronavirus, worsen marginalized workers' social stigma as "super spreaders", persistent suffering and the crises that go along with it (Guadagno, 2020). The pandemic made already-existing intersectional inequality and disparity, as well as marginal people's susceptibility, worse (Mia & Griffiths, 2020). Separating the locals from the marginalized (migrants) through the dichotomy of "we versus they" and the social labelling of outsiders breed prejudice and greater marginalization, which can be dangerous to oneself (Bhattacharya et al., 2020). Separation and marginalization progress more quickly when their psychological anguish and alienation result from the disadvantaged group's lack of sociocultural capital, which limits their everyday cultural expression space. Many negotiation techniques are being used to address the sense of cultural displacement (Storey, 2014). Furthermore, migrants enter a disruptive phase of transition that fractures their information systems as a result of information marginalization brought on by information resistance, a loss of traditional social networks, poor language proficiency, and mistrust of strangers in a new metropolitan setting (Lloyd, 2017). A contrasting message of hope and resiliency is told by the literary and empirical evidence of the marginal life story of reconnecting with the native country and returning home. The sense of belongingness, social connectedness, community living, and specific cultural and social factors like engagement with family and friends positively contribute to the wellbeing of returnees (Verma et al., 2021).

Midlife and Marginalization

A wide range of socioeconomic shifts and difficulties, including changes in identity, status and finances, are all part of the backdrop to the midlife journey. The voyage is made special by these events, especially for those who are living apart from family. As a result of the midlife transition, their sense of accomplishment in life is diminished in middle age due to sentiments of social rejection, recurrent sets of obstacles, declining health and increased economic pressure (Donnell & Richardson, 2018). Additionally, Donnell and Richardson (2018) noted that the midlife transition is linked to a strong feeling of a socially created position, confronting the failure of unfulfilled objectives, and cumulative psychosocial tasks that push middle-aged persons to the margins of masculinity. The limitations on leisure time that come with being a migrant have a detrimental effect on psychological health and wellbeing. Recent studies on middle-aged female migrants who take on caregiving roles after relocating from rural to urban regions have shown the beneficial effects of leisure on migrants' lives, supporting their overall wellbeing, adaptation and identity-building. (Monica & Monika Stodolska, 2018). Furthermore, leisure time enhances adult life satisfaction, self-esteem, and ethnic identity development and maintenance (Kim et al., 2011). Additionally, middle-aged working-class urban migrants feel like "outsiders" and are unwilling to ask for psychosocial support at work due to gender conventions and a lack of social support. Due to continuing gender norms and societal attitudes toward males, a study on middle-aged men investigating the triggering causes of high suicide rates in Ireland found that seeking social support for men had achieved saturation in middle age (Donnell & Richardson, 2018). Traditional societal and gendered ideals, such as being independent, self-sufficient, patient and responsible, are frequently instilled in middle age. This idea contrasts with the perception that asking for help may make one appear weak or burdensome (Donnell & Richardson, 2018). Due to gender bias and disparate productivity metrics that underpin society, people of post-reproductive age, particularly middle-aged women, see themselves as distinct entities, feel neglected in the gender discourse, and as a result, marginalize themselves in many spheres of life (Hussain, 2021). However, socioeconomic status is the primary factor influencing midlifers' mental health and wellbeing. According to a study on middle-aged immigrants, economically marginalized groups are less protected from health issues than higher-income groups (Assari, 2020). They enter crises when they experience discrimination, low status, low self-esteem and the social stigma linked to occupations over time. Thus, along the voyage toward middle age, the path of marginalization and other characteristics of crises frequently interact with one another.

Experience of Sexual Marginalization

The shades of love and its sexual expression are not binary. However, the heteronormative narrative always dominates the discourse, shifting non-heterosexual narratives to the margin. Thus, marginality and discrimination are not always limited to those experiencing a resource crunch. Experiences of marginality can originate from liminal identity as well. Shifts in attitudes towards non-heterosexuals in a positive direction are evident in recent psychosocial research, which also indicates the stability of the changed attitudes (Ekstam, 2023). However, an in-depth look at the overall scenario reflects a different picture of discrimination toward sexual minorities (Rosenbaum et al., 2021). This discrimination is not limited to a particular culture or society, but is a global phenomenon and is present in Indian societies as well (Karala et al., 2010).

In India also, for persons possessing non-heteronormative sexual orientations (in a predominantly heteronormative traditional society), pains and complexities coexist with life. Deep-seated societal discrimination percolates and gets mirrored in everyday life, and even permeates into intimate family relations (Ranade, 2018). Pre-existing psychosocial taboos about homosexuality, marginalized sexual orientations and gender identities (Karala et al., 2010) truncate the thriving, expressive psychosocial space of LGBTIQAA+ individuals. Consequentially the threatened expression of self-identity to a great extent lessens the possibilities of coming out. The agonies accompanied with fear of stigma, social rejection and discrimination, (Griffith & Hebl, 2002) are possible predictors of reducing the likelihood of coming out. It is well archived and narrated through oral history that incidents of violence in accordance with gender and sexual identity are prevalent in patriarchal social systems (Narrain & Chandran, 2016). In a recent study, the participants asserted the significance of coming out and the genesis of entitativity (Biswas et al., 2022). The participants felt that the loss of agency by being queer can only be surmounted by overcoming minority stresses on individuals in terms of hope, wellbeing, and meaningful life (Biswas et al., 2022).

Marginalization Due to Stigmatized Profession

In the wake of socio-politico-cultural determiners, professions can be stigmatized. Stigmatized identity, both concealable and non-concealable, leads to perilous professional consequences. Women in a stigmatized profession (such as sex workers) experience double marginalization because of their intersectional marginality. Poor women involved in sex work face moral stigma, social exclusion and shame. The dual play of poverty and stigma shapes identity formation and reformation in the context of female sex workers in India. The reshaping of identities in to positive orientation consequentially reconfigures and guards personal identity and self-esteem against vulnerability (Mitra et al., 2022).

While the shades and varieties of marginality are numerous, so are the ways of negotiating marginality. The socio-politico-cultural epistemic ways to deal with vulnerabilities and directing and reshaping of identity in constructive and efficacious direction pave the path to wellbeing. Policy decisions and recognition of diversity and inclusivity are the precursors of a rightful democratic society promoting wellbeing for all.

References

Aassve, A., Alfani, G., Gandolfi, F., & Le Moglie, M. (2021). Epidemics and trust: The case of the Spanish Flu. *Health Economics, 30*(4), 840–857. https://doi.org/10.1002/hec.4218

Altay, T., G. Yurdakul, & Cortège, A. C. (2021). Crossing borders: The intersectional marginalisation of bulgarian muslim trans* immigrant sex workers in Berlin. *Journal of Ethnic and Migration Studies, 47*(9), 1922–1939. https://doi.org/10.1080/1369183X.2020.1862646

Assari, S. (2020) Income and mental well-being of middle-aged and older Americans: Immigrants' diminished returns. *International Journal of Travel Medicine and Global Health, 8*(1), 37–43.

Bai, Y., Lin, C. C., Lin, C. Y., Chen, J. Y., Chue, C. M., & Chou, P. (2004). Survey of stress reactions among health care workers involved with the SARS outbreak. *Psychiatry Services, 55,* 1055–1057. https://doi.org/10.1176/appi.ps.55.9.1055

Banks, N., Roy, M., & Hulme, D. (2011). Neglecting the urban poor in Bangladesh: Research, policy and action in the context of climate change. *Environment and Urbanization, 23*(2), 487–502. https://doi.org/10.1177/0956247811417794

Benson, M., & Jackson, E. (2013). Place-making and place maintenance: Performativity, place and belonging among the middle classes. *Sociology, 47*(4), 793–809. https://doi.org/10.1177/0038038512454350

Bhattacharya, P., Banerjee, D., & Rao, T. S. S. (2020). The "untold" side of COVID-19: Social stigma and its consequences in India. *Indian Journal of Psychological Medicine, 42*, 1–5.
Biswas, D., Chaudhuri, A., Mitra, N., & Roy Chaudhuri, H. (2022). Pride or closet? Unpacking experiences of minority stress, coping, and resistance among gender and sexual minorities in India. *Journal of Homosexuality*. https://doi.org/10.1080/00918369.2022.2071662
Cacioppo, J. T., Hawkley, L. C., Norman, G. J., & Berntson, G. G. (2011). Social isolation. *Annals of the New York Academy of Sciences, 1231*(1), 17–22.
Chaplin, D., Twigg, J., & Lovell, E. (2019). *'ntersectional approaches to vulnerability reduction and resilience building: A scoping study*. Resilience Intel. BRACED and ODI.
Chomsky, N. (2000). *Rogue states: The rule of force in world affairs*. Pluto Press.
Chu, E., & Michael, K. (2019). Recognition in urban climate justice: Marginality and exclusion of migrants in Indian cities. *Environment and Urbanization*, 31(1), 139-156.
Collins, P. H., & Bilge, S. (2020). *Intersectionality*. John Wiley & Sons.
Crenshaw, K. (1989). Demarginalizing the intersection of race and sex: A Black feminist critique of antidiscrimination doctrine, feminist theory and antiracist politics. *University of Chicago Legal Forum, 140*, 139–167.
Davis, K. (2008). Intersectionality as buzzword: A sociology of science perspective on what makes a feminist theory successful. *Feminist Theory, 9*(1), 67–85. https://doi.org/10.1177/1464700108086364
Dutta, M., Agarwal, D., & Sivakami, M. (2020). The "invisible" among the marginalised: Do gender and intersectionality matter in the Covid-19 response? *Indian Journal of Medical Ethics, 5*(4), 302–308. https://doi.org/10.20529/IJME.2020.086
Ekstam, D. (2023). Change and continuity in attitudes toward homosexu-ality across the lifespan. *Journal of Homosexuality, 70*(5), 851–875. https://doi.org/10.1080/00918369.2021.2004795
Fisk, M. (1992). Poststructuralism, difference and marxism. *Praxis International, 12*(4), 323–340.
Flynn, M., & Kay, R. (2017). Migrants' experiences of material and emotional security in rural Scotland: Implications for longer-term settlement. *Journal of Rural Studies, 52*, 56–65. https://doi.org/10.1016/j.jrurstud.2017.03.010
Frisen, A., Hasselblad, T., & Holmqvist, K. (2012). What actually makes bullying stop? Reports from former victims. *Journal of Adolescence, 35*(4), 981–990. https://doi.org/10.1016/j.jrurstud.2017.03.010
Fylling, I., & Melboe, L. (2019). Culturalisation, homogenisation, assimilation? Intersectional perspectives on the life experiences of Sami people with disabilities. *Scandinavian Journal of Disability Research, 21*(1), 89–99. https://doi.org/10.16993/sjdr.575
Giddens, A. (2001). *Sociology* (4th ed.). Polity.
Griffith, K. H., & Hebl, M. R. (2002). The disclsure dilemma fr gay men and lesbians: "Cming-ut" at wrk. *Journal of Applied Psychology, 87*(6), 1191–1199. https://doi.org/10.1037/0021-9010.87.6.1191
Guadagno, L. (2020). *Migrants and the COVID-19 pandemic: An initial analysis*. Migrant Research Series No. 60. https://publications.iom.int/books/mrs-no-60-migrants-and-covid-19-pandemic-initialanalysis
Hussain, S., (2021). The transcending age: A study of psycho-social wellbeing of elderly women in India. *Journal of Sociological Research, 12*(1). ISSN 1948-5468.
Kagan, C., & Burton, M. (2005). Marginalization. In G. Nelson & I. Prilleltensky (Eds.), *Community psychology: In pursuit of liberation and wellness* (pp. 293–308). MacMillan/Palgrave.

Karala, G., Gupta, S., & Bhugra, D. (2010). Sexual variation in India: A view from the west. *Indian Journal of Psychiatry, 57*(7), 264–268.
Kim, J., Dattilo, J., & Heo, J. (2011). Taekwondo participation as serious leisure for life satisfaction and health: Cross-cultural contact and serious leisure experiences. *Journal of Leisure Research, 43*(4), 545–559.
Kuran, C., Morsut, C., Kruke, B. I., Krüger, M., Segnestam, L., Orru, K., Nævestad, T.-O., et al. (2020). Vulnerability and vulnerable groups from an intersectionality perspective. *International Journal of Disaster Risk Reduction, 50,* 101826. https://doi.org/10.1016/j.ijdrr.2020.101826
Kurtz, G., Amichai-Hamburger, Y., & Kantor, J. (2009). Psychosocial well-being of Israeli students and attitudes toward open and distance learning. *International Review of Research in Open and Distributed Learning*, 10(2).
Lloyd, A. (2017). Researching fractured (information) landscapes: Implications for library and information science researchers undertaking research with refugees and forced migration studies. *Journal of Documentation*, *73*(1), 35–47.
Messiou, K. (2012). Collaborating with children in exploring marginalization: An approach to inclusive education. *International Journal of Inclusive Education, 16*(12), 1311–1322.
Mia, M. A., & Griffiths, M. D. (2020). The economic and mental health costs of COVID- 19 to immigrants. *Journal of Psychiatric Research*, 128(September), 23–24. https://doi.org/10.1016/j.jpsychires.2020.06.003
Mitra, N., Hill, R. P., Roy Chaudhuri, H., & Chaudhuri, A. (2022). Identity management as a coping strategy for stigmatization: The case of indian sex workers in a libidinal market. *Journal of Public Policy & Marketing,* 1–17. https://doi.org/10.1177/07439156211058097
Monica, Z. L., & Stodolska, M. (2018). Leisure as a constraint and a Manifesto for empowerment: The life story of a Chinese female migrant worker. *Leisure Sciences*. https://doi.org/10.1080/01490400.2018.1483854
Mowat, J. G. (2015). Towards a new conceptualisation of marginalisation. *European Educational Research Journal*, *14*(5), 454–476.
Narrain, A., & Chandran, V. (2016). *Nothing to fix: Medicalisation of sexual orientation and gender identity*. SAGE. https://us.sagepub.cm/en-us/nam/nthing-t-fix/bk251842#descriptin
O'Donnell, S., & Richardson, N. (2018). *Middle-aged men and suicide in Ireland.* Men's Health Forum in Ireland. https://doi.org/10.13140/RG.2.2.25196.46724
Osborne, N. (2015). Intersectionality and kyriarchy: A framework for approaching power and social justice in planning and climate change adaptation. *Planning Theory*, *14*(2), 130–151. https://doi.org/10.1177/1473095213516443
Phinney, J. (1990). Ethnic identity in adolescents and adults: A new scale with diverse groups. *Journal of Adolescent Research*, *7*, 156–176.
Phinney, J. (1993). A three-stage model of ethnic identity development. In M. Bernal & G. Knight (Eds.), *Ethnic identity: Formation and transmission among Hispanics and other minorities* (pp. 61–79). State University of New York Press.
Ranade, K. (2018). *Growing up gay in urban India: A critical psychosocial perspective.* Springer. https://www.springer.cm/us/bk/9789811083655
Razer, M., Friedman, V. J., & Warshofsky, B. (2013). Schools as agents of social exclusion and inclusion. *International Journal of Inclusive Education, 17*(11), 1152–1170.
Rosenbaum, M. S., Ramirez, G. C., & Kim, K. K. (2021). From overt to covert: Exploring discrimination against homosexual consumers in retail stores. Journal of Retailing and Consumer Services, 59, 102426.
Salagame, K. (2016). Meaning and well-being: Indian perspectives. *Journal of Constructivist Psychology, 00*(00), 1–6.

Schlossberg, D. (2004). Reconceiving environmental justice: Global movements and political theories. *Environmental Politics, 13*(3), 517–540.

Singh, O. P. (2020). Mental health of migrant laborers in COVID-19 pandemic and lockdown: Challenges ahead. *Indian Journal of Psychiatry, 62*, 233. https://doi.org/10.4103/psychiatry.IndianJPsychiatry_422_20

Sreedharan, N., & Murale, D. V. (2018). Social integration of migrant workers in kerala. *International Journal of Pure and Applied Mathematics, 118,* 631–636.

Standing, G. (2014). *The precariat: The new dangerous class.* Bloomsbury Academic.

Storey, J. (2014). From popular culture to everyday life. In *From popular culture,* 1-160. *Routledge.*

Swader, C. S. (2019). Loneliness in Europe: Personal and societal individualism-collectivism and their connection to social isolation. *Social Forces, 97*(3), 1307–1336. https://doi.org/10.4324/9780203077023

Vasas, E. B. (2005). Examining the margins: A concept analysis of marginalization. *ANS. Advances in Nursing Science*, 28(3), 194–202. https://doi.org/10.1097/00012272-200507000-00002

Verma, K., Mujawar, Z., Mujawar, S., & Banerjee, A. (2021). Mental health impact of the COVID 19 pandemic on reverse migrant workers in Uttarakhand: A cross-sectional study. *Indian Journal of Social Psychiatry, 37,* 407–412.

Young, R. (2000). Continuity and change: Marginality and later prehistoric settlement in the northern uplands. *British Archaeology Reports, 302*, 71–80.

13 Community Intervention, Support and Wellbeing in Midlife

Rudrani Chatterjee and Rudra P. Goswami

At the age of 49, Parul could not believe her ears when she was diagnosed with diabetes. She had watched her weight ever since she could remember. Her octogenarian father Madhav, who lived with her since his wife passed away, felt worried. How would he be able to ask her for help with his monthly hospital visits for dialysis? Parul's level-headed husband Rahul comforted her from his distant work site. He had faith in her that she would pull through. He'd be around in another year now. Parul, a tech executive, had passed up on promotion for two consecutive years; she had been going to accept it this time now that Shiuli, their daughter was leaving for Germany and her father had been stable for some time. Would she? Things had been finally going her way, and then they were not.

Midlife happens to be a life transition where care takes new forms and dimensions. The way toward wellbeing is an ongoing conversation among individuals, their bodies, their social-occupational being and their caregiving responsibilities. Much like us, wellbeing looks different at different ages. It is a journey from being held to being able to hold oneself and others; from looking for appreciation to learning to appreciate; from achieving new heights to rediscovering purpose, perspective and meaning; from holding on to letting go.

Adulthood is a much-awaited dream of a lot of children. We hope to acquire in adulthood the limits and boundaries which were denied to us as children. Yet the liberty of adulthood is but an illusion. Never is the lifting of the veil from that illusion more apparent than when an individual gravitates toward middle adulthood. A time when, to all appearances, we have become all that we could have become. A time when we have reached the limits of our achievements and failures. Or at least are in a position to envision how our lives would look like without an astrologer's help. A realisation that "every compromise is at the same time a renunciation" (Hall, 1954) and that the liberty of adulthood comes with the cost of responsibility, and accountability sinks in with deepening maturity. Recent decades have seen an increasing rise in chronic health conditions in the form of diabetes, cardiovascular problems, obesity and arthritis, originating in midlife and contributing to early-onset functional impairment previously noted in older adults. One-fifth of middle-aged adults have mental health problems. After being the object

DOI: 10.4324/9781003568360-16

of derision for years, "midlife crisis" (Jacques, 1965) seems to have found ministration in midlife's "nadir" in wellbeing recognised as a reality. Which explanation is convincing – age or cohort, cross-sectional or longitudinal inquiry?

Is community intervention an answer to midlife's woes? Where lies the redemption? These are a few pathways we explore in this chapter.

Perspectives about Midlife, Support and Wellbeing

Theoretical Conceptualisation

In the early theorisations of human development, midlife rarely found a place. Physical, cognitive, emotional and moral development were held to have been completed by late adolescence, and adulthood was considered the ultimate stage of maturity. The lifespan perspective, however, acknowledges the developmental processes across biological, historical, sociocultural and psychological factors on human behaviour from conception to death (Lerner, 2018). In essence, midlife encompasses both gains and losses, as elaborated by the Selective Optimisation with Compensation (SOC) Theory. It is also about striking a balance; be it in relationships or workplace demands. Ergo, by being extremely stressful, it calls on more skills pertaining to emotion regulation which holds true in later life (Magai & Halpern, 2001).

A few classic theorists like Jung and Erikson emphasised middle age in their conceptualisations. Midlife, according to Jung (1971), calls for greater individuation, implying integration of various aspects of the psyche, dealing with the physical and psychological changes. and balancing the masculine (animus) and feminine (anima) aspects. The latter has been investigated, but without conclusive evidence (Lachman, 2001; James et al., 1995; Helson et al., 1995; Parker & Aldwin, 1997), albeit there is some indication of the emergence of certain characteristics of opposite sex roles (James et al., 1995).

The pivotal point for Erikson's theory based on the principle of epigenesis is generativity. The "widening commitment to *take care of* the persons, the products, and the ideas one has learned to *care for*" (Erikson, 1998) which emanates from the strengths acquired from overcoming the hurdles that lead up to midlife is the redemption for self-absorption and stagnation, argues Erikson. Social relationships are considered the single greatest cause of happiness (Argyle, 2013). The multifaceted and multidimensional view of generativity in the domains of parenting, caregiving and societal involvement reflects the crucial role that commitment to others plays in the development of wellbeing in midlife (McAdams, 2001; McAdams & de St. Aubin 1998).

Wellbeing

Wellbeing can be understood in two paradoxical frameworks. The bottom-up framework presumes that objective situations in life, like health and social relationships, predict wellbeing, and the top-down perspective presumes that individuals' perception of life circumstances determines wellbeing. In the bottom-up framework, then, wellbeing is expected to decline with age-related losses (Diener, 1984). However, the lifespan literature reveals that individuals are capable of maintaining their wellbeing until late adulthood. The SOCn theory (Baltes & Baltes, 1990), a meta-theory with lifespan perspective, holds that people maximise gains and minimise losses throughout life by harnessing self-regulatory strategies. In synchrony with SOC, Socioemotional Selectivity Theory (SST; Carstensen et al., 1999) states that older adults give precedence to emotional gains as they perceive their time as delimited. Yet the dominant strategy for regulating emotions may differ across cultures. While maximising positive emotions might be a hallmark of individualistic cultures, those in collectivistic ones seek to maintain a balance between positive and negative emotions, thereby seeing negative life experiences in perspective, and accept, rather than avoid, negative affect when it happens (Nakagawa et al., 2021).

In the midlife literature, wellbeing is confusing, to say the least. On one hand, Ulloa et al. (2013) suggest a U-shaped, inverted-U-shaped or linear relation between ageing and subjective wellbeing; on the other hand, Lachman (2015) argues that the dip, even if present, is significant enough to warrant mention. Blanchflower (2021) vigorously argues against such assumptions, claiming that even small-sample-sized studies did show a U shape. His empirical study, across 145 countries including developing countries, re-examined the relationship between various measures of wellbeing and age in individuals below 70 while controlling for the mediational effects of education, marital and employment status. The study found evidence of "the nadir in happiness" in all the countries examined. It is interesting that the curve's trajectory holds good in countries irrespective of high or low median wage and high or low life expectancy. Blanchflower and Graham (2020a) reanalysed previously analysed Eurobarometer files and found that without controls in a life satisfaction equation, there was a well-defined nadir in wellbeing in age when controlling for year and nation that reached a minimum at 48 years age. Also, an equation which controlled for gender, education, marital status and employment status minimised at 43 years of age. He found that 48.3 was the mean age at which the U shape minimised across the 477 country-level estimates irrespective of the nation's wealth status (Blanchflower, 2021). The study declared that well-being has a U shape in ageU.

Mental Health

The picture of mental health in midlife is a contrast. Satisfaction, stability and the richness of the exploits of midlife are accompanied by a preponderance of psychiatric diagnoses, be they depression, anxiety or psychological distress. In this, too, women, the economically weaker and those with alternate identities (LGBTQ+) have been reported to be particularly vulnerable (Fredriksen-Goldsen et al., 2015; Brody et al., 2018). Therefore, unsurprisingly, use of antidepressants and seeing a mental health professional increase in midlife compared to other stages of adulthood. The findings hold truer for those with limited formal education and women (Blanchflower & Oswald, 2016). A study based on the British Birth Cohort found associations between early-life mental health and biomarkers in midlife as well as premature mortality, implying that effective interventions on early-life mental health have the potential to shift the distribution of risk and may have additional benefits, reducing future risk of premature mortality and improving multiple physical health outcomes (Ploubidis et al., 2021)

The shrinking social milieu (Fredrickson & Carstensen, 1990) coupled with increased responsibility in midlife may make social and emotional support harder to find, or seek for that matter, because midlife is the worst time to present vulnerability. It is the time when people are expected to have reached their "full potential". Shame and isolation therefore may add on to the effects of the stressors at a midlife low. Adverse life circumstances adversely affect diversity in the form of people with disabilities, less education, in broken families or who have lost their jobs. Downward spirals as age and life circumstances interact may become evident. Yet the psychosocial changes experienced in midlife, mentioned earlier in this section, are usually associated with positive changes. These may include "better emotional regulation" (Magai & Halpern, 2001), "increased wisdom and practical intelligence" (Baltes et al., 1999) or "a strong sense of mastery" (Lachman & Bertrand, 2001). This is because in general, midlife signifies a summit in terms of earnings and standing at work, and the authority experienced in the family and decision-making, hence the impact it has on self-confidence (Lachman 2015).

The evolving picture of mental health may well be a threat to wellbeing. The concept of "deaths of despair" has been emerging, whereby middle-aged individuals undergo risk of mortality, particularly deaths by suicide, especially by poisoning and chronic liver disease (Case & Deaton, 2015). These seem to emanate from stress related to work, family and social relationships, with the scales tipping and the situation jeopardised due to ready access to narcotics (Case & Deaton, 2015; Masters et al., 2018).

Physical Health

The onset of midlife sees the onset of non-communicable diseases like hypertension, cardiovascular ailments, metabolic syndrome (Masters et al., 2018) or musculoskeletal diseases (Chen & Sloan, 2015). These chronic ailments, largely manageable but in general never curable, signal ageing, which is frowned upon in most cultures and hence can cause distress. Possible contributory factors are increase in obesity, increased calorie intake, consumption of processed food and sedentary lifestyle with insurance crisis of sections of individuals in the US (Crimmins & Zhang, 2019). Again, these findings are more applicable to those with limited formal education (Kirsch et al., 2019), the marginalised (Hispanics and Blacks) (Hales et al., 2017) and those with non-mainstream identities (LGBTQ+) (Fredriksen-Goldsen et al., 2013).

There is longitudinal evidence of extreme distress in middle-aged adults across countries, with those in countires with high gross domestic product) reporting more sleep disturbances, chronic headaches, struggles with attention span and alcoholism compared to younger or older adults. These individuals are close to their peak lifetime income with no prior experience of serious ailments (Giuntella et al., 2023).

Thus, middle aged adults en route to older age are burdened with chronic physical ailments or conditions like obesity, often compounded by prescription drug use or substance use shall be finding it necessary to relegate parental duties to other family members and suffer the thrust of health insurance.

Scope of Community Intervention

The discipline of community psychology thrives on the pre-emptive. Those who are on the receiving end of intervention need to be active in the delivery thereof. It stands on the foundation of:

- Identification of unmet needs or unsolved problems in a population in question;
- Scientific understanding thereof;
- Empirical understanding of the risks and protective factors;
- Ecological changes that need to happen;
- Readiness in the said community to bring about the change;
- Active participation of community members in planning and implementation of the programme;
- Community dynamics that will help or hinder.

Designing effective programmes for community intervention is a challenge, especially because the effectiveness of such programmes depends on the participation and involvement evoked in the participants. randomised controlled trialss can help assess the feasibility of designs on outcome expectation.

So can community-based participatory research (CBPR). It is a person-centred, community-driven and collaborative research approach to address growing health disparities. It acknowledges the strengths of community members, researchers and other stakeholders in the research process. CBPR sets out to unite knowledge and action to generate and sustain the required social change. It creates involvement and increased ownership, crucial for the success of a community intervention. A review of the existing literature shows that CBPR, though widely used for health promotion paradigms, has had limited implementation in psychological research in spite of being embedded within similar ethical principles.

Philosophy of Community-based Research

The relationship between the researchers and the researched (members of the community) is of prime importance. Historically, in a top-down fashion, university or government researchers collected data on communities by conducting surveys and interviews, collecting documents and keeping records for projects. Although community-based, this method did not necessarily warrant the intimation or participation of community leaders, officials and residents.

In the 1970s, educators, researchers, community organisers and social movement activists started using strategies which led to participatory action research.

§ Embedded in the strategy was a philosophy that research needs be done with or by those being researched, rather than their being mere objects of observation and scrutiny by those who were not.
§ Research would be a collective and democratic emergent endeavour addressing the community's felt needs.
§ That a critical reflexive step paving the way toward social and political action, policy changes and then back to conversations on community needs and data collection, reiteratively.

The resulting process became an approach whereby community members and researchers engaged in collaboration and partnerships with mutual benefits. CBPR is one such "bottom-up" approach conceptualised into three models:

Model 1: Single-themed collaboration between a university-based centre and a community organisation;
Model 2: Targeted, area-based collaboration between academic researchers and a small group of community organisations;
Model 3: Broad-based coalitions of grassroot organizations.

Across models successful CBPR partnerships go out with problems looking for solutions, build a relationship and leave something of value to the community.

To optimise the wellbeing of middle-aged adults, Infurna et al. (2020) suggest some avenues to promote:

§ Interventions targeting physical health;
§ Interventions reducing caregiver-related stress;
§ Interventions targeting mental health through social engagement;
§ Policy changes.

The systematic review in the following section will examine community intervention studies hitherto conducted to improve wellbeing and support in midlife.

Systematic Review

We conducted a systematic review on December 3, 2023 searching psychINFO, PubMed, Scopus and Embase databases and platforms with the keywords "community based participatory research", "participatory research", "midlife", "middle aged" and "older adults", in various combinations. Only English-language articles were selected, and articles published before the year 2000 were pruned. We excluded review articles, systematic review articles, single case reports, newspaper articles and editorials. The combined search result was uploaded into the software package Covidence (Figure 13.1).

After full-text review of 21 studies, ten were selected for further discussion based on relevance (Table 13.1).

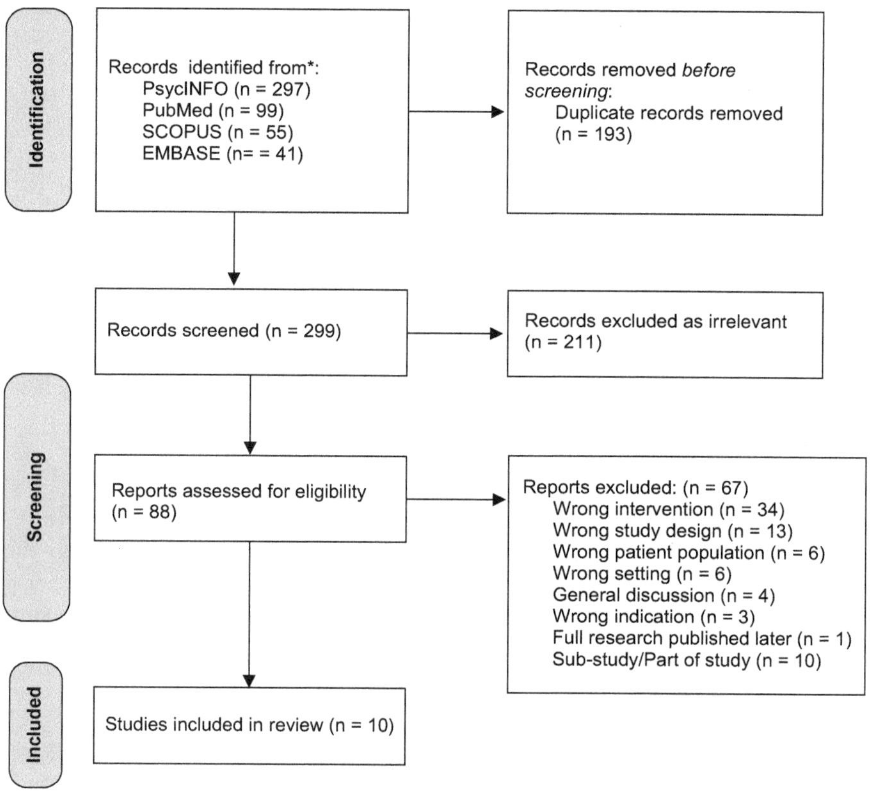

Figure 13.1 PRISMA flow diagram

Table 13.1 Systematic review of community-based participatory research on middle-aged adults: feasibility and outcome studies

Study	*Objective*	*Target group*	*Intervention and data collection*	*Results*	*Strengths*	*Limitations*
Sharpe et al. 2010), USA	To increase physical activity among irregularly active or inactive middle-aged women (35–54 years)	Three groups: full-intervention, women living in the media-exposed county but not enrolled and no exposure to either	A year-long media campaign versus an intensive, 24-week, minimal-contact behavioural intervention. Data for random digit dialled telephonic survey in 2003 (control n=234; media only n=245) and in 2005. Programme enlisted were given questionnaires (pre, n=430; post n=234).	Significant weight loss, more physical exercise and outdoor exercise, exercise with partners and other "exercise-like" behaviours more prominent in the intervention group only.	Focus group approach; identification of target groups' attributes; positive results.	Significant attrition; the three groups are only historically comparable; very small effect size; temporal variability; racial differences in participation.
Lattimore et al. (2010), USA	Individually adapted health behaviour change programmes	Midlife and older adults who were irregularly active	The two physical activity programmes were Active Choices (AC, Stanford University, telephone-delivered, home-based) and Active Living Every Day (ALED, Cooper Institute, Dallas, TX, group-based physical activity programme); total n=2,796.	Challenges and adaptations emerged in three categories: (1) programme logistics, (2) programme theory and (3) programme philosophy.	Challenges, with some level of adaptation, were overcome and effective delivery was possible.	Qualitative study.
Norberg et al. (2010), Sweden	Reducing morbidity from cardiovascular disease and diabetes through the Västerbotten Intervention Programme	All subjects in the county who attain the ages 40–60 are invited yearly	Comprehensive questionnaire followed by information about the results and advice, dialogue and motivational interviews; with updating of methodology and communication from 1985 through 2005.	Overall, 113,203 health examinations conducted and 6,500–7,000 examinations yearly; ~27,000 subjects have participated twice (rate 48–67%); Multiple publications and theses have been done and basic studies from the stored biological samples.	Feasibility of community-based intervention through integration with public health system.	Whether this has reduced morbidity or simply increased the number of newly identified cases remains to be seen

(*Continued*)

Table 13.1 Continued

Study	*Objective*	*Target group*	*Intervention and data collection*	*Results*	*Strengths*	*Limitations*
Studts (2012), USA	To increase Papanicolaou (PAP) test use among middle-aged and older women	Women aged 40–64 overdue for PAP smear	Single-blind two-armed randomised controlled trial (Faith Moves Mountains) over four years. Participants chosen from churches, randomised. Intervention group (n=176) received home visits from lay health advisors, and others waitlisted (n=169).	Significantly more participants in the intervention arm received a PAP smear.	Religious gathering-based recruitment was a novel method of community intervention; well-defined target population	Generalisability limited; self-reported outcome measure; method of randomisation not clear; information may have been shared between the two groups.
Lee et al., (2011), USA	Effectiveness of a group cohesion intervention to increase physical activity and improve dietary habits	"Women of colour	Based on Ecological Model of Physical Activity (EMPA) and group dynamics theory, "women of colour" were screened and randomised to physical activity group and fruits and vegetables group. Lay health advisors.	Feasibility attained. Multiple sub-studies published.	Community engagement with continued recruitment for sub-studies from the original participants over a decade.	No clear-cut outcome defined. Ecological study. Generalisability not possible.
Scarincini (2014), USA	To promote healthy eating and physical activity	African-American women aged 45–65, rural	Group randomised controlled trial (n=565). Two arms: (1) promotion of healthy eating and physical activity; (2) promotion of breast and cervical cancer screening.	Retention: 54.7%; higher in active arm with significant positive changes.	Culturally relevant intervention, can improve (and maintain) healthy eating.	High variability of retention rates. Control arm which looked at cancer screening is a form of healthy life, thus promoting better outcomes.

Lin et al. (2014), China	Community-based lifestyle intervention on blood pressure and glucose levels	Middle-aged and older Chinese population	Cluster randomised trial (n=474), intensive health education and behavioural intervention, versus conventional education. Intervention consisted of two stages of group-based information and counselling sessions and six individual education sessions.	Intervention group had significantly lower blood pressure and blood glucose at 12th month which sustained until 24th month	Strong participation of primary health system a key to success.	Insufficient power. Low effect size. Very homogeneous population. Possible fluidity of information.
Mendes et al. (2015), Portugal	Impact of a long-term community-based combined exercise programme	Middle-aged patients with type 2 diabetes	Participants were engaged in Diabetes em Movimento®, a community-based exercise programme developed in Portugal (three times a week for nine months). 43 participants completed the programme.	While test performances improved, habitual non-supervised physical activity did not change over nine months.	Long-term intervention (nine months), integrative exercises, use of low-cost exercise	Supervision needed; niche population; adherence moderate.

(Continued)

Table 13.1 Continued

Study	*Objective*	*Target group*	*Intervention and data collection*	*Results*	*Strengths*	*Limitations*
Ralston et al. (2017), USA	Longitudinal church-based intervention to reduce cardiovascular disease risk in midlife and older African-Americans	Middle-aged African-Americans at risk of cardiovascular disease	Health for Hearts United CBPR church-initiated programming (treatment only), joint church-project staff programming (treatment only), project staff-initiated standard programming (treatment only), and data collection and health promotion (treatment and com parison). Four health messages: Eat Better, Move Around More, Reduce Stress, and Take Charge of Your Health.	Providing consistency in programming even during participant absences, providing structured activities to assist health ministries in sustainability, and addressing changes at the church level.	Collaborative approach. Culturally appropriate.	Niche population.
Lee et al. (2018), UK	To work in a neighbourhood with poorer health outcome measures while developing insights into perceptions of ageing well	Middle-aged community at risk for poor health outcomes	Connected for Cognitive Health in Later Life (CHILL) project, used CBPR methodology to extend research information regarding risk factors of dementia to engage communities to develop insight their livelihoods.	Two public engagement activities: (1) to garner information on knowledge and interest in the topic; (2) to extend research findings in interesting ways. Both objectives were met.	Delved into causes of failure of CBPR.	Recruitment, especially driven working group development, was difficult. The study ended up only as a scoping project rather than a comprehensive one.

Jones et al. (2022), USA	To determine employability of a culturally adapted, eight-week group intervention leveraging stress reduction and goal-setting	Midlife Black women recruited from a large Midwestern metropolitan city	Randomised feasibility trial (B-SWELL). Two groups: B SWELL and Wellness (WE), n=25 each. B-SWELL session: guided meditation, module content and case study, breakout groups for goal-setting, and special topic presentations/ demonstrations about stress reduction and/or lifestyle strategies. WE group: all similar to B-SWELL, except content about stress, stress reduction strategies and goal-setting were not included.	Both B-SWELL and WE groups had low attrition and navigated the online platform well. Further, both groups experienced lower perceived stress, reduced depressive symptoms and greater perceived general health from baseline to eight weeks.	CBPR through online mode is an added benefit. Randomised controlled trial design.	Very low sample size. Not reflective of community setting. No definitive conclusion about content over intent could be shown.

Opportunities and Barriers

The systematic review brings to light that the body of CBPR in midlife has focused on studying the feasibility and outcomes of physical health and lifestyle interventions up to the present. Although community-based participatory research provides a fertile conceptual and methodological framework for collaborative community research and advocacy, the approach faces several barriers in the forms of time and money (Brydon-Miller, 2008; Giles and Giles 2012; Lake & Wendland, 2018). Establishing and maintaining successful collaborative relationships between researchers and community members requires time and patience, especially in the initial stages when mutual trust may be fragile. Also, few universities committed to academic principles (Arrieta et al., 2017; Giles & Giles, 2012) or, conversely, personnel-strapped community-based organisations (CBOs) fight against time in attending to immediate community needs. Without the scope for collaboration between CBO leaders and staff and researchers, CBPR is left with little hope of success. The review brought to light issues of attrition (≥50% lost to follow-up on follow-up visits in the majority of studies), low sample sizes (reflecting difficulty in reaching out to the target audience), niche patient population (only a well-defined homogeneous population responds well and comes back for repeat assessments), and perhaps most importantly, the need for integration with public health systems or congregational systems (Lin et al., 2014; Ralston et al., 2017) for not only outreach but sustainability over decades.

Concluding Remarks

This chapter has discussed the predicament of midlife with the balances that need to be struck and the compromises that need to be made. It took a look at the conceptualisation of wellbeing in the current midlife literature and arrived at a disturbing scenario whereby researchers agree on a "nadir in wellbeing" in middle age which holds true after controlling for gender, education, marital status and employment status. I found that psychological and social changes experienced in midlife are usually positive, yet antidepressant medication use and regular visits to mental health professionals are highest in midlife (late forties to early sixties) compared to earlier or later in adulthood. Also, this was more prominent in women and individuals with fewer years of education. Metabolic conditions giving rise to chronic illnesses, and disability coupled with longitudinal evidence of extreme distress in middle-aged adults across affluent nations compared to those in young adulthood and old age paint a distressing picture of physical health attributable to lifestyle and economic factors. Recognising the need for involvement of the people in question, community-based participatory research paradigms have emerged to promote healthy behaviours, mostly targeting physical health. A systematic review of the literature showed that the challenges are great and the stakes are high. Feasibility and outcome studies in small, often niche, marginalised populations revealed the need for greater resources in terms of funding, time and investment in forming effective collaborative relationships for CBPR to weave its magic.

References

Argyle, M. (2013). *The psychology of happiness* (0 ed.). Routledge. https://doi.org/10.4324/9781315812212

Arrieta, M. I., Fisher, L., Shaw, T., Bryan, V., Hudson, A., Hansberry, S., Eastburn, S., Freed, C. R., Shelley-Tremblay, S., Hanks, R. S., Washington-Lewis, C., Roussel, L., Dagenais, P. A., Icenogle, M., Slagle, M. L., Parker, L. L., & Crook, E. (2017). Consolidating the academic end of a community-based participatory research venture to address health disparities. *Journal of Higher Education Outreach and Engagement*, *21*(3), 113–134.

Baltes, P. B., & Baltes, M. M. (1990). Psychological perspectives on successful aging: The model of selective optimization with compensation. In *Successful aging: Perspectives from the behavioral sciences* (pp. 1–34). Cambridge University Press. https://doi.org/10.1017/CBO9780511665684.003

Baltes, P. B., Staudinger, U. M., & Lindenberger, U. (1999). Lifespan psychology: Theory and application to intellectual functioning. *Annual Review of Psychology*, *50*, 471–507. https://doi.org/10.1146/annurev.psych.50.1.471

Blanchflower, D. G. (2021). Is happiness U-shaped everywhere? Age and subjective well-being in 145 countries. *Journal of Population Economics*, *34*(2), 575–624. https://doi.org/10.1007/s00148-020-00797-z

Blanchflower, D. G., & Graham, C. L. (2022). The mid-life dip in well-being: A critique. *Social Indicators Research*, *161*(1), 287–344. https://doi.org/10.1007/s11205-021-02773-w

Blanchflower, D. G., & Oswald, A. J. (2016). Antidepressants and age: A new form of evidence for U-shaped well-being through life. *Journal of Economic Behavior & Organization*, *127*, 46–58. https://doi.org/10.1016/j.jebo.2016.04.010

Brody, D. J., Pratt, L. A., & Hughes, J. P. (2018). Prevalence of depression among adults aged 20 and over: United States, 2013–2016. *NCHS Data Brief*, *303*, 1–8.

Brydon-Miller, M. (2008). *The SAGE handbook of action research*. SAGE Publications Ltd. https://doi.org/10.4135/9781848607934

Carstensen, L. L., Isaacowitz, D. M., & Charles, S. T. (1999). Taking time seriously. A theory of socioemotional selectivity. *The American Psychologist*, *54*(3), 165–181. https://doi.org/10.1037//0003-066x.54.3.165

Case, A., & Deaton, A. (2015). Rising morbidity and mortality in midlife among white non-Hispanic Americans in the 21st century. *Proceedings of the National Academy of Sciences of the United States of America*, *112*(49), 15078–15083. https://doi.org/10.1073/pnas.1518393112

Chen, Y., & Sloan, F. A. (2015). Explaining disability trends in the U.S. elderly and near-elderly population. *Health Services Research*, *50*(5), 1528–1549. https://doi.org/10.1111/1475-6773.12284

Crimmins, E. M., Zhang, Y. S., Kim, J. K., & Levine, M. E. (2019). Changing disease prevalence, incidence, and mortality among older cohorts: The health and retirement study. *The Journals of Gerontology Series A: Biological Sciences and Medical Sciences*, *74*(Suppl 1), S21–S26. https://doi.org/10.1093/gerona/glz075

Diener, E. (1984). Subjective well-being. *Psychological Bulletin*, *95*(3), 542–575. https://doi.org/10.1037/0033-2909.95.3.542

Erikson, E. H & Erikson, J. M (1998). The Life-Cycle Completed. WW Norton.

Fredrickson, B. L., & Carstensen, L. L. (1990). Choosing social partners: How old age and anticipated endings make people more selective. *Psychology and Aging*, *5*(3), 335–347.

Fredriksen-Goldsen, K. I., & Kim, H.-J. (2015). Count me in: Response to sexual orientation measures among older adults. *Research on Aging*, *37*(5), 464–480. https://doi.org/10.1177/0164027514542109

Fredriksen-Goldsen, K. I., Kim, H.-J., Barkan, S. E., Muraco, A., & Hoy-Ellis, C. P. (2013). Health disparities among lesbian, gay, and bisexual older adults: Results from a population-based study. *American Journal of Public Health*, *103*(10), 1802–1809. https://doi.org/10.2105/AJPH.2012.301110

Giles, H., & Giles, S. (2012). Negotiating the boundary between the academy and the community. In D. W. Butin & S. Seider (Eds.), *The engaged campus: Majors, minors, and certificates as the new community engagement* (pp. 49–67). Palgrave Macmillan US. https://doi.org/10.1057/9781137113283_4

Giuntella, O., McManus, S., Mujcic, R., Oswald, A. J., Powdthavee, N., & Tohamy, A. (2023). The midlife crisis. *Economica*, *90*(357), 65–110. https://doi.org/10.1111/ecca.12452

Hales, C. M., Carroll, M. D., Fryar, C. D., & Ogden, C. L. (2017). Prevalence of obesity among adults and youth: United States, 2015–2016. *NCHS Data Brief*, *288*, 1–8.

Hall, C. S. (1954). The development of personality. In *A primer of Freudian psychology* (pp. 72–115). New American Library. https://doi.org/10.1037/10640-004

Helson, R., Stewart, A. J., & Ostrove, J. (1995). Identity in three cohorts of midlife women. *Journal of Personality and Social Psychology*, *69*(3), 544–557. https://doi.org/10.1037//0022-3514.69.3.544

Infurna, F. J., Gerstorf, D., & Lachman, M. E. (2020). Midlife in the 2020s: Opportunities and challenges. *The American Psychologist*, *75*(4), 470–485. https://doi.org/10.1037/amp0000591

James, J. B., Lewkowicz, C., Libhaber, J., & Lachman, M. (1995). Rethinking the gender identity crossover hypothesis: A test of a new model. *Sex Roles*, *32*(3), 185–207. https://doi.org/10.1007/BF01544788

Jaques, E. (1965). Death and the mid-life crisis. *The International Journal of Psycho-Analysis*, *46*(4), 502–514.

Jones, H. J., Butsch Kovacic, M., Lambert, J., Almallah, W. R., Becker, R., de Las Fuentes, L., & Bakas, T. (2022). A randomized feasibility trial of the midlife Black Women's Stress and Wellness intervention (B-SWELL); A community participatory intervention to increase adoption of life's simple 7 healthy lifestyle behaviors. *Translational Behavioral Medicine*, *12*(11), 1084–1095. https://doi.org/10.1093/tbm/ibac075

Jung, C. (1971). *Collected works of C. G. Jung, Volume 6 by Carl Jung (Ebook)—Read free for 30 days*. Retrieved December 25, 2023, from https://www.everand.com/book/233048654/Collected-Works-of-C-G-Jung-Volume-6-Psychological-Types

Kirsch, J. A., Love, G. D., Radler, B. T., & Ryff, C. D. (2019). Scientific imperatives Vis-à-vis growing inequality in America. *The American Psychologist*, *74*(7), 764–777. https://doi.org/10.1037/amp0000481

Lachman, M. E. (Ed.). (2001). *Handbook of midlife development*. Wiley.

Lachman, M. E., & Bertrand, R. M. (2001). Personality and the self in midlife.

Lachman, M. E. (2015). Mind the gap in the middle: A call to study midlife. *Research in Human Development*, *12*(3–4), 327–334. https://doi.org/10.1080/15427609.2015.1068048

Lake, D., & Wendland, J. (2018). Practical, epistemological, and ethical challenges of participatory action research: A cross-disciplinary review of the literature. *Journal of Higher Education Outreach and Engagement*, *22*(3), Article 3.

Lattimore, D., Griffin, S. F., Wilcox, S., Rheaume, C., Dowdy, D. M., Leviton, L. C., & Ory, M. G. (2010). Understanding the challenges encountered and adaptations made by community organizations in translation of evidence-based behavior change physical activity interventions: A qualitative study. *American Journal of Health Promotion: AJHP*, *24*(6), 427–434. https://doi.org/10.4278/ajhp.081024-QUAL-252

Lee, C., Mellor, T., Dilworth-Anderson, P., Young, T., Brayne, C., & Lafortune, L. (2018). Opportunities and challenges in public and community engagement: The connected for Cognitive Health in Later Life (CHILL) project. *Research Involvement and Engagement*, *4*, 42. https://doi.org/10.1186/s40900-018-0127-x

Lee, R. E., Medina, A. V., Mama, S. K., Reese-Smith, J. Y., O'Connor, D. P., Brosnan, M., Cubbin, C., McMillan, T., & Estabrooks, P. A. (2011). Health is power: An ecological theory-based health intervention for women of color. *Contemporary Clinical Trials*, *32*(6), 916–923. https://doi.org/10.1016/j.cct.2011.07.008

Lerner, R. M. (2018). *Concepts and theories of human development* (4th ed.). Routledge. https://doi.org/10.4324/9780203581629

Lin, A., Zhang, G., Liu, Z., Gu, J., Chen, W., & Luo, F. (2014). Community-based lifestyle intervention for reducing blood pressure and glucose among middle-aged and older adults in China: A pilot study. *International Journal of Environmental Research and Public Health*, *11*(11), 11645–11663. https://doi.org/10.3390/ijerph111111645

Magai, C., & Halpern, B. (2001). Emotional development during the middle years.

Masters, R. K., Tilstra, A. M., & Simon, D. H. (2018). Explaining recent mortality trends among younger and middle-aged White Americans. *International Journal of Epidemiology*, *47*(1), 81–88. https://doi.org/10.1093/ije/dyx127

McAdams, D. P. (2001). The psychology of life stories. *Review of general psychology*, *5*(2), 100-122.

McAdams, D. P., & de St Aubin, E. D. (1998). Generativity and adult development. Washington, DC American Psychological Association

Mendes, R., Sousa, N., Almeida, A., Subtil, P., Guedes-Marques, F., Reis, V., & Themudo-Barata, J. (2015). Lifestyle intervention in type 2 diabetes: Diabetes em Movimento® community-based exercise program: Romeu Mendes. *European Journal of Public Health*, *25*(suppl_3), ckv170.040. https://doi.org/10.1093/eurpub/ckv170.040

Nakagawa, T., Nishita, Y., Tange, C., Tomida, M., Kinoshita, K., Otsuka, R., ... & Shimokata, H. (2021). Stability and change in well-being among middle-aged and older Japanese. International Journal of Behavioral Development, 45(1), 78–88.

Norberg, M., Wall, S., Boman, K., & Weinehall, L. (2010). The västerbotten intervention programme: Background, design and implications. *Global Health Action*, *3*. https://doi.org/10.3402/gha.v3i0.4643

Parker, R. A., & Aldwin, C. M. (1997). Do aspects of gender identity change from early to middle adulthood? Disentangling age, cohort and period effects.

Ploubidis, G. B., Batty, G. D., Patalay, P., Bann, D., & Goodman, A. (2021). Association of early-life mental health with biomarkers in midlife and premature mortality: Evidence from the 1958 British Birth Cohort. *JAMA Psychiatry*, *78*(1), 38–46. https://doi.org/10.1001/jamapsychiatry.2020.2893

Ralston, P. A., Young-Clark, I., & Coccia, C. (2017). The development of health for hearts united: A longitudinal church-based intervention to reduce cardiovascular risk in mid-life and older African Americans. *Ethnicity & Disease*, *27*(1), 21–30. https://doi.org/10.18865/ed.27.1.21

Scarinci, I. C., Moore, A., Wynn-Wallace, T., Cherrington, A., Fouad, M., & Li, Y. (2014). A community-based, culturally relevant intervention to promote healthy eating and physical activity among middle-aged African American women in rural Alabama: Findings from a group randomized controlled trial. *Preventive Medicine*, *69*, 13–20. https://doi.org/10.1016/j.ypmed.2014.08.016

Sharpe, P. A., Burroughs, E. L., Granner, M. L., Wilcox, S., Hutto, B. E., Bryant, C. A., Peck, L., & Pekuri, L. (2010). Impact of a community-based prevention marketing intervention to promote physical activity among middle-aged women. *Health Education & Behavior: The Official Publication of the Society for Public Health Education*, *37*(3), 403–423. https://doi.org/10.1177/1090198109341929

Studts, C. R., Tarasenko, Y. N., Schoenberg, N. E., Shelton, B. J., Hatcher-Keller, J., & Dignan, M. B. (2012). A community-based randomized trial of a faith-placed intervention to reduce cervical cancer burden in Appalachia. Preventive medicine, 54(6), 408-414.

PART IV

The Creative Portrayal of Midlife

14 Midlife Transitions in Men and their Representations in Literature across Centuries

Sukanya Saha

Midlife Crisis: An Overview

Elliott Jaques' introduction of the concept of "midlife crisis" in the social and psychological spheres of knowledge shaped Western conceptions of it. This leads to the understanding of the whys and hows of middle-aged men feeling bewildered and frustrated in their professions, uninterested in relations, detached from familial ties, and other unique symptoms of personal crises. Individual variations in degrees and behavioural patterns are very evident too. Post-war studies viewed biological and psychological changes among midlifers as triggers of anxiety in them as they started feeling the dread of death. Literature and films may have dismissed midlife crisis as myth or undermined its presence with satirical representations, yet they could never deny its occurrence. The concept has thrived through stereotypical portrayals in literary characters. Specific social, physical and emotional battles each character undergoes are manifestations of the varying aspects of crisis in midlifers. Emergence of this theory was in no way a coincidence, rather a close observation of symptomatic behaviours. Long before 20th-century psychology could take up the argument about validity of the midlife crisis, oddities evident in several famous literary characters from the history of Western literature established midlife crisis as a recognised phenomenon among authors.

Since antiquity, the critical age of 50 is associated with physical and mental decline in men. Man's desire for superior intellectual accomplishments, emotional support or virility is augmented in his middle years. This makes transitions in his psychology too complex for theoretical specifications. Emotional turmoil introduces deliberate changes in midlifers' lifestyle, and they may adopt noticeably strange pursuits. David Bainbridge, in *Middle Age: A Natural History*, argues that "incline towards irresponsible and immature things" in midlife should be seen as a liberation, not as crisis (Bainbridge, 2013). Jung counsels that rejecting one's old self and assuming new motives are signs of "successful midlife transition" (Rendall, 2010). These, however, seem meagre forces in dousing the flames that this crisis arouses through unique psychic transformations in individuals.

DOI: 10.4324/9781003568360-18

Jaques propounded that the typical features of midlife crisis in men surface when they assess themselves as unsuccessful in fulfilling the demands of marriage and occupation. This explains their clichéd behaviour of disillusionment – desperation, and dissatisfaction along with physical decline. Such a depressive scenario drives individuals around 35 years of age toward immature behaviour.

Midlife Crisis in Literature from the 13th to 19th Centuries

Dante's *Inferno* and *Divine Comedy*

Dante introduced "midlife crisis" 700 years before Elliot Jaques' formal naming of it in his 1965 essay "Death and the Mid-life Crisis". In addition to Jaques' analysis of his subjects, the reading of Dante's *Inferno* prompted him to convincingly conclude it existed. Jaques later wrote that Dante's "beautiful lines melded with my own inner experiences of the midlife struggle with its vivid sense of the meaning of personal death" (Jackson, n.d.). Dante's *The Divine Comedy,* written in the 13th century, is another work believed to be born out of his midlife crisis. This in fact, made him "its poet laureate" (Hawkins, n.d.). At 37 years of age, Dante appears perplexed with self-questioning and is not only uninterested in the future but also dissatisfied with the past. Most importantly, he appears visibly anxious about the approach of death. In such great astonishment he shows wasted in bleak and menacing dark wood. Dante writes how in the middle of his days in the mortal plane, he found life gloomy and directionless. Life's savage wilderness with its robust and rough growth was making it an uphill task to live, "Which to remember only, my dismay / Renews, in bitterness not far from death" (Alighieri, 1995).

Dante's melancholia bears similarities with what men experience today during their middle years. Jaques was certain that it is "the reality and inevitability of one's own eventual personal death that is the central and crucial feature of the mid-life phase" (Liqun, 2012) and that "No-one believes in his own death. In the unconscious everyone is convinced of his own immortality" (Hushidari, 2007). Fear of the inevitability of death has thus been pronounced a major contributing factor in influencing midlifers' psyches. Once this fear starts hovering over them, the mounting distress manifests itself in varied and unprecedented ways. Jacques' (1965) emphasis on prospective death as central and crucial to midlife crisis, Brim's (1976) association of declining hormonal levels and physical powers with midlife crisis, and Levinson's (1986) theory about unfulfilled dreams of youth resurfacing during midlife signify that "changes in midlife as primarily internally motivated, rather than being triggered by external life events" (Liqun, 2012). Kieran Setiya acknowledges similar fears. He writes that despite a perceptibly content life, "there was something hollow". "Decline" and "death" troubled him as he "felt a disconcerting mixture of nostalgia, regret, claustrophobia, emptiness, and fear" (Setiya, 2017).

Cervantes' *Don Quixote*

Cervantes in early 1600s created the middle-aged Don Quixote, who ushered himself into a kind of fake reality and displayed proneness to hallucinations. Deeply misled by medieval legends of knights of the round table, his own identity was lost. Quixote's case demonstrates how during midlife, men seek escape from their dreadful surroundings and opt for oblivion in falsities. In "From Midlife Crisis to Regeneration and Personal Growth: Cervantes' *Don Quixote* as a Psychotherapeutic Rehabilitation Tool", Danielle Gurevitch initiates the discussion with a popular notion that Cervantes' Don Quixote is "the eternal archetype of the ageing loser" (Gurevitch, 2014). However, Gurevitch later argues that through Quixote, Cervantes teaches how to deal with crises and overcome despair, and live with optimism, humour and *joie de vivre*. Donald Capps in "Don Quixote as Moral Narcissist: Implications for Mid-career Male Ministers" identifies Quixote's paranoia, melancholia, and his fictive personality as prominent traits in midlifers. Capps uses these to examine midlife crisis in many male ministers (Capps, 1999).

William Shakespeare' Sonnet 138 and *King Lear*

The dynamics of midlife crisis are more involved than mere assumptions based on superficial observances. During their middle years, men tend to claim to have acquired wisdom of a higher order and superior insights into others' deceptions. This knowledge, however, may in turn exacerbate their restiveness. Shakespeare's Sonnet 138 is a monologue of a man, adequately aware to fathom the infidelity of his mistress. Shakespeare writes that when his beloved claims truthfulness, he believes her though he knows that she is deceitful. He is aware that she takes him to be naïve, uninformed about pretentious, two-faced people: "Thus vainly thinking that she thinks me young, / Although she knows my days are past the best."

Karl F. Zender writes that Shakespeare's depictions of midlife experiences are inclined toward "an interiorized understanding". Zender finds that the representations of human life in literature during Shakespeare's time were attaining more "historical and psychological" orientations (Zender, 2008, p. 2). In the chapter "Lear's Age" of his book *Shakespeare, Midlife, and Generativity*, Zender argues that elderly Lear fears geographical distancing from Cordelia after she is married as he seeks her continued care and is jealous of her future husband. Also, Lear's cursing of Goneril, Zender believes, is expressive of his "rage at the transfer of power and identity implicit in having children old enough to become parents themselves" (Zender, 2008, pp. 15–16) Lear's agitation here is linked to Erik Erikson's theory of "generativity", which Zender develops further. Zender's compendium is an exhaustive analysis of Shakespeare's "engagements with the dilemmas and challenges of middle years ... guilt, denial, marriage, and violence; the texture of life subsequent to the midlife crisis" (Zender, 2008, p. 37).

During the 18th century, studies show that the boundaries between midlife and old age were not marked distinctly. This lack of clarity persisted in much of the 19th century too, and ambiguity in literature was evident. Kay Heath and Karen Chase have explored the fiction works by Charles Dickens, Anthony Trollope, Elizabeth Gaskell, Oscar Wilde and H. Rider Haggard. Personal and collective experiences of ageing in cultural construction along with fictive characters formed the basis for discussions (Martin, 2011).

Literature of the 20th Century and Midlife Crisis

Thomas Mann's *Death in Venice*

In Thomas Mann's novella *Death in Venice* (2001), the ageing Aschenbach grows obsessed with a 14-year-old boy, Tadzio. He turns into a degraded slave of passion and is stripped of self-restraint and dignity. Leah Davidson in a paper presented at a Meeting of the American Academy of Psychoanalysis, relates Aschenbach's case. She writes that the central character, a 50-year-old man with a successful writing career, "has developed a work inhibition that he does not understand". Inspired by a stranger (symbolic), he travels to Italy for a vacation. During his sojourn on a remote island, he fails to relax and decides to move to Venice. Mann writes: "When one wanted to arrive overnight at the incomparable, the fabulous, the like nothing-else-in-the-world, where was it one went? Why obviously; he had intended to go there, what ever he was doing here?" (Davidson, 1976).

In Venice, his destiny is revealed, as Aschenbach, the hero, meets Tadzio. That adolescent Polish boy's beauty on the brink of his youth fascinates Aschenbach. Tadzio's position in his family and among his peers is another factor that adds to Aschenbach's obsessing over him. As the days roll by, Aschenbach starts weaving narratives around Tadzio, idolising him and harbouring deeper feelings for him. Tadzio and his family are now being discreetly followed by Aschenbach all over Venice. His obsession for Tadzio's love, as he admits to himself, is leading him toward his own degradation, yet he revels in it. The story ends with Aschenbach dying of cholera as when Venice is marred by the epidemic, he finds it impossible to leave the boy there (Davidson, 1976).

The middle-aged Aschenbach visualised in Tadzio his own youth. At this juncture, growing wary of failures and imminent death, Aschenbach obsessively pursued Tadzio so that he could entrust him with his life's unaccomplished aspirations. This aligns with Jaques' identifier – "infidelity with a younger, more athletic accomplice" (Jackson, n.d.). Aschenbach's midlife crisis is energetically masked in his "manic determination to thwart advancing years" as Jaques proposed (Jackson, n.d.). With his time now limited, Aschenbach desires attainments far more than humanly possible, and thus hopes to continue living through Tadzio. Davidson also explains how "Von Aschenbach reduces himself, through several regressive manoeuvres to an enamoured elderly buffoon" in 12 steps (Davidson, 1976). Aschenbach's midlife crisis endorses Daniel J. Levinson's conception of the same:

> In the Mid-life Transition, as a man reviews his life and considers how to give it greater meaning .... Knowing that his own death is not far off, he is eager to affirm life for himself and for the generations to come.
>
> (Levinson, 1991)

Somerset Maugham's *The Moon and Sixpence*

Calvin A. Colarusso and Robert A. Nemiroff (1981) discuss complexities in Charles Strickland's marital and occupational life. Strickland, the protagonist in Somerset Maugham's novel *The Moon and Sixpence* (2023), is called a "great narcissistic villain of literature" by them. At the age of 40, without any warning, abandoning his family and a successful stockbroking career, Strickland goes to Paris to pursue painting. His life in Paris is full of hardships. However, such circumstances hardly affect him. Drowned in painting and canvas, he becomes oblivious of discomforts. He neither wants fame nor wealth, and therefore never sells his paintings. He lives in an illusion, and reality is blurred for him. Strickland may appear selfish, cruel, cold and sceptical to readers. He ruins the lives of his children and his wife, who nursed him during severe illness. Misfortunes dawn on all those who come in contact with him. Such oddities are typically cited as occurring in individuals undergoing midlife crisis.

T.S. Eliot's "The Love Song of J. Alfred Prufrock"

T.S. Eliot's disorientated, middle-aged Prufrock is unable to communicate emotions coherently. His indecisiveness about the need for visions and revisions indicates a profound crisis. With a bald patch on the head and thin arms and legs, he is despondent about his physical appearance. This arouses social anxieties and deep insecurities in him. Loneliness and life's meaningless pursuits are bewildering for him. He visualises death and is horrified by it. The old man is petrified as he is losing youth and vigour. The spectral image haunts him:

> And I have seen the eternal
> Footman hold my coat, and snicker,
> And in short, I was afraid.
>
> (Eliot, 1952)

As a desperate measure to come to terms with the fact of ageing and impending death, Prufrock wants to adopt the idiosyncrasies of the aged. As he grows old, he will fold the bottoms his trousers, and he wonders about parting his hair from behind and eating peaches. Perhaps the white flannel trousers will be comfortable for beach walks.

Prufrock's discontentment about life's meaninglessness leads him to derangements. He is constantly plagued by questions and suffers internally due to confusion and disorderliness. Self-questioning is a significant indicator of his crisis. As another such occurrence, Kieran Setiya in *Midlife: A Philosophical Guide* cites Albert Camus's *Myth of Sisyphus* and points out how Camus's absurd man, aged 30, after reckoning with the end of his life's journey, is horrified and finds his body revolting against his longing for tomorrow (Setiya, 2017).

Midlife Crisis in Contemporary Literature

J.M. Coetzee's *Disgrace*

Like Prufrock, David Lurie in J.M. Coetzee's *Disgrace* also appears troubled by self-questioning. David is unsure about happiness. He is not finding his job as a teacher meaningful, and contemplates death. Dissatisfied with an unfulfilled life, he is obsessed with younger women. He has failed in his roles as husband, father and teacher, which results in inner chaos. Men at middle age equate decline in sexual potency with the end of youth and vigour. The fear brings forth a desperation to hold on to youth. Midlifers thus want to do things which will reinstate youthful vigour in them. Added to this is David's loneliness, which intensifies his crisis. His leaning toward poetry could be seen as his way of running away from a lousy life and a wish to set up an imaginary world. Being tired of criticism and measured for his prose, he takes resort in music, "Byron in Italy, a meditation on love between the sexes in the form of chamber opera". Like his colleagues of the same age, he feels more out of place now – more so because these men are not brought up trained to perform certain tasks. It is the burden of their upbringing which impacts them negatively(Coetzee, 2000).

Borrowing from Jaques, Hushidari writes, "David's escape from daily life to a world of literature is a way of externalizing his crisis, writing enables him to distance himself from his inner chaos ..." (Hushidari, p. 15, 2007). David's comment, "After a certain age, all affairs are serious, like heart attacks",(Coetzee, 2000, pg 42) precisely puts across how society perceives transitions in midlife – insane and irrational:

> You're what – fifty-two? Do you think a young girl finds any pleasure in going to bed with a man of that age? Do you think she finds it good to watch you in the middle of you? ... Don't expect sympathy from me, David, and don't expect sympathy from anyone else either. No sympathy, no mercy, not in these days and this age .... You are too old to be meddling with other people's children. You should have expected the worst.
>
> (*Coetzee, 2000, pg 44-45*)

James Joyce's "The Dead"

The conflicting forces of an ageing body, perturbed psyche and society's assessments start exerting unsettling pressures on a midlifer. Thomas Rendall in his essay "Joyce's 'The Dead' and the Midlife Crisis" also claims that "major personality adjustments are common in middle age" (Rendall, 2010). He traces much-agreed-upon descriptors of midlife crisis assimilated into Joyce's narrative "The Dead". Rendall identifies reasons that build up Gabriel's midlife crisis:

1. Gabriel's university degree (a clear indicator of him being endowed with greater intellect);
2. His escapist tendencies;
3. Emotional turmoil due to the death of both his parents at a young age;
4. Anxiety associated with approaching death;
5. Loss of youthful passion in marriage with Gretta;
6. Irritability due to Gretta's revelation of her first love;
7. Gretta's assertiveness (in which she reveals herself as a wilful woman).

Rendall thus cites ample evidence from this short story to provide for his beliefs.

Midlife Crisis in Postwar Fiction

Escapist tendencies in midlifers have been made evident in literary narratives. In David Ely's *Seconds* (1963), the protagonist, Antiochus Wilson, engages which would help him change his identity so that he can break away from the sociocultural conventions that stifle him at home and work. Sloan Wilson's protagonist in *Man in a Gray Flannel Suit* (Wilson, 2009) is tired of family life and his corporate job after returning from the war. He starts seeking pleasures elsewhere to find comfort and excitement. In another such instance of escape, David Nobbs' character fakes his own death to escape from work and wife in *The Death of Reginald Perrin* (Nobbs, 1975).

Martin Amis's *The Information* (1996)

The midlife crisis of Richard Tull in Martin Amis's *The Information* also conforms to similar attributes. Richard is envious of his friend Gwyn Barry's success in his writing career, wealth and marriage. He is jealous, stressed, anxious and constantly under pressure to evade accountability for his own failures. Amis writes that Tull woke up at 6 a.m. and did not need an alarm as he was already "comprehensively alarmed. He was tired, and his tiredness had no cure in sleep. Amis captures middle-aged Tull's restlessness and paints an image of him that perfectly fits into the frame of midlife crisis in men.

Tull was unsure of the kind of tiredness that bothered him. Sleep might give some momentary respite; however, the tiredness was somewhere above and beneath him, wrapping him from all around. His tiredness was not limited to defined specificity. It was the outcome of his days lived, of "gravity, which wants you down there in the center of the earth" (Amis, 1995, p. 4). The burden of his tiredness was growing steadily with no sign of leaving him, and neither a nap nor a cuppa could make it better. His tears had long dried up, and now he could not recollect those nights he spent crying in desperation:

> Now his eyes were dry and open. He was in a terrible state – that of consciousness. Some while ago in his life he had lost the knack of choosing what to think about. He slid out of bed in the mornings just to find some peace. He slid out of bed in the mornings just to get a little rest. He was forty tomorrow, and reviewed books.
>
> (Amis,1995, pg, 4,))

Contemporary authors are rather articulate about the midlife crisis, and incorporate the phrase directly into their texts without reserve. Richard Tull, for instance considers, "Poor circulation, unhappy childhood, midlife crisis, ozone depletion, unpaid bills, overpopulation" (Amis, 1995, p. 151) as palpable excuses for his frustrations.

Salman Rushdie's *Quichotte*

Salman Rushdie's *Quichotte* (2019) features a mediocre spy-thriller writer, Sam DuChamp, who creates Quichotte, a travelling pharmaceutical salesman. Several key attributes of midlife transitions proposed so far are also observable in Quichotte as symptoms of midlife crisis in him. Quichotte, as Rushdie introduces him, is a man whose mental powers are receding due to advancing age. He is obsessed with mindless television and has spent countless days in cheap hotels rooms watching an excess of TV shows under their yellow lights. Quichotte also suffers "a peculiar form of brain damage as a result" (*Rushdie, 2019, p. 3*). Rushdie thus rationalises Quichotte's behaviour through the circumstances that led to such derangements in him, exactly in line with what Cervantes did for his Don Quixote.

Quichotte's "hopeless", "unwholesome" and "entirely one-sided" passion for a TV star, Miss Salma R, forms the core of the novel. This love was developed at an unknown point of time of his life. His infatuation with the beautiful and witty, he misconstrued as love. However, Quichotte understands that Salma R "would not simply keel over with joy at the first declaration of *amour fou* from a total stranger", and Rushdie is also wise enough to acknowledge the same – "He wasn't as crazy as *that*" (*Rushdie, 2019 p. 6*) – otherwise the credibility of Quichotte's portrayal would be forfeited. The sincerity and depth of Quichotte's affection is hence reinforced. Love in

Quichotte's case is not projected as romantic, but strange. Rushdie portrays him as a loner in search of love. It is not meant as joke, but as creating the vision to see the world strangely. Rushdie plays with the notion of reality and fantasy through Quichotte's entangled perceptions. Obsessed with television, Quichotte is rendered delusional and seems to have lost his sanity, fed with content that claims to be true, but is absurdly untrue, manipulated and essentially fictionalised. His ability to distinguishl facts from lies is seriously affected under the impact of junk television and the internet, in addition to his ageing self. The boundaries between truth and fantasy have become blurred for him.

Rushdie writes that with time, the quicksand of this illusion of love is drowning Quichotte further. The unreality of what his delusional persona assumes as the real world is consuming him: "he felt himself becoming emotionally involved with many of the inhabitants of that other, brighter world, membership in which he thought of as his to claim by right .... (Rushdie, 2019, p. 4)

Quichotte is in no way melancholic, though, or perhaps he is oblivious of his crisis. He is rather a dreamer. Pursuing a dream for Quichotte is about living a belief. Believing with conviction will turn things true for him. He visualises a son, Sancho, a fabrication of his lonely self, and embarks on a quest with the latter across America intending to prove his worth to Salma R. To prove himself worthy of her becomes his foremost concern. He finds it necessary to constantly strive for it. He is optimistic and believes that the world will carry him toward his goal, and that love will find its way. He is losing his sanity in believing that a beautiful celebrity might miraculously fall for him, making him triumphant in romance. Quichotte's is a story of hope and love. The old man stays hopeful about loving and being loved.

Recognition of midlife crisis as a paradigm in *Quichotte* is led by Rushdie himself. Sam and Quichotte's emotional expressiveness during their individual quests establishes that midlifers' psychology needs to be understood considering the factors that have caused such upheavals in them and led them to such delusional behaviours or beliefs. Rushdie in an interview admitted that both he and Quichotte suffered the detriments of ageing in some way or other, "and they are both thinking about the end of the line, the subject of facing the end, a subject which the book takes on very centrally"(p. 6). In his seventies, Rushdie is right in saying that thinking about the end is the most obvious behaviour. Quichotte is actually partly him, "trying to face up to those things. The work ahead of you is much shorter, much briefer period than the work behind you. It concentrates the mind" (Rushdie, 2019, p. 4).

Sam and Quichotte are perspicuous representations of Rushdie himself, who raises questions about transformed virtues of the times in which anything can happen. Rushdie intends to underline the disintegrating insanity of living in a world drifting away from reality. Daniel Levinson inferred that midlifers create a motivating image for themselves, and he suitably termed this image "the dream" (Lifespan Development, n.d.). For Quichotte, the pursuit of love thus motivates him to direct his energies with absolute conviction, "his sincerity, the depth of his affections, and the lengths to which he was ready to go to gain her hand" (*Rushdie, 2019, pg 6*) and that "He would be Lancelot to her Guinevere, and carry her away to Joyous Gard" (*Rushdie, 2019 p. 6*):

> Having a midlife crisis is equivalent to acting on the dream. Acting on a dream generates a crisis-like situation ... the benefits from dream realization tend to be ... individual-specific, therefore often intangible to others ... acting on the dream disrupts a "normal" life ....
>
> (Liu, 2012, p. 52)

Sam DuChamp, "the ostensible author" as Rushdie calls him, is old and ponders about mortality. His own family problems and loneliness echo in his invented Quichotte's narrative. Rushdie articulates the common pointers of midlife crisis in Sam DuChamp and Quichotte with precision. Both were of the same age, an age when most are orphaned. Their own generation was on its way out too. Their physical complaints were worsening: "Brother's aching back, Quichotte's dragging leg"(Rushdie, 2019, pg 22) Sam and Quichotte were both alone and childless. Sam's son has left him long ago without any trace, and his wife was gone too. They were both living in precarious financial situations. Quichotte had an imaginary son and was hoping for a romantic involvement. The cardinal symptoms of midlife crisis – hallucinations and delusions – are evident in Sam. He hallucinates about something following him:

> of dark-windowed cars parked on the corner of his block with their motors running, footsteps that stopped when he stopped, then started up again when he walked on, clicking noises on the phone, strange problems with his laptop, telemarketing messages with, he thought, a menace behind the banal words, threats on his Twitter feed, murmurs from his publishing company that mid-list Authors like himself might have difficulty being published in the future.
>
> (*Rushdie, 2019, pg 23*)

Rushdie continues to add to Sam's miseries – his credit cards have issues and his social media account is hacked too often. This has become a random thing. Once he had come home at night, and although nothing had been disturbed, yet he was sure that his apartment had been broken into.

The control over self, motives, eagerness and obligations toward activities in Quichotte are manifested as acquiring new attitudes and beliefs. Also, his crisis is a precipitation of "personal review and revaluation of one's past" (Aiken, 1993, p. 289). Aiken, under the title "Narcissistic Personality Disorder", writes that middle-aged adults,

> are in excessive need for attention and admiration and an exaggerated sense of self-importance and personal accomplishment. These

> individuals frequently make grandiose plans and set impossible goals, most of which cannot be realised .... they are interpersonally exploitative and have a defective conscience. They see things only through their own eyes and from their own viewpoint.
>
> (Aiken, 1993, p. 289)

Levinson held the belief that midlifers encounter "deillusionment" consequent to the "individual's unavoidable comparison between his youthful dreams and his sobering present reality" (Bering, 2011 pg 1). A strong desire to escape from the present and relive youth characterise midlife transition. Instead of reverting to reality, the brain tends to build up delusions to accommodate the phantasmagoria that enable individuals to cruise through stark and painful reality and fuel their life-sustaining goals. Delusions also tend to stretch into new dimensions in response to the information acquired. Quichotte's mind is supposedly deranged by the junk culture of the present, and his crisis manifests itself in the transformations of his awareness of reality. He embarks on a journey in pursuit of an impossible goal. Through his dysfunctional conscience, he sees things only through his own viewpoint, thus reality for him lies in his interpretation of it and the significance he attaches to it, guided by erroneous beliefs. Quichotte has one well-organised delusion surrounding which he has spun deep seated-convictions:

> A person who is deluded that he is loved by a celebrity approaches the world with this certainty and knowledge and acts accordingly by writing to, telephoning or attempting to visit the celebrity. This erroneous belief invests the patient's world with new meanings. In these terms *reality* lies in the interpretation of, or the significance attached to, events that occur interpreted in the light of the primary erroneous belief.
>
> (Oyebode, 2018, p. 119)

Delusions are manifestations of judgements. Quichotte's "statements are expressed with conviction and certainty and not subject to discussion and inquiry" (Oyebode, 2018, p. 112):

> in delusional disorder cases, in other words paranoia, we do not see a significant loss of functionality or destruction of personality. However, the delusions affect every aspect of the patient's life, as in line with delusions the patient may misinterpret many things. The delusions often serious ones, the person may believe that he is a very important person or has made an important discovery...delusional disorder generally sets in during midlife and has a chronic progression.
>
> (Arikan, 2022, p. 1)

However, despite deranged minds and socially dysfunctional behaviours, "these individuals appear to have normal cognitive personal and occupational functioning" (Tampi, 2019, p. 2). Rushdie claims the same in the opening pages of his book. Quichotte's past had "damaged his memory" and he had not many memories left about the middle period of his life. Most of them had been filled up or erased, replaced largely with stuff seen on TV. Physically, he was fit for his age and in good shape overtly, with the charming manners of a gentleman and a cheerful smile.

The composition of the content of Quichotte's delusion is also a reflection of his environment. Added to these are his individual choices and decisions about what to do with life and how to invest his time and resources. Cervantes created Don Quixote 400 years ago as an archetype of an adventure-seeking, ageing dud misled by the romances he read. Rushdie models his Quichotte on Cervantes' Quixote. Is Quichotte aware of the development of his inner world? Has Rushdie penned a comic character? If yes, then with what intent and at whose expense? One plausible argument is that reading *Quichotte* is therapeutic. If there is humiliation, ridicule and misery, it is cathartic. Living through the present is a constant striving to retain the sanity, and Quichotte not only does that, but also upholds the virtues of joy, hope and love. There is no despair in Quichotte's hopeless pursuit. Rushdie communicates a universal philosophical message about mental health, about how to deal with midlife crisis and overcome despair, behavioural disorders and sleeplessness. Rushdie's own world and his eventful life find reflections in this therapeutic journey of Quichotte. Behind the façade of ridicule and laughter settles a calming sense of optimism. Rushdie's *Quichotte* is thus a psychoanalytic case study of midlife crisis of Quichotte and Sam.

Literature and Midlife Crisis in Men: Concluding Arguments

Theories about midlife crisis are inconclusive: "the psychological picture of persons going through midlife crisis or transition seems to be incomplete" (Oles, 1999, pp. 1059-1069). What exactly transpires as midlife crisis in individuals and how it is manifested needs consolidation. Sollod in *An Introduction to Theories of Personality* writes: "Human nature has long been a matter of curiosity and great interest. People have always wanted to be able to understand and predict the behaviour of others" (Sollod, 2009, p. ix), and literature has offered tangible images of human behaviour. Emotional turbulence that midlifers experience provides plotlines for many narrative accounts depicting personal, marital and social crises. Incidentally, "psychoanalysts seldom get a chance to study healthy reactions to the problems of living" (Davidson, 1976, p. 204). Literary accounts illustrate how crises were triggered by realisations of physical decline and impending death.

Transitions or crises – what middle-aged adults will eventually experience is arguable, yet undeniably, midlife happens. Whether the fear of eventual mortality, as Elliott Jaques identified, is basic and inherent or is derived from other more fundamental emotions and stages of being, must be the subject of debate. Adult development experts hold that "midlife crisis has been exaggerated" (Santrock, 2011, p. 545). Also, there is no dearth of misconceptions and false narratives (Infurna, 2021). Despite this, psychologists maintain that "midlife is a crisis in development" (Santrock, 2011, p. 545).

The observable and somewhat common traits in middle-aged adults have generated generalised perceptions or stereotypes. Literature has strengthened these perceptions by moulding characters who exhibit acute angst about personal death, declining physical powers or intellect, and society's pronounced prescriptive norms. The conscious choices or unconsciously motivated impulses in them in their middle years are subjected to constant psychological scrutiny. If Quichotte was lost "in the deranged logic of his private universe ... to be able to function properly, or even grasp what was really going on in the actually existing world around him" (*Rushdie, 2019, p. 4*), his Cervantine counterpart had displayed the same derangements. Dante and Prufrock dreaded death. Aschenbach and Lear became subjects for generativity propositions. David Lurie, Gabriel and Richard Tull serve as examples of midlife as an intensive and complex transition.

The interplay of multiple roles a man plays and his ageing self make midlife a complex phenomenon. This discussion has tried to present how authors have portrayed salient features of midlife crisis through their protagonists. The physical and psychological changes in these characters project images and define attributes of midlife crisis. Personality changes, emotional reactions, disturbed familial relations, declining health etc. are most commonly found among them.

References

Aiken, L. R. (1993). *Personality: Theories, research, and applications.* Prentice Hall.

Alighieri, D. (1995). *The Divine comedy: Inferno; Purgatorio; Paradiso (Everyman's Library)* (A. Mandelbaum, Trans.). Alfred A. Knopf.

Amis, M. (n.d.). *The information.* Harmony Books.

Bainbridge, D. (2013, Summer). midlife. *RSA Journal, 159*(5554), 50.

Brim, O. G. (1976). Theories of the Male Mid-Life Crisis. The Counselling Psychologist, 6(1), 2-9. Retrieved from https://doi.org/10.1177/001100007600600102

Capps, D. D. (1999). Quixote as moral narcissist: Implications for mid-career male ministers. *Pastoral Psychology*, *47*, 401–423.

Coetzee, J. M. (2000). *Disgrace.* Vintage.

Davidson, L. (1976). Midlife crisis in Thomas Mann's "death in Venice". *The Journal of the American Academy of Psychoanalysis,* 4(2), 203–214.

Delusional disorders (Paranoia). (n.d.). Retrieved December 15, 2022, from Prof. Dr. Kemal Arıkan psychiatrist: https://www.kemalarikan.com/en/delusional-disorders-paranoia.html

Eliot, T. (1952). *The complete poems and plays.* Faber and Faber.

Ely, D. (1963). Seconds. David Ely: Harper Voyager; Reprint edition (January 22, 2013).

Gurevitch, D. (2014). From midlife crisis to regeneration and personal growth: Cervantes' "Don Quixote" as a psychotherapeutic rehabilitation tool. *Academic Journal of Creative Art Therapies,* 4(2).pg- 447

Half Dead: Men and the "Midlife Crisis". (2011, October 3). Retrieved December 14, 2022, from Scientific American: https://blogs.scientificamerican.com/bering-in-mind/half-dead-men-and-the-mid-life-crisis/

Hawkins, P. S. (n.d.). *Dante's commedia: From despair to hope to glory*. Retrieved February 8, 2023, from https://berkeleydivinity.yale.edu/sites/default/files/dr_peter_hawkins_pitt_lecture_2019.pdf

Hushidari, M. (2007, Fall). *Midlife crisis or male wound? A psychoanalytical study of the Protagonist's behaviour as midlife crisis in J M Coetzee's Disgrace*. Södertörn University College, English Department.

Infurna, F. J. (2021, May 1). *Midlife in the 2020s: Opportunities and challenges*. https://doi.org/10.1037/amp0000591

Jackson, M. (n.d.). Life begins at 40: The demographic and cultural roots of the midlife crisis. *Notes and Records:The Royal Society Journal of the History of Science*. https://doi.org/10.1098/rsnr.2020.0008

Levinson, D. J. (1986). The Seasons of a Man's Life: The Groundbreaking 10-Year Study That Was the Basis for Passages!. Ballantine Books.

Levinson, D. J. (1991). For the man at midlife. In J. A. Zweig (Ed.), *Meeting the shadow: The hidden power of the dark side of human nature* (p. 262). Jeremy P. Tarcher, Inc.

Lifespan Development Chapter 8: Middle Adulthood. (n.d.). Retrieved from midlife crisis? https://courses.lumenlearning.com/suny-lifespandevelopment/chapter/midlife-crisis/

Liqun, L. A. (2012, January 13). A rational choice theory of midlife crisis. *Economics Bulletin, 32*(1), 51–58.

Liu, L. A. (2012, January). A rational choice theory of midlife crises. *Economics Bulletin, 32*(1). Retrieved 19, 2022, from https://www.researchgate.net/publication/227410506_A_rational_choice_theory_of_midlife_crises

Mann, T. (2001). Death In Venice and Other Stories. Vintage Classics.

Martin, M. (2011). Aging by the book: The emergence of midlife in Victorian Britain, by Kay Heath The Victorians and Old Age, by Karen Chase. *Victorian Studies, 53*(2), 375–378. https://doi.org/10.2979/victorianstudies.53.2.375

Maugham, W. S. (2023). The Moon and Sixpence. The Project Gutenberg. Retrieved September 30, 2024.

Nemiroff, C. A. (1981). Male midlife crisis: The Gauguin syndrome, myth and reality. In *Adult development. Critical issues in psychiatry* (pp. 119–128). Springer Science+Business Media New York. https://doi.org/10.1007/978-1-4899-3656-1_7

Nobbs, D. (1975). The Death of Reginald Perrin. Gollancz

Oles, P. K. (1999). Towards a psychological model of midlife crisis. *Psychological Reports, 84*, 1059–1069.

Oyebode, F. (2018). *Sim's -symptoms in the mind: Textbook of descriptive psychopathology* (5th ed.). Elsevier.

Rendall, T. (2010). Joyce's "The Dead" and the midlife crisis. *Joyce Studies Annual*, 263–272. Retrieved December 15, 2022, from http://www.jstor.org/stable/26288764

Rushdie, S. (2019). *Quichotte*. Penguin Random House India.

Rushdie, S. (2019, September 7). *Salman Rushdie on his latest novel, "Quichotte"* (W. Isaacson, Interviewer). Amanpour and Company. https://www.youtube.com/watch?v=SBIBcp5OcJ0&t=630s

Rushdie, S. (2019, November 4). *Salman Rushdie: Quichotte* (J. Day, Interviewer). Chigago Humanities Festival. https://www.youtube.com/watch?v=fSNOVrmj16w&t=2712s

Santrock, J. W. (2011). *Life-span development.* McGraw Hill Higher Education.
Setiya, K. (2017). *Midlife: A philosophical guide.* Princeton University Press.
Sollod, R. N. (2009). *Beneath the mask: An introduction to theories of personality* (8th ed.). John Wiley.
Tampi, R. R. (2019, October 16). *Psychotic disorders in late life: A narrative review.* https://doi.org/10.1177/2045125319882798
Wilson, S. (2009). The man in the gray flannel suit. Da Capo Press.
Zender, K. F. (2008). *Shakespeare, midlife and generativity.* Louisiana State University Press.

15 Midlife, Stereotypes and Agencies in *English Vinglish* (2012), *The Lunch Box* (2013) and *Three of Us* (2022)

Subham Dutta and Nabamita Chakraborty

Cultural texts have always been replete with concerns and anxieties about ageing. However, the academic interventions that interrogate the relationship between ageing and the ideological functions of a particular society remain meagre. With a thrust on middle age, this chapter intends to read three Bollywood films, *English Vinglish* (2012), *The Lunch Box* (2013) and *Three of Us* (2022) in terms of the psychological and social factors that underpin the representation of midlife in them. Ageing in Bollywood has predominantly revolved around a duality where the youth and the old-aged are represented as complimentary to each other. While old age with the embodiments of physical frailty and the vast remit of experience is delineated in the light of guidance and nurturance, the younger generation, contrarily, is invested with the aspects of vigour, vitality and the audacity to carry forward a tradition already instituted by the older generation. In this traditional dialogue and dichotomy between the old and the young, what becomes inconspicuous is midlife and the issues associated with it. Bollywood, a gentrified version of the Hindi film industry, based in Bombay, has remained a key site of cultural and social productions in India. Multiple studies (Prasad 2000; Dwyer and Patel 2002) have unravelled the relationships between state ideology and film productions, in which the cinematic space acts as a potent site for the interplay of different social and ideological forces. Although this chapter highlights some common tropes and motifs in the representation of midlife, what we contend here is that midlife, far from being a homogeneous, crisis-laden phase, operates in a socially and psychologically heterogeneous manner. The objective of this chapter is to trace how the Bollywood films of recent times deal with the divergent aspects of midlife going beyond the dominant tropes and formulas. Academic inquiries that interrogate midlife through the lens of cinematic representation are meagre. This chapter seeks to fill that gap by addressing the socio-political and cultural dynamics of midlife, and their reverberations within the cinematic space.

DOI: 10.4324/9781003568360-19

What Is Midlife?

Middle adulthood as a distinct life phase seems to be dynamic and strongly subject to age-related, socio-cultural, gender-related and history-graded influences such as demographic, political and cultural transitions (Wahl & Kruse, 2005). The idea that the life course can be broken down into multiple distinct developmental phases had already prevailed for a while, although that did not allow narrowing them down or circumscribing them to definite age boundaries. Purposeful attempts to define midlife reveal its opacity and fuzziness as a concept.

With a clear lack of consensus consistently leading the way in terms of the exact time span of midlife, the most accepted age range for the phase seems to be 35–60 years (Santrock, 1997; Willis & Martin, 2005; Chakraborty et al., 2012). Some popular variations claim that the phase begins at 40 years of age and extends into the seventies (Kohli Meyer, 1986), while many others, claim that the middle years tend to halt at 60 years of age. Considering the possibility of a young midlife and a late midlife may add a higher degree of precision to the boundaries and their understanding.

Midlife, Gender and Representation

The co-relation between midlife, gender and representation opens up a less discussed, yet highly problematic field of social and cultural inquiry. Midlife and ageing, being integral conditions of life, not only register changes in the human body, but they also create different geographies of belonging. In *Geography and Ageing* (2008), Gerald Hodge traces the relationship between "ageing" and social geography. Studying elderly people's life trajectories, Hodge shows how ageing contributes abidingly to the re-negotiation of their relationship with the environment. Ageing, here, is measured through an individual's response to the environment, underscoring the role that the spaces perform in shaping individual subjectivity.

Hodge's observation is crucial to our reading of the relationship between midlife and gender. Hodge's idea of the geography of spaces could be effectively linked with the Lefebvrean paradigm of space, in which he looks at the ideological field of power and representation in the shaping of spaces. This chapter probes into an intersectional field where ageing as a biological process closely shares spaces with the ideologies of ageing.

Andrew. B. Wister (2020) demonstrates that ageing as a social category can be seen from multiple perspectives. Considering it to be an important tool of social analysis, he demonstrates how ageing could be categorised differently: chronological, biological, psychological and social. His contention testifies to the evolving relationship between ageing and its multiple impacts. It categorically underlines that ageing is not just about chronological progress in terms of time or embodying biological changes, it is also about the psychological and affective changes instrumental to the development of our personality. This interrelation impels one to ask as to how it shapes our social and cultural identity. Furthermore, it is interesting to look at how this interaction between the different aspects of ageing propagates ideologies and stereotypes of ageing.

Gender and midlife intersect in ways that perpetuate gender differences and double standards in midlifers' age identity constructs and mediated constructions of extended midlife. Research on gender and midlife suggests that the negative consequences of ageing are greater for women as ageing, along with the stereotypical socio-biological milestones (e.g. marriage, childbearing, nursing and menopause) take a heavier toll on their physical attractiveness. During and after childbearing and the climacteric, usually scheduled for onset around midlife, a majority of women will experience weight gain. Changes in their oestrogen levels will lead to a redistribution of body fat from the hips and back to the stomach. Such changes depart from the dominantly desirable version and fantasy centred around the body of the woman, thereby leading to social devaluation due to the pre-existing cultural weight assigned to youth, attractiveness and reproductive potential.

Ben Hutchinson (2020) demonstrates the cultural, philosophical and psychological aspects of midlife. Hutchinson's intervention is important because it sheds light on the complex intersections between "how we age" and "how we see ourselves as ageing". It also delves deeper into the discursive nature of the perceptions of ageing to trace their embeddedness in dominant norms and cultural traditions. Hutchinson offers an overall trajectory of midlife, tracing the areas of crisis and vulnerability. Delving deeper into the fields of perception and representation, he argues that midlife "crystallizes not just our dawning sense of personal mortality, but the way we come to question the very meaning of our lives as we reach middle age" (Hutchinson, 2020, p. 1-16). He also traces how gender remains embedded as an important category of negotiation in this conceptualizion of midlife, marked by a form of "sculpted creativity", drawing on Jaques' psychoanalytic intervention of midlife crisis. He propounds the dominant field of perception about midlife by putting forth the cultural platitudes that treat the inevitability of ageing in a gendered manner: "Men merely pause where women menopause."

Midlife and Cultural Theories

Cultural theories on midlife focus on understanding how indigenous social norms and expectations shape human maturity cross-culturally. Cultural studies encompass several areas, such as media representations of women midlifers and how such portrayals and cultural narratives influence societal perceptions of midlife women, including beauty standards, achievements and challenges. Studies on body image and ageing are invested with how cultural attitudes toward ageing and physical appearance impact a midlife woman's body image and self-esteem. Role transitions include studying cultural expectations related to transitions such as empty-nesting, caregiving for ageing parents, and redefining professional and personal identities during midlife.

Empowerment and resistance studies examine instances of empowerment and resistance within cultural contexts where midlife women challenge stereotypes and redefine societal expectations. These theories contribute to a more nuanced understanding of how diverse cultural factors shape the experiences, challenges and opportunities that women encounter during this life stage.

Jung introduced a concept that deals with norms from a different perspective. He observed that at midlife the "body and values tend to undergo a reversal into the opposite" (1934/2001), a "gender crossover". According to this line of thought, men in midlife have used up their supply of masculine resources and have a small amount of "feminine" substance left over. Women in midlife discover their masculine side. This reversal has implications for needs and motivations. Men at this time relinquish their competitive endeavours, and women show an uncommon indecisiveness which pushes the feelings and the heart aside. Interpreted in the context of a larger framework, older individuals are allowed a greater sense of independence and autonomy over choices and roles than the young, who are offered a unitary society-driven sex-role orientation.

Laura Cartensen's *Socio-emotional Selectivity Theory* (2021) suggests that as individuals age, their priorities shift toward maximising emotional well-being and maintaining important social relationships. Her work on ageing and emotion has highlighted the significance of social connections during middle adulthood. As an expert in adult development, Susan Krauss Whitbourne examined topics such as gender identity in midlife and the impact of societal expectations on the well-being of individuals in middle adulthood. Her research on adult development documented support for the theory of Erikson (1963), in that adults continue to grow and mature throughout their lifespan. However, age-graded conflicts and their resolution continue beyond the age frameworks prescribed by Erikson. Chrisler's research on women's health and wellbeing has explored the unique challenges and experiences faced by women during middle adulthood, including issues related to body image, menopause and social expectations.

Indian Perspectives on Midlife

Each culture has its way of representing developmental trajectories, and such trajectories form significant parts of its members' worldviews. In the Indian culture, midlife is viewed often through a holistic lens that incorporates physical, emotional and spiritual dimensions. Concepts from several philosophical and religious traditions contribute to understanding this life phase. With an exclusive sample of men, ancient Hindu conceptions divide the life course into Brahmacharya, Garhastya, Vanaprastha and Sanyasa. Middle age supposedly coincides with the third stage (Kakar, 1998). The idea of Vanaprastha in Hinduism suggests a gradual withdrawal from worldly responsibilities to focus on spiritual pursuits during middle age. In this phase, ideally Hinduism prescribes a certain non-attachment and not being bound to the fruits of one's labours. Such non-attachment will lead to *moksha* or a certain self-refinement and cleansing of all desires, and thereby a subsequent release from *samsara*.

Nivedita Menon in her book called *Seeing like a Feminist* (2012) writes about sexual division of labour that makes women primarily responsible for housework, child-rearing, cooking cleaning and such other duties day after day, even when performing labour outside the home and earning wages or salary. Men escape such duties and cannot be held accountable for them, being an equal or higher authority in the household, though they are equally capable of doing them and though their biological constitution does not explain any difference of proficiency at such tasks. The performance of these tasks is intrinsically bound to a woman and entrenched into her personal belief system as not being tasks to demand remuneration for, but rather responsibilities to accept unquestioningly.

Through her poetry, Kamala Das criticises the patriarchal structures and systems that subjugate women. The universe of her poems is India. She challenges the unequal power dynamics in society and advocates for gender equality. She questions the role of traditions and religious dogma in shaping women's lives and identities and their struggles in a patriarchal society. Her poetry rejects the traditional notion of women's role as passive or submissive. She rejects traditional expectations placed on women related to marriage, motherhood and domesticity. Her work criticises the social structures that limit women's opportunities and autonomy. Das's poetry examines the domestic sphere and its impact on women's lives. She reflects on the confines of marriage and motherhood and how they often become traps for women. Her poetry thus offers insights into the struggles and aspirations of women in a patriarchal world, and powerfully explores the complex relationships between women, society and gender roles.

Uma Chakravarty, an eminent historian, in her work *Conceptualizing Brahminical Patriarchy in India* has traced the frailty in the understanding of how social processes have shaped men and women in early India as being restricted to questions of marriage, law, property rights and rights related to religious practices. She claims that the extent and form of subordination faced by women have been conditioned by the social and cultural environment in which women have been placed.

Her book reveals the historical trajectory of the woman's role in society and how it is determined by the men conceptualizing her as innately sinful, adulterous, having an insatiable lust and uncontrolled sexuality governing her promiscuous nature. Such a projection of the fear of the woman's uncontrolled sexuality became the background to the obsession with creating an effective system of control and the need to guard women constantly in order to maintain the purity of the caste and blood.

The original attitude of prehistoric societies to women and their power of reproduction had posed no problems and accepted their sexuality as inherent. This was later replaced by stringent control systems – the maternal power had to be organised and ordered by paternal power. They were subordinated and controlled by the ideology of *streedharma* and *pativratadharma*, to be internalised by women to live up to the ideal notion of womanhood. Thus was resolved the tension between nature and culture, and women themselves volunteered to become paragons of virtue by becoming ideal wives to men and restricting themselves to a life of dedicated service to the household.

Leela Kasturi: Kasturi, in her work *Development, Patriarchy and & Politics: Indian women in the Political Process 1947–1992*, focuses on the lack of uniformity in the problems faced by women. Marked by differences of rural and urban residences, occupational and gender role diversities across caste, class and community, and separate systems of law across religions, the problems become increasingly complex and diversified. in her book, she points out inter-state and inter-region variations in women's status. Such variations are dominated by a number of interlinked historical, ideological, economic and cultural factors. There is a marked gender disparity in labour-force participation rates for rural and urban areas.

Kasturi, in her research, mentions how relations in the family, class status and the ideology of the social group to which they belong, that of patriarchy, govern social and gender relations in India, in an ideology based on the power of men. Women are socialised to "fit in" to these norms. Such an arrangement hinders women's progress and development. Though there may be class and caste segregations among women in India, male strength, authority and power oppress them at all levels, as is visible in all indicators of women's status – education, economic and political participation, legal status and so on.

The wide variety of theoretical along with practical insights offered by the multidisciplinary perspectives from psychology, sociology, biology and cultural studies converge to create an ambivalent concept of the phase of middle adulthood. A complex interplay of quite a number of critical factors shapes the adult developmental trajectory during this phase of life. It is to decipher and recognise such intersectionality that a dialogue between cultures and representations becomes relevant and insightful in the journey of an adult through the middle years.

Midlife and Cinema

The genres of films and fiction have provided audiences with varied representations of the phase of middle adulthood and thus created a prototype or stereotype of this life phase in their minds. Such prototypes represent socio-culturally standardised identity-related aspirations, milestones and practices, and such ideals are commonly held and significantly contribute to personal well-being. In his 1972 work "Ways of Seeing", English art critic and novelist John Berger commented "...men act, women appear. Men watch, women watch themselves being watched" (pg- 67) in his analysis of the representation of women across media (see Marwaha, 2020).

In a report by the Green Davis Institute (Shah & Kapoor 2018), only one in ten Bollywood directors is a woman. According to other statistics, women receive a mere 31.5% of screen time in comparison to a whopping 70% received by male actors. With the rare adoption of offscreen roles by women, those involving intellectual reasoning, thought and problem-solving, creativity and decision-making, such as the roles of directors, scriptwriters and film-makers, women are portrayed largely from the man's perspective, and fail to overcome the barriers imposed by patriarchy.

Both Hollywood and Bollywood portrayals of women have been rich in their objectification of women as agents of fantasy and sexual pleasure. They are mostly characterised in supposedly nurturant roles as a doting mother, a loving wife or a devoted daughter-in-law. Surprisingly, a woman's portrayal is autonomous, sexually expressive, intelligent and confident only when holding harmful intentions toward innocent others.

Using midlife as a social category of ageing, this chapter seeks to trace the cultural co-ordinates around which ageing is represented in dominant cultural discourses. The ideologies and stereotypes of ageing become crucial to our quest as it deals with cinema, an important vector of public opinion and cultural dissemination. The spaces of representation constitute an important field of power. This chapter explores how the film texts engage with these fields of power using the lens of midlife. As a result, it is pertinent to probe into the difficult question of how ageing and its dominant perception share a mutual relationship and shape discourse.

English Vinglish, Midlife and the Politics of Gender

English Vinglish is another significant Indian film that deals with the representation of midlife. A comedy-drama directed by Gauri Shinde, *English Vinglish* marks the silver screen return of the diva Sree Devi. In the role of Sree Devi, the film portrays the story of a middle-aged homemaker Shashi who occasionally sells *laddus* to earn her living. Shashi's business gives her a source of sustenance in an otherwise hostile marriage.

As a family drama, this narrative ventures into the power dynamics of the family. Despite her efforts to eke out a living, and live a life satisfactorily through her creative pursuits of sweet-making, Shashi suffers humiliation in the family because of her lack of English. Alongside her husband, even her daughter participates in the process of discrimination.

In contrast to *The Lunch Box*, where one finds an intimate representation of the mother–daughter relationship, *English Vinglish* shows how, without the support of the daughter, the mother feels even more lonely and vulnerable. Under the circumstances, Shashi's sister becomes her saviour, inviting her to come to America to make arrangements for her daughter Meera's wedding.

From this point onwards, the narrative delineates Shaishi's journey to America. Interestingly, this journey does not remain restricted to its physical sense, but rather opens up a new vista of self-discovery for Shashi. In the multicultural world of America, Shashi enrols herself in an English language training course with the paltry amount of money she has accumulated by selling sweets.

This shift in the narrative offers it a much-needed upthrust foregrounding a transition from the family melodrama to a coming-of-age narrative in which Shashi finds herself in a global family, the microcosmic representation of multicultural America. Her friendships with students from other countries portray America as a liberating cultural melting pot. However, Shashi's emancipation is only partial, and the narrative fails to decolonise her mind of the ingrained Indian value system about the sanctity of marriage.

At an important turning point in the narrative, the film portrays a growing friendship between Shashi and Fischer. Despite Fischer's romantic inclinations, Shashi upholds the sanctity of marriage and does not pursue this. The nub of the matter is that even after exposing herself to the Western value system and its liberating pursuits, Shashi, as a woman, remains firmly grounded in her Indian ethos which valorises the institution of marriage.

The fact that Shashi remains inextricably rooted in the tradition of marriage is illustrated through a long speech she delivers during the wedding of her sister's daughter. Even after grappling with a hostile marriage, her speech delivered in English resonates with the values of love, hope, optimism and fulfilment, which an ideal and companionate marriage should embody. She also mentions how an ideal marriage enables the growth and expansion of the nation. Shashi's speech serves as an eye-opener for her family, and she returns to India, learning the magical language of power.

The film holds an interesting premise of a woman's liberation from the stereotypes of gender through creativity and education. However, in the end, the re-articulation of the tropes and ideas associated with the sanctity of marriage and its values as an institution seems to undercut the emancipatory potential the film ordinarily seeks to espouse through Shashi's exposure to Anglicised, multicultural America. Even after reaching the land of self-fulfilment, Shashi does not repudiate her rootedness within the Indian ethos. In a way, this rootedness paves the way for a "rooted cosmopolitanism" (Appiah, 2017) which "finds a way to accommodate prejudice without really challenging us to uproot ourselves and forge a new world community with an enlarged sphere of concern" (Leib, 2006, p. 89).

Shashi's identity constructed through the archetypes of nationalism undercuts her agency as an individual. The film's representation of her as an embodiment of the Indian value system resonates with deeper cultural politics. The projection of Shashi as an archetype undermines its intersectionality with her gender and the roles specified by it. While Shashi's assimilation into global cultural fields opens up a space of dialogue, what remains unresolved is why Shashi upholds marriage, among other aspects, to be the sole marker of the Indian value system, even while grappling with an uneasy, hostile marriage. Even being humiliated as a mother, she advocates the glories of motherhood, continuing with her role. The film, at a subliminal level, seems to endorse the stereotype that an Indian woman's social value remains grossly incomplete without a successful marriage, family and motherhood. Jyotsna Kapur writes extensively on the politics of the Bollywood cultural industry and its imbrication with the dominant modes of Indian nationalism (2009 p. 221-233). In her study of how "global capital is most intimately experienced and lived", Kapur focuses on the "ideological redefinition of nationalism/citizenship as both acts of consumption and the re-enactment of patriarchal and caste-based identities" (2009, p. 221-233).

Tejaswini Ganti demonstrates how patriarchal politics remain predicated on the construction of an ideal female beauty. She shows how this becomes an important ingredient in the representation:

> The intense colourism that plagues Indian society, where fair skin is extremely valorised as the ideal of beauty, manifests itself most blatantly in the Hindi film industry where, throughout much of its history, actresses have been disproportionately lighter skinned than the majority of the population.
>
> (Ganti, 2016, p. 263)

The casting of Sridevi, the first female superstar of Bollywood (Roychoudhury, 2024), in the role of middle-aged Shashi is not devoid of this cultural politics of representation. Kareen Khubchandani highlights Sridevi's rise into prominence as a "snake woman" and how she became a sex symbol in Bollywood, establishing "intimate and embodied relationships" (2016 pp. 69-85) with her audiences.

The casting of Sridevi in the role of Shashi in this film in the role of a middle-aged woman seems to affirm this cultural politics of sexism. Shashi's mentor's attraction to her reiterates the idea of ageless beauty and unfading charm that she possesses even in her midlife. Shashi (the fictionalised representation of Sridevi), as an epitome of Indian beauty, does not lose her charm, beauty and ability to impress her mentor. The cinematic space thereby unravels a representational site where the onscreen identity of Sridevi as Shashi and her real identity as an epitome of ageless beauty intersect. This intersection articulates a complex cultural paradox of the Indian idea of beauty, negotiated through the retention of ageless charm even in midlife on the one hand, and a scrupulous adherence to the typical ideological markers of Indian femininity, marked by the values of chastity and motherhood, on the other. *English Vinglish*, despite focusing on the necessity of a woman's independence and self-tutoring, does not emancipate the protagonist from the binary of playing the gender roles: either as an evasive object of desire or as a socially conformist object clinging on to motherhood and wifehood, and the institution of marriage at large, even seeing the seamy side of it.

Food, Desire and the Creative Entanglements of Midlife in *The Lunch Box*

Food as a metaphor and a trope has shaped the cultural and social imaginaries of Indian cinema in multiple ways. Film-makers have negotiated its cultural significance, nutritional values and emotional attributes to render food a major vector of representation both socially and culturally. Critics have shed light on the "pleasures, dangers, and implications of consumption" Baron et al., 2012) in the aesthetic registers of film. Steve Zimmerman traces the genealogy of food representation in films to demonstrate how the representation of food in films captures "attention", and enriches the storytelling in "distinctive ways" (2009, p. 25-34). *The Lunch Box*, by Ritesh Batra, brings to the foreground the rich imbrication between food and storytelling. Batra's film weaves an intimate tapestry of life in the bustling city of Mumbai, around a misplaced lunch box that brings together feelings of love, affection and crisis.

The Lunch Box is not a film about midlife and its crises. However, midlife remains an important subtext in the plot, forging connections between two lonely individuals trapped in their worlds. Revolving around a misadventure associated with a lunch box, the narrative shares a delicate yet poignant story of emotional cadences. Mumbai with its cultural dynamics and social markers, becomes an important site in the narrative through the mediations of tastes, memories, crises and a relentless urge to overcome them.

In the story, the lunch box works as a major objective co-relative. With its frequent transit from one hand to another, it becomes a dominant motif in the story, being always in motion. Like the lunch box, the characters in the story also remain in motion throughout the story, without being able to reach their desired destinations. This being-in-transit of the lunch box depicts an unpredictable openness around which the identities of the characters are woven in the story. It symbolizes an openness that resonates with the open-endedness of the story. It is a story about a young, lonely housewife Ila and Saajan Fernandes, a strict widower who works as an accountant in an office.

Following the suggestions of Mrs Deshpande (Bharati Achreka), Ila adds spice to her husband's lunch in a desperate attempt to get his attention. However, by a quirky turn of events, it gets delivered to a middle-aged grumpy man, Saajan Fernandes. This serendipity leads to a series of events that hold the story of The Lunch Box. Realising the mistake, Ila informs Saajan about it in a letter. However, the ensuing exchange of letters ignites their friendship and offers forays into their respective emotional spaces. The creative exchanges of food and letters, tinged with affection and creative nurturance, rejuvenate their zeal for living, continuing with their lives, despite their despondency. It is reflected through Saajan's gradually growing friendship with Aslam Sheikh, a young trainee who works as an apprentice under him. Ila, too, ponders leaving Mumbai for Bhutan on discovering her husband's extramarital relationship. The two plan to meet for the first time, but Saajan, coming and looking at Ila from a distance, decides to leave considering, himself a mismatch for her youthfulness and beauty. In the end, the narrative leaves their destinies tantalisingly open to negotiations without offering any closure to them.

The Lunch Box, set in Mumbai, meticulously, maps the socio-spatial landscape of Mumbai. The claustrophobic spaces of the local trains, the lonely kitchen space of Ila, her interactions with older women of her locality, and the spaces of the office remain juxtaposed against each other in the narrative. The delineation of a city in relentless transit and movement situates Mumbai at the crossroads of multiple forces and spaces a heterotopia – at once "real" and "virtual" (Foucault, 1967). While the *dabbawalas*' constant mobility across spaces lends a sense of place to the story and works as a cultural marker, its impact on the characters – the intricate matrix of emotional and social relationships it builds – demonstrates its casual and inadvertent subversion of the everyday logic of temporality. The timeless "mythic city" (Prakash, 2010) inhabited by the timeless images of the *dabbawalas* is constantly altered, and rewritten by the temporality of their relentless mobility. The relationship between the two midlifers grows out of this tension between the timeless and the temporal rhythms of Mumbai that continually rewrite it as a space.

This subversion of the everyday logic of temporality comes as a breath of fresh air into the lives of the two midlifers in the story. The portrayal of midlife in this story is stereotypical and routine-bound. It is evident from the mechanical nature of Saajan's job, and the way he handles it with austerity and abstinence. For Ila, the routinised existence is measured by her frenetic attempts to patch up a crumbling marital relationship through a helpless enactment of the domestic chores. Unlike the other two films in our discussion, this film evocatively depicts midlife through the quotidian banality and slowness of the urban space. In this milieu, the characters also remain struck with relentless self-questioning about their worth in a rapidly changing universe.

Apart from the fields of crisis and indeterminacy, *The Lunch Box* also weaves narratives of creativity and sustenance around midlife. In a world of technology and immense visibility, the romance between Saajan and Ila thrives completely in anonymity, without a physical meeting. Their interactions transform their lives quite significantly. Saajan's growing friendship with Aslam, crossing the barriers of age and religion, also testifies to a phase of generativity that midlife brings in. On the other hand, Ila's decision to disentangle herself from an unhappy marriage marks the gradual yet steady emergence of her autonomy. In its intimate portrayal of the vulnerabilities, rigidities and desires for creative bonding beyond the social and institutional barriers, the film seems to capture the spirit of midlife in its multiple aspects. The dilemma with which the film ends, becomes emblematic of the dilemma of a particular generation. The dilemma comprises an invitation to start afresh in a new life with hopes, zeal and optimism on the one hand and the restrictive pulls of embittered memories and social learning on the other. As a result, the characters and their relationships in the narrative remain tantalisingly open and fluid.

The subtext of midlife invokes an ambivalence in the representation of gender in this film. The cultural industry thrives on stereotype building even around midlife. Predominantly, middle-aged male characters are presented either in roles that desperately try to communicate a message of social heroism (as evident in films like *Taare Zamin Paar*, *Bajrangi Bhaaijan*, *Chak De India* and *Raaez*) or as villains driven by vested interests as evident in the role of Gabbar Sing. Female characters are stereotyped as mothers and grandmothers (as is evident in *Mom*, *Badhai Ho* and *English Vinglish*). Such stereotypes, being very superficial, hardly explore the emotional and affective changes associated with midlife. Going against the grain, this film treats midlife and its problems as a separate ontological category. It delves deeper into the affective complexities of midlife and demonstrates how they create an intricate mesh of creative desire and a resistant force that engages in a constant conflict with it. This open-ended and ambivalent representation of midlife, both in the portrayal of Ila and Saajan, makes the film profound in its portrayal of midlife.

Love, Loss and the Longing of Midlife in *Three of Us*

Midlife becomes an important crossroads where emotional, social, and neurological crises meet in *Three of Us*. The film poignantly explores the relationship between memory, midlife and accompanying problems. Revolving around Shailaja's dilemma, the story brings together a wonderful tapestry of memories, longing, and desire.

It narrates the story of Shailaja, a middle-aged woman on the verge of losing her memory due to dementia. The overwhelming sense of loss around herself and her identity impels her to revisit the traces of her past to relive the moments that will soon be lost in the quicksand of forgetfulness. Shailaja, the protagonist of the movie, finds herself in a position of psychological dilemma suffering from an acute crisis owing to dementia. Her dementia aggravates to such an extent that she, in fact, becomes sceptical about her ability to remember her son after some years. This awareness of vulnerability, however, does not deter her from embracing the lost threads of life by reconnecting with them. Her exploration of the spaces outside her home and immersion in creative practices not only renew her affinities with the world, but also offer resistance to the debilitating forces of life. The scene in which she launches into a conversation with her childhood friend and how they relive the moments becomes poignantly painful.

Shailaja's character demonstrates a strong engagement with the present, however banal or painful it appears. Midlife and the vulnerability here do not compound each other by engaging in an intricate mesh of sentimental pessimism. Instead, the narrative shows a relentless urge to hold onto a vanishing time by finding news of "dwelling" within it. A renewed engagement with time and the memories comes with a different form of self-discovery and realisation with an inherent openness to time, where the past and the present remain inextricably tangled.

Shailaja's husband, a middle-aged man, is also left with the drudgery of his personal and professional life. He feels overwhelmed by the tedious nature of his job. In his personal life, with his son settled far from home for higher studies and his wife grappling with the anxieties and problems of dementia, he finds himself in the crucible of circumstances. His crisis and vulnerability, although not as apparent and explicit as Shailaja's, becomes evident through his helplessness in the face of the dreadful inevitability of his life. His wife's longing to revisit her childhood spaces and people is gracefully supported by him. Despite the understandable sense of insecurity lying within him, he does not allow it to get the better of him. Being in a liminal space in this relationship without much agency, he demonstrates incredible resilience in his role as a midlifer, and thereby drifts far away from the traditional role of a husband.

Revisiting her native village, Shailaja rediscovers the spaces that impacted her upbringing. This retreat becomes a way to rediscover herself as this journey ignites her lost desire for her lost sweetheart Pradeep Kamat. Pradeep, a middle-aged bank manager, revives her creative self when they meet after the long gap. Shailaja and Pardeep's voyages through the alleyways of their unspoken pasts become a channel through which they negotiate their selfhood and identities.

However banal the nature of Pradeep's job is, his creative engagement keeps him moving. His character seems to be a foil to Shailaja. Whereas Shailaja struggles to keep the threads of her memory intact, Pradeep creates a world of his own through his creative impulses. When they meet again after 28 years, their exchanges and revisits to the "sites of memory" about their shared past make them part of the same threshold from which they re-map and renegotiate their selves and identities. Pradeep's journey with Shailaja becomes an emotional retrospection filled with innocence and genuine care. Traversing the paths of nostalgia, the narrative delves into psychological and emotional profundities, which do not remain confined to a painful longing for the past, but resonate with an active agency for making it a tangible weapon of survival and self-discovery.

Foraying into the psychological conflicts of midlife, this film embarks on an emotional journey to re-inhabit the "sites" of childhood and adolescence. The narrative portrays an evocative landscape of Konkon, which apart from the human characters, becomes intrinsic to the plot. The deft use and presentation of cinematic *mise-en-scène* enables the characters in the film to navigate the emotional complexities of their selves and lost relationships. Apart from the space, time becomes crucial here, underlining how the presence of an "uncanny", spectral past dislodges the apparent coherence of the present.

Three of Us seems to be an interesting representation of midlife in Indian cinema. What sets this apart is not the representation of vulnerability, but the urge a creative transcendence of it. The film portrays an irresistible urge for retaining autonomy, creativity and selfhood even while recognising the dreadful inevitabilities of life. At a superficial level, the film portrays midlife as a crisis-laden situation, but in hindsight it charts out a profoundly meditative portrayal of midlife with the cultivation of philosophical strength and resilience against the dreadful inevitability of loss and longing. A frenetic desire to reignite the bonds with the past and entrenched love for life within the characters overturns the stereotypes of sterility, and crisis that shape the general discourse of midlife. Navigation of spaces, physical, social and psychological, and their social structures remains integral to the characters' movements and their meanderings across lives. Through these paths of navigation, the film never falls short in lending a new perspective to midlife, projecting it as a site of resistance to time, friendship and care, and thereby forging genuine connections, identifying a shared site of pain and pleasure.

The relationship between midlife and its cinematic representation is understandably complex. However, it is interesting to see that film-makers in Bollywood are increasingly focusing on it. Despite the predominance of stereotypical representations, films like *The Lunch Box* and *Three of Us* depart from popular tropes and discourses to offer renewed engagements with the emotional complexities of midlife. The varieties in representation underscore how midlife is lived, perceived and conceived across spaces and cultures.

References

Appiah, K. A. (2017). Cosmopolitanisms. NYU Press.

Baron, C., Carson, D., & Bernard, M. (2012). Appetites and anxieties: Food, film, and the politics of representation. Wayne State University Press.

Chakraborty, N., Chatterjee, T., & Das, S. (2012). Midlife and the life-course: The associated shifts in life perspective and societal obligations. *Indian Journal of Positive Psychology*, *3*(4), 388.

Erikson, E. H. (1963). *Childhood and society* (Vol. 2). Norton.

Foucault, M. (2008). Of other spaces*(1967). In Heterotopia and the City (pp. 25-42). Routledge.

Ganti, T. (2016). Fair and lovely: Class, gender, and colorism in Bollywood song sequences. In The Routledge Companion to Cinema & Gender (pp. 276-285). Routledge.

Hodge, G. (2008). The geography of aging: Preparing communities for the surge in seniors. McGill-Queen's Press-MQUP.

Hutchinson, B. (2020). The Midlife Mind: Literature and the Art of Ageing. Reaktion Books.

Jung, C. G. (1997). *Visions: Notes of the seminar given in 1930-1934 by CG Jung* (Vol. 99). Princeton University Press.

Kakar, S. (1998). The search for middle age in India. Welcome to middle age, 75-98.

Kapur, J. (2009). An "Arranged love" marriage: India's neoliberal turn and the bollywood wedding culture industry. Communication, Culture & Critique, 2(2), 221-233.

Kohli, M., & Meyer, J. W. (1986). Social structure and social construction of life stages. *Human Development*, *29*(3), 145–149.

Khubchandani, K. (2016). Snakes on the dance floor: Bollywood, gesture, and gender. The Velvet Light Trap, (77), 69-85.
Leib, E. J. (2006). Rooted cosmopolitans. Policy Review, 137, 89.
Marwaha, P. (2020). The Portrayal of Gender Inequality in Selected Female Oriented Bollywood Movies. SMART MOVES JOURNAL IJELLH, 8(5), 23-35.
Prakash, G. (2010). Mumbai fables. Princeton University Press.
Roy Chowdhury, A., & Khan, A. A. R. (2024). 'South Asian'Diaspora Theatre in Sydney: Cultural Politics of the Proscenium and Transforming the Mise-En-Scène. *Journal of Intercultural Studies*, 45(2), 190-207.
Santrock, J. W. (1997). *Life-span development Madison*. Brown and Benchmark Publishers.
Shah, G. R., & Kapur, M. (2018). Changemakers: Twenty Women Transforming Bollywood from Behind the Scenes. Penguin Random House India Private Limited.
Wahl, H. W., & Kruse, A. (2005). Historical perspectives of middle age within the life span. In *Middle adulthood: A lifespan perspective* (pp. 3–34). Sage.
Willis, S. L., & Martin, M. (Eds.). (2005). *Middle adulthood: A lifespan perspective*. Sage.
Wister, A. V. (2020). Multimorbidity resilience: Conceptual, theoretical, and measurement developments. Resilience and Aging: Emerging Science and Future Possibilities, 81-105.
Zimmerman, S. (2009). Food in films: A star is born. Gastronomica, 9(2), 25-34.

16 The Socio-political Canvas of Middle Adulthood

An Analysis through Tagore's Literary Lens

Tanaya Roy Chowdhury and Rudrani Chatterjee

Middle adulthood is a stage of the human lifespan that encompasses various psychological and physiological characteristics and developments. This phase of life can be described from different perspectives. Middle adulthood is not only the stage of cherishing memory of childhood, it is also a stage of creating memories to enjoy throughout one's lifetime.

In the field of psychology, many eminent psychologists have explained different characteristics of adulthood in their own ways. According to Erik Erikson, a prominent developmental psychologist, a psychosocial stage known as generativity versus stagnation typically occurs during middle adulthood. "Generativity" refers to the desire and ability to contribute to the wellbeing of future generations and society as a whole. On the other hand, "stagnation" occurs when individuals become self-centered and fail to engage in generative activities. Stagnation can lead to feelings of unfulfillment, a lack of purpose, and a sense of being disconnected from one's larger community or society. Carl Jung, a Swiss psychiatrist and psychoanalyst, believed that inner exploration, integration of diverse psychological elements and a quest for wholeness and self-realization are the basic elements of middle adulthood. According to him, the process of individuation is the central goal at that time. Another influential Austrian psychiatrist and founder of individual psychology, Alfred Adler, explained middle adulthood in different way. He emphasized that individuals have the power to shape their own lives through the choices they make. He believed that each person develops a unique lifestyle, which includes their patterns of thinking, feeling and behaving. Overall, adulthood presents opportunities for individuals to reflect on their lifestyle and make conscious decisions to change or adapt their behaviors and attitudes to lead more fulfilling lives. Urie Bronfenbrenner, in his ecological system theory, explained that in adulthood individuals are shaped by cultural expectations, societal norms and broader contextual factors that contribute to their behaviors, beliefs and attitudes. The ecological perspectives acknowledge the dynamic nature of the person–environment relationship which influences individual wellbeing. Glen Elder suggests that each

DOI: 10.4324/9781003568360-20

life stage influences the next, and together the social, economic and physical environments in which we live have a profound influence on our health and the health of our community. In his Life Course Theory, he talked about a turning point, which involves a particular event, experience, or awareness that results in changes in the direction of a pathway or persistent trajectory over the long term.

In Bengali culture, middle adulthood is the most popularly discussed stage of life, which is reflected in different Bengali literary genres. Bengali literature, with its long and diverse tradition, huge range of authors and themes, offers a comprehensive exploration of middle adulthood, depicting the joys, struggles and complex relationships that individuals in this stage of life encounter as well as reflecting cultural, social and psychological aspects of middle-aged individuals in various ways. The first Bengali Nobel laureate, Rabindranath Tagore, became a living institution in the field of literature. During his lifetime he created a huge number of poems, novels, short stories, dramas, paintings and songs. The most alluring aspect of his novels is their multi-layered psychosocial issues as literary themes. He was also a social reformer on the basis of his philosophy, which was influenced by Brahmo Samaj, a socio-religious reform movement originated in 19th-century India, founded by Raja Ram Mohan Roy and later led by other prominent figures like Debendranath Tagore. The chief aim of Brahmo Samaj was the worship of the eternal God. It was opposed to priesthood, rituals and sacrifices. It focused on prayers, meditation and reading of the scriptures. Bramo Samaj had considerable success with its programs of social reform, but never had a significant popular following at that time.

Psychoanalytically, it is said that literature is the mirror authors' minds, how they perceive their surroundings and how they deals with them. At the same time, any form of literature is influenced by contemporary socio-political scenarios. So it is obvious that contemporary socio-political influences would be prominent in the writings of such a socially aware legend as Rabindranath Tagore. His three popular novels, *Chokher Bali*, *Ghore Baire* and *Shesher Kobita*, are not directly political novels, but the influence is very clear. This chapter delves into the intricate landscape of middle adulthood through the lens of these three timeless novels.

Chokher Bali was published in 1903 in colonial India, two years before the first partition of Bengal. The impact of British rule was felt across all aspects of Indian society, including politics, economy, education, culture and gender roles. In this era, India was witnessing the rise of various socio-political movements that aimed to challenge British dominance and work toward independence. Bengal was a prominent center of cultural and intellectual activity at that time. The Bengal Renaissance, a period of sociocultural reform and intellectual awakening, was in full swing. It was characterized by efforts to modernize society, promote education, women's empowerment, and challenging prevailing social norms and practices. In this period, women's issues and the status of women in society were important topics of discussion. At that time abolition of child marriage and widow remarriage was gaining momentum. Tagore himself was a strong advocate for women's rights and empowerment. He championed the cause of education for women and was against oppressive social customs like the seclusion of widows. The whole picture was very extensively reflected in Tagore's literary works.

Ghore Baire is a novel written in 1916, set against the backdrop of the Swadeshi movement in Bengal during that time. While the novel itself is not an explicit commentary on contemporary socio-political events, it does reflect the broader context of the time in which it was written. At that time, significant socio-political and economic movements in India aimed to promote indigenous industries and products while opposing British colonial rule.

Sesher Kobita was first published in 1929. During the early 19th century, there was a growing sentiment of nationalism and resistance against British rule in India. Tagore's idea of nationalism was closely tied to humanism. He believed that the wellbeing and development of individuals were essential for the progress of a nation. He was critical of narrow, aggressive nationalism that promoted divisions among people. Tagore also emphasized the importance of cultural nationalism, where a nation's identity is rooted in its cultural heritage, arts and literature. He believed that India's strength lay in its rich cultural traditions and diversity, and that these should be celebrated and preserved.

The socio-political scenario in which *Chokher Bali* is set is reflective of the tensions and transformations of that time. The novel portrays a society grappling with changing social norms and the clash between tradition and modernity. It explores themes of love, desire, marriage, societal expectations, individual freedom and women's rights, particularly through the experiences of women. The female characters, mainly Binodini, in *Chokher Bali* challenge traditional gender roles and expectations. She navigates her desires, personal aspirations and relationships within a conservative society. The novel addresses themes of widow remarriage, extramarital affairs and the struggles faced by women in a patriarchal society. Overall, the socio-political scenario of colonial India during the early 19th century serves as a backdrop for the themes and conflicts depicted in *Chokher Bali*. It captures the complexities of a society in transition, grappling with the influences of British rule, changing social norms and the evolving role of women. In conclusion, while the immediate socio-political scenario of the time may not have had a direct impact on the plot of *Chokher Bali*, the broader context of the Bengal Renaissance and the evolving status of women in society provide a backdrop that influences the themes and portrayal of characters in the novel.

Ghore Baire is set during a time when India was struggling for independence from British rule, and the Swadeshi movement, which aimed to boycott foreign goods and promote indigenous products, plays a significant role in the narrative. Tagore examines the impact of nationalism on individuals and the nation as a whole. The characters in this novel grapple with the clash between traditional values and modern ideas, and tensions between old and new, particularly through the characters. *Ghore Baire* examines the individual's quest for self-realization and the pursuit of personal ideals. In this novel, different characters represent different facets of individualism and idealism, and their interactions reflect the broader societal struggles. Manipulation of ideologies for personal gain is a prominent feature of this novel.

Sesher Kobita is set against this backdrop of nationalism and political awakening. It portrays the conflicts and dilemmas faced by its characters in a changing socio-political landscape. The novel reflects the contemporary social and political scenario of the time, which was marked by the Indian independence movement and the rise of nationalism. Furthermore, *Sesher Kobita* highlights the changing roles of women in society. The struggle for independence from British colonialism was a dominant theme in the socio-political landscape. Intellectuals and writers, including Tagore himself, played a significant role in advocating for national consciousness and cultural identity. The dynamics of relationships portrayed in this novel reflect the changing attitudes and aspirations of the contemporary generations, influenced by new ideas and values brought about by the impact of British colonialism and the Bengal Renaissance. Furthermore, *Sesher Kobita* reflects Tagore's own views on nationalism and internationalism. Tagore was a staunch advocate of cultural exchange and harmony between nations. Through his characters and their interactions, Tagore expresses his belief in the importance of universal human values and the need to go beyond narrow nationalist sentiments. It is essential to note that while *Sesher Kobita* is not a directly political novel, it is deeply influenced by the socio-political climate of its time. *Sesher Kobita* explores the tension between the ideas of nationalism and individual freedom.

This chapter will discuss central female characters in these three novels, Binodini, Bimala and Labanyalata. Personality is a complex and multifaceted construct influenced by both nature (genetics and biology) and nurture (environment and social context). While social context plays a significant role in shaping personality, it interacts with other factors to form a unique individual identity. The attractiveness of three characters like Binodini, Bimala and Labanyalata in Bengali literature can be attributed to their complexity, their portrayal as progressive women in that conservative time frame, the intricacies of their relationships, the exploration of desire and passion, the timeless themes they embody and their cultural significance. These factors combine to make them enduring and compelling adult personalities in literature.

In the context of these socio-political developments. Tagore's portrayal of Binodini, a widow who challenges societal norms by asserting her independence and desires, can be seen as a reflection of the changing role of women in Bengal during the Bengal Renaissance. The protagonist Binodini's character represents a departure from the traditional docile and submissive widow archetype, as she dares to express her desires, seeks personal fulfillment and independence, and actively pursues her own happiness. In *Chokher Bali*, through Binodini's character, Tagore portrays the struggles and aspirations of women in a conservative society. Binodini exhibits emotional resilience in the face of various challenges. Despite her status as a widow and societal expectations, she possesses a strong will and refuses to conform to traditional norms. On the other hand, Binodini experiences a significant amount of emotional turmoil throughout the narrative. Her conflicting emotions, particularly regarding her relationships, create internal tension and psychological distress. Tagore expresses her inner struggles as a reflection of complexities of human emotions during middle adulthood. Binodini has intellectual curiosity, but at that time it was not socially accepted. After all, Binodini might influence other women in her surroundings through her knowledge of foreign languages and through her in a lifestyle which was strictly prohibited for a widow. According to Adler, striving for individuality is at its peak during middle adulthood. Binodini craves independence and longs for a life beyond the limitations imposed on widows in the society at that time. She strives to assert her individuality and seeks personal fulfillment, often at odds with societal expectations. The character of Binodini also represents the darker and more complex aspects of the themes of the novel. She manipulates everyone to achieve her own desires. To satisfy her unfulfilled needs, she may make a choice which may be considered morally questionable. Her pursuit of her own happiness and desires can be seen as a betrayal of trust and friendship, which is followed by sense of guilt and unhappiness. Tagore creates a mid-adult personality in Binodini, who leads a unique lifestyle, which includes her patterns of thinking, feeling and behaving. Tagore enables the mid-adult to reflect personal choices in her lifestyle and make conscious decisions to change or adapt her behaviors and attitudes to lead a more fulfilling life. The popular concept of middle adulthood of Erikson is reflected in this character. Binodini, as an adult, follows her personal choices and selects the path of generativity, which is fulfilling for her own life. Binodini's journey involves a search for her identity, both as a woman and as an individual. She grapples with her desires, societal expectations and the consequences of her actions. This search for identity reflects psychological processes such as self-exploration and self-definition.

Bimala, the central character of *Ghore Baire*, is portrayed as a complex and evolving character throughout the novel. This character is initially depicted as a traditional and sheltered woman whose life revolves around her domestic duties. However, as the story progresses, Bimala undergoes a significant personal and ideological transformation. She becomes influenced by the nationalist fervor of the Swadeshi movement and is drawn toward the charismatic nationalist leader Sandip, another prominent character in the novel. Bimala's character represents the tension between tradition and modernity as well as conflict between personal desires and social obligations. Her internal struggles mirror the larger societal challenges faced by India during that period. As she navigates her way through love, politics and self-discovery, Bimala embodies the complexities of identity and agencies in a rapidly changing socio-political landscape. In *Ghore Baire*, Tagore skillfully explores Bimala's journey as a powerful metaphor for the dilemmas faced by individuals and the nation at large during a time of social and political upheaval. Bimala possesses many admirable qualities, but there are negative aspects of her character as well. Bimala is portrayed as a somewhat naïve and idealistic character, especially in the beginning of the novel. These traits lead her into a situation that has negative repercussions for herself and those around her. It is seen throughout the novel that Bimala tends to avoid confrontation and conflict, even when it is necessary. Instead of addressing issues head-on, she often internalizes her feelings, leading to internal turmoil and exacerbation of conflicts. Sometimes, her lack of lack of determination, which prominently features in the novel, contributes to her vulnerability and susceptibility to external influences. It is important to note that Tagore's portrayal of Bimala is nuanced, and her flaws contribute to the overall complexities throughout the novel. At the same time, negative aspects of her character highlight the challenges and conflicts faced by individuals in such a changing socio-political landscape.

In *Shesher Kobita*, Labanyalata's character is so popular because of ambiguity and complexities. Labanyalata exhibits emotional depth and sensitivity. She is capable of experiencing a wide range of emotions, from joy and passion to vulnerability and insecurity to confidence and sadness. Her emotional sensitivity allows her to connect deeply with others and empathize with their experiences, contributing to her complex and nuanced psychological makeup. Emotional stability is a prominent feature of middle adulthood, and Tagore presents it very well. Labanyalata embodies a strong sense of individuality and independence. She refuses to conform to societal expectations and seeks to create her own path in life. Her independent thinking and actions reflect a psychological need for self-determination and a desire for personal freedom. These middle adulthood traits of self-determination and autonomy are also influenced by the contemporary socio-political background. Her motivations often appear multifaceted, making it challenging to decipher her true intentions. This complexity adds depth to her psychological portrayal as a midlifer. Labanyalata is portrayed as an intellectually curious character. She is well-read, expressive and engages in philosophical discussions. Her intellectual curiosity reflects a psychological inclination toward seeking knowledge, understanding and exploring life's deeper meaning. Labanyalata resists conformity and the idea of settling for a conventional, predictable life. She expresses a fear of losing her individuality and becoming trapped in societal norms and expectations. This fear indicates a psychological desire for authenticity and a reluctance to compromise her values and dreams. Like many midlifers, Labanyalata is on a quest for meaning and purpose of life. She reflects on her past, contemplates her future, and seeks a more profound understanding of love and life. But her idealism sometimes leads to frustration and disappointment when reality doesn't align with her lofty ideals. Throughout the novel, Labanyalata's perspective on love evolves. Initially, she appears to be skeptical of romantic relationships, favoring intellectual connections over emotional attachments. However, as the story progresses, she experiences personal growth and begins to embrace the transformative power of love and gains the capacity for emotional growth as a midlifer. Labanyalata, as a midlifer, represents a woman in a transitional phase of life where she is no longer in her youth, but has not yet reached old age.

This chapter aims to reveal different shades of middle adulthood which are reflected in the three different types of novels, *Chokher Bali, Ghore Baire* and *Sesher Kobita*. Growth of adult personality, ego strength, autonomy, purposefulness and lastly the journey toward generativity are depicted very well in these novels. The main female characters Binodini, Bimala and Labanyalata are reflections of the status of females in contemporary society. It would be more appropriate to say that these creations are reflections of Tagore's respect toward women as well as progressive thoughts regarding women's empowerment. Tagore was born in a family where the women in particular played a significant role in promoting women's empowerment in India during the late 19th and 20th centuries. Since before Tagore's birth, women of his family had been role models for contemporary society. They used to pursue education, personal growth, professions and entertainment as well as sustaining family life smoothly. Tagore's protective childhood was influenced by his socially aware and culturally rich family. Throughout his life, in his personality as well as in his creations, these influences are seen very clearly. From various letters to Tagore's wife, Mrinalini Devi, his expectations from his life partner arte very clear. He writes many times about the importance of mutual respect, equality and companionship in a marital relationship. At that time, when women were so oppressed in Bengali society, Tagore sought help from his wife in all his activities, even in her various regular cultural activities. But he always insisted that she not lose her own choices, thoughts, independence and moreover her individuality. He wanted his partner to be equal and free to pursue her aspirations, dreams and most importantly happiness during middle adulthood. In these popular novels, the interpersonal as well as intrapersonal conflicts experienced by the characters are prominent. In *Chokher Bali*, Binodini tries to live independently by her own choice, but there are multilayered obstacles in her family and society. Bimala is portrayed as more complex in *Ghore Baire*. But Labanyalata in *Shesher Kobita* is portrayed as an independent and strong-willed woman who is determined to live her life on her own terms. Throughout the novel, she seeks to find her own identity and purpose in a society that has certain expectations and constraints for women. Binodini also wants the same, but she fails to establish herself in broader society, whereas Bimala is perplexed in dealing with personal and social conflicts. So it can be said that Labanyalata's journey is a sociocultural extension of Binodini's through Bimala. In these novels, Tagore extensively expresses his concerns about and awareness of the sociocultural situation of women as well as their psychological structure in middle adulthood.

The characters Binodini, Bimala and Labanyalata are not typically considered middle-aged individuals. Each character represents different aspects of life, experiences and stages of development. Binodini in *Chokher Bali* is a young widow facing complex relationships and societal norms. She is not a middle-aged character, but is a young woman dealing with many challenges and life tasks that are similar to those of middle age. In *Ghore Baire*, the central character Bimala, a young woman, becomes entangled in political and personal conflicts. Though in terms of biological age she is young adult, her dealings with complex circumstances mean she can easily be included in a discussion regarding midlife. Labanyalata is also a young adult whose psychological makeup is very much similar to that of middle adulthood. All three characters are young in biological age, but their life tasks, emotional stability and complexities as well as emotional wellbeing, relationship dynamics, the psychosocial structure of their personalities and their journeys toward generativity help to understand and analyse them as midlifers.

These three novels were written when Tagore was aged 42 years, 55 years and 67 years respectively. Tagore experienced his journey of adulthood along with his characters. In the novel *Chokher Bali*, Tagore primarily focuses on the growth and development of young adults, particularly through Binodini, Mahendra, Asha and Bihari. Tagore depicts the transition from innocence to maturity as the characters grapple with their own emotions and relationships, laying the foundation for his exploration of adulthood. In *Ghore Baire*, Tagore examines the tension between individual aspirations and collective identity. The characters in the novel struggle with the idea of balancing personal desires with the greater good of the nation. the novel also explores different forms of love, including marital love, platonic love as well as love for one's country. The relationships between the characters reflect the emotional complexities that are the prominent features of midlife. *Sesher Kobita*, is also a reflection on love and relationships in the later stages of adulthood. The characters Amit and Labanyalata represent the maturation of love and the wisdom that comes with age. This novel is a contemplative exploration of adulthood in the context of mature, long-lasting relationships. During this period, Tagore's works became more reflective and philosophical, exploring the multifaceted dimensions of middle adulthood, from the youthful struggles and desires depicted in *Chokher Bali* to the emotional complexities in *Ghore Baire* to mature and enduring love portrayed in *Sesher Kobita*. Tagore's writing evolved in its depth and complexity, addressing the psychological, emotional and intellectual aspects of growing into adulthood. His works during this period offered profound insights into the development of individuals as they navigated the changing landscapes of their lives and society.

Chokher Bali, *Ghore Baire* and *Sesher Kobita* provide rich insights in the complexities of middle adulthood. These literary works showcase the clash between individual desires and societal expectations, the consequences of one's choices and the importance of self-realization and emotional maturity from young adulthood to middle adulthood. They serve as timeless reflections on the challenges and dilemmas faced by midlifers as they navigate the intricate tapestry of life, love and relationships. Through the characters and narratives crafted by Tagore, readers gain a deeper understanding of complexities and nuances that define this significant stage of human development. From the introspective journey of *Chokher Bali* to the spiritual quest depicted in *Ghore Baire* and finally the journey toward generativity in *Sesher Kobita*, this chapter has uncovered the richness of Tagore's storytelling to illuminate the challenges, triumphs and transformations inherent in the middle adulthood phase.

Reference

Banerjee, A. K. (2020). Ghare Baire: An eco-critical perspective. *South Asian Review, 42*(1), 48–67. https://doi.org/10.1080/02759527.2020.1799674

Data, P. K. (2005). *Rabindranath Tagore's the home and the world: A critical companion*. Anthem Press (An imprint of Wimbledon Publishing Company).

Dutta, K., & Robinson, A. (1995). *Rabindranath Tagore: The Myriad man*. Saint Martin's Press. https://thedoglife.home.blog/2020/06/09/women-of-tagore-bimala/

Johri, M. (2023). Dimension of culture, gender and society in Tagore's Chokher Bali. https://www.researchgate.net/publication/374919454_DIMENSIONS_OF_CULTURE_GENDER_AND_SOCIETY_IN_TAGORE'S_CHOKHER_BALI

Jung, C. (1933). *Modern man in search of soul* (W. Dell & C. Baynes, Trans.). Harcourt Harvest (August 4, 1955).

Morgan, C., King, R., Weisz, J., & Schopler, J. (1986). Introduction to psychology (7th ed.). Tata McGraw-Hill Publishing Company Limited.

Ray, S. (1996). Sesher Kabita: Tagorean ideals towards the man – woman relationship. *Analecta Husserliana, 49*, 165–175.

Sadock, B., & Sadock, V. (2007). *Kaplan and Sadock's synopsis of psychiatry: Behavioral sciences/clinical psychiatry* (10th North American ed.). Lippincott Williams & Wilkins.

Sengupta, M. (2012). Shesher Kobita: Punopather Prostabona. *Paidhwani the Echo, 1*, 1–11.

Tagore, R. N. (1938). *Shesher Kobita*. Shantiniketan Press, Biswabharati Gronthon Bibhag; 4th reprint.

Tagore, R. N. (1948). *Chokher Bali*. Shantiniketan Press, Biswabharati Gronthon Bibhag; 8th reprint.

Tagore, R. N. (1948). *Ghore baire*. Shantiniketan Press, Biswabharati Gronthon Bibhag; 8th reprint.

Tagore, R. N. (2015). *Nationalism* (2nd ed.). Fingerprint Publishing House.

Tagore, R. N. (2020). *Jibansmriti*. Shantiniketan Press, Biswabharati Gronthon Bibhag; 28th reprint.

17 Cinematherapy

A Sustainable Way to Overcome Midlife Woes in Women

Sukanya Saha

Crises in women during midlife seem manifold compared to men. Middle-aged women consciously or unconsciously are trapped inside a mundanity, a saturation point, where they are not left with any choices but to carry on. They may feel depressed as their teenaged children no longer need their mother, distracted at work as it holds no purpose and meaning except paying bills and dodging boredom, dreading reunions as everyone else looks in good shape and happier, being indecisive about what they really want toundefined become and who they are now, and perplexed because old parents, husbands, in-laws, children and bosses never appear content. Torn between relations and career, anxiety seeps into their bloodstream which combines with menopausal hormonal changes to produce a crisis.

Mary Lynn Crow precisely identifies the core of this crisis in women. She says that in women, awareness about being trapped in life and fast-approaching death precipitate the feeling that not much time is left for desired accomplishments and there is no escape from circumstances. For working women, their personal lives and careers together weigh them down:

> Women may feel trapped much earlier than midlife – trapped by a relationship, a career, children, or life circumstances – but in their twenties and even in the early thirties, they can always believe that there is time to get out. "There's always an advanced degree I can earn," or "When the children are older ...." At midlife, this optimism may be gone; time is no longer the great escape.
>
> (Crow, 1987, p. 413)

Physical ageing (Li Ping Wong, 2012) concerns women the most: "Men are 'allowed' to age, without penalty, in several ways that women are not" (Susan Sontag, quoted in Schmidt, 2018). Women who take up the responsibilities of supporting their families in the ways men traditionally do seem less purturbed during their middle years. The masculine and feminine roles performed by women protect them from acute crisis (Lieblich, 1986). Factors such as annual family income, the company of other women of the same age,

DOI: 10.4324/9781003568360-21

close friends and confidants, prospects for a better future, positive self-esteem, good health and appearance etc. help evade crisis in women (McQuaide, 1998). Women need to identify those factors which will enable them to live through this critical period. This establishes the need to define and study midlife crisis in women more deeply (Mihailova Lilia, 2022).

In a study of middle-aged Malay women, it was found that they were dissatisfied with their ageing bodies and looks, which they thought were making them undesirable. The influence of the media had a large part to play, in that they fixated their minds on conforming to Western ideals of youth and beauty. They had spent a lot of money to retain youth and vitality (Diah, 2018). In another study, marital satisfaction was considered a crucial factor compared to others in preparing women for midlife and emotional wellbeing. It assumed that other factors were not so significant (Lee, 2014). Clausen (1990) aptly called midlife a "psychological turning-point" which imparts insights into one's own self and others, and thus leads to significant changes or new directions. This turning point proposition was reviewed by Wethington and her colleagues, leading to the finding that "women were more likely than men to report turning points at mid-life (Moen & Wethington, 1999)" (Wethington, quoted in Aldwin, n.d.)

An ageing body, its gradual ailments and dwindling mental peace have no apparent cure, unless one chooses to undergo psychotherapy to ease the tensions. In cases where persisting conditions become painfully intense and beyond control, women may resortn to antidepressants or alcohol, which may bring some temporary relief. Sustainable practices with assured outcomes that will heal without harming are most sought after. One such way to help overcome the distress is cinematherapy. This therapeutic technique has shown some promising results over the past few decades in helping with mental illnesses and has been studied extensively. Elena Sacilotto and colleagues analysed 38 studies and found that 36 of them reported positive outcomes from the treatment (Sacilotto, 2023). Judy Kuriansky and colleagues also reviewed and evaluated cinematherapy as a tool and technique for therapy, counselling and coaching for individuals and couples, to help them deal with real-life problems such as, dating, divorce or abuse. They also included specific issues, particular settings and varying client populations. They highlighted the need for cautious handling of the technique and further research to maximise its impact (Kuriansky, 2009). In cinematherapy, therapists select movies for their clients to watch alone or in groups. The films either address the issues directly or work as stimulants to orient patients toward specific problems. The viewing sessions are followed by further interventions as needed. This technique is an extension to bibliotherapy – treatment through prescribed readings (Berg-Cross, 1990).

Scenes from films have been proven to leave lasting impressions in our lives in some way or other. Cinema is a powerful medium. It opens up a wide spectrum of emotions, ranging from elation to intense grief. The qualitative insights that films impart about human minds have great potential in contributing towards psychiatry. Cinema and psychology have a lot in common. Both disciplines delve into the complexities of human emotions (Orchowski, 2006). Through cinema, mental illness in subjects can be understood inside-out. Humans seek escape through entertainment, which makes cinema a perfect method to draw in patients who may otherwise be reluctant in trusting therapies prescribed for their problems. Films engage, entertain and also empower. Pleasure, concentration and inspiration are the three factors that make cinema a potential medium to address and treat psychological issues (Niemiec, 2020). In movies, watching relatable characters grappling with similar circumstances, having the same desires and fears, may help subjects believe that their crisis is not unique and there are workable solutions available to overcome their problems. Brie Turns and Porter Macey presented case studies to discuss the effectiveness of cinematherapy, its clinical implications and usefulness for future uses. They suggest how externalisation of movie characters' issues and their qualities help in overcoming problems in subjects (Turns, 2016).

The discussion in this chapter highlights some movies from international cinema to explore how these plots address crises, specifically in women, and bring out practicl solutions.

The Bridges of Madison County (1995)

Francesca's diaries reveal her brief romantic tryst with Robert to her adult children after her death. Torn between desires and responsibilities, middle-aged Francesca opens her heart in her narration and is honest in her account, with no regrets. Seeing herself again in a new light through the eyes of a complete stranger and longing forassionate lovemaking drove her toward Robert. This short affair transformed her.

Like Francesca, women at middle age apprehend that a large part of their lives has just passed them by, watching it haplessly, lost amidst mundanity, a husband and teenaged children. Francesca pined for passionate romance, which she found during four days and three thrilling nights with Robert when her family were away. She let her guard down and surrendered to the bliss that episode offered. In the posthumous letter to her children, her confessions mirror those thoughts that most women of this age probably nurture yet consciously dodge, wary of embarrassment.

Francesca and Robert's torrid affair does not have a fairytale ending. Loyalty toward her family binds Francesca's conscience, though her love for Robert remains. An incredible, transcendant and powerful experience, as she describes their lovemaking, makes her now-adult and married children realise that their own marriages and loyalties are casual and immature compared to their mother's selfless sacrifices. Francesca's story underlines that essential dilemma in which the middle-aged women perched on the top of the fence wrestle with indecisiveness about dropping themselves on any one side. Francesca no longer finds passion in her marriage, yet is unable to abandon her teenaged children and doting husband. Her narrative brings up the question of how long a spontaneous relationship lasts and if a woman seeks new avenues to look forward to in life, how much she should be subjected to societal judgements.

Eat, Pray, Love (2010)

Liz has been married for eight years. She chose that life for herself, and made it with dreams. Despite a successful career and beautiful house, she seems lost. Unsure of what she wants from life, she files for divorce, which her husband does not want. She also gets romantically involved in a fling. This too, however, does not bring her happiness. She is aware of the crisis that is building up in her. She confesses that as she wakes up in the morning, she has "No passion, no spark, no faith, no heat. Absolutely nothing." The consoling idea that she is probably having a "a bad moment" is no longer working. It is a crisis way beyond that. This is terrifying for her, and even worse than death that most people dread above all. She has to bring about changes in herself because she feels she has no pulse left, as if her spirit is lost: "I used to have this appetite for food, for my life, and it is just gone. I wanna go someplace where I can marvel at something. … I have not given myself two weeks of a breather to just deal with, you know, myself."

Confounded by overwhelming emotions, Liz sets out on a year-long trip during which she is to stay in three destinations: Italy, India and Bali. She embarks on the journey of discovering her true self and meaning in life. In Italy, savouring pasta, pizza and gelato to her heart's content, she is unfazed about her dreaded "muffin top". Her expanding waistline does not affect her. It is important how she shuns self-loathing. The next four months she is to spend in an ashram in India, where the power of praying restores her faith in love and life. During her Bali sojourn, Liz finds love but panics and withdraws. Following the advice of a soothsayer, she finally embraces love and finds her inner peace.

Liz's narrative brings up travel as an effective mode of unwinding one's self from complexities that tie women down in entangled mesh of societal expectations. Liz ponders over motherhood, pines for an understanding partner and is bewildered about her present. Her journey to three destinations and meeting new people impart her with new purposes to live a happy life.

A Man Wanted (2017)

This romantic comedy from Egypt, intended as lighthearted entertainment, highlights one significant problem among middle-aged women: a ticking body-clock. Despite being a successful banker, Sham's ageing self does not let her be at peace. Urgency to become a mother before the age of 40 forces her to find a man whose sperm she can use for in vitro fertilisation treatment. She plans to enter into a contractual marriage which entails divorce as soon as the child is conceived successfully. Bahgat, a veterinarian, agrees to enter into the contract, attracted by the huge amount of money on offer. Although the movie does not directly deal with midlife crisis in women, it does address middle age and its imperative – childbearing before a certain age. She refers to an ominous fear which creeps-in while conforming to the precise social mould. Despite fears and frustrations, women keep on living and try finding ways to cope. When stereotypes are broken, people are shocked, even those who are closest. Sham says that it is the point when one must start distancing one's self from life itself, because if this is not done, the fear of breaking boundaries consumes you: "I wonder, can you keep on living with that fear?"

In her exchanges with her doctor, one may find how important society makes it for women to get pregnant before they reach their forties. Likelihood of pregnancy decreases once a woman leaves the thirties. There is an alarm bell that has to be paid attention to:

> Doctor: Women of your age have a 70% chance of giving birth. Your chance is 40%. This means one thing. If you want to have a baby, you must hurry. … Seriously, you must hurry. Every passing month reduces your chances of being a mother.

Although Sham's is a love story, her desperation to give birth to a child under societal pressure is a much-remarked phenomenon. Affluent career-oriented urban women like Sham will relate to her drive to embark on crazy means to attain their goal of motherhood.

Wine Country (2019)

In this American comedy film, six middle-aged women – Abby, Rebecca, Naomi, Catherine, Val and Jenny – go on a weekend getaway to Napa Valley in California. They have been friends since they were all young waitresses in a pizzeria, and have come together to celebrate the fiftieth birthday of Rebecca. This movie addresses crucial symptoms of crisis in women during their middle years, and concludes on a cheerful note.

All of them have their own middle-age woes and problems, yet at the end they choose to reconcile with their present and live through what life throws at them. They are shown strengthening their bond with each other. Each of them has her own fears and frustrations, which are revealed in short episodes during the film. In the swimming pool, Naomi confesses to Jenny about her fear of death. She says that life has not been easy for her, as if the whole universe is making her realise that her idols are dying and she is getting older as well, destined to die too sooner or later. For her, dying is the worst nightmare: "If anything … happened to me … I just think about … I just think about my poor kids. Like, my babies. You know? Like … I know. No one's gonna love my babies like I do."

Since Abby planned the entire trip, she becomes overtly controlling. When Rebecca urges her to let go of control as "everything will fall into place" on its own, she cannot contain herself and retaliates, saying that for her nothing has fallen into place so far. As she grows older, will someone spare time to take care of her, or she will be left to survive on her own. So far, to her, everyone who has come into her life has been selfish. Her broken marriage was distressing, and added to that was her midlife crisis, where she found herself unable to cope with anything. Abby lashes back at Rebecca by inquiring about Rebecca's marriage and ageing body: "Maybe the therapist should go to therapy." Abby goes on venting about her negative impressions of life gathered so far. Her career has not been a respite either. She has lost her job, blabbers about random things, and feels stupid wailing about the loss of a job. Middle-aged women are torn between expressing emotions openly and staying poised in extreme agitation to safeguard their dignity:

> Shit, I mean, people are starving in the world and there's earthquakes, ... people are shooting at each other. I'm crying about my stupid poor job. ... Plus, what are we doing to the environment? ... There's no fish anymore! All the plastic is ... filling up in the ocean. ... There's like one rhinoceros left!

Abby has lost her job for not being comfortable with technology: "One time I can't figure out how to get on Snapchat. One time. And everybody saw." Anxiety and depression take hold over her conscious mind. The ever-evolving technological world add to the woes of midlifers who feel left out or lagging behind in the race. For their children or younger colleagues, they are identified as "boomers". For not being sufficiently up-to-date, their children or colleagues find them dispensable, and thus the crisis of incompetence deepens.

Midlifers evaluate their past and find their present agonising. Random bewildering thoughts hinder rational thinking. Rebecca is not happy in her marriage with Brian. Until an epiphany, she has been in denial that her husband is a "world-class ding-dong". Her friends know it well and already hate him. At night, she falls on the floor and cannot straighten her back. Naomi comes to wish her happy birthday and finds her there. In their exchanges, Rebecca narrates about her realisation of truth of life. She appears delirious. She says that she has been lying on the floor all night and has realised that Abby was right about her in saying that she needs a good look at the mirror or the door in this particular scenario. Rebecca hallucinates about a raccoon family. She looks into the eyes of a dead raccoon and discovers the truth about herself. She feels as she could connect with those raccoons more that anyone else during this weekend trip: "They helped me see what I really am. An old lady. ... Yes, it's true. I'm old, 50. That's half a fucking century." Naomi tries to bring Rebecca back to her senses by lecturing that they all getting older and their bodies are not working as before. Paying no heed to that, Rebecca goes on about her enlightenment that she must bring drastic changes, firstly by stopping lying to herself: "I'm ready to tell like it is. ... It's later than we think ...."

The realisation that fifty years is a long time and that the time left is too short to continue living inside a bubble is a common occurrence at this age. Women endure the taken-for-granted state of living for a considerable amount of time in their adult lives. They find comfort in this zone, feeling wanted, important or dependable. However, as midlife approaches, a sense of redundancy descends over them. Their feeling of self-worth starts dwindling. Making changes that bring uplift from perpetual anxiety becomes essential. Rebecca thus decides to shrug off her miserable present and embrace positivity.

Each of them has her own miseries. Val seeks love and pins her hopes on a young waitress and artist, Jade, and flirts with her. Jade, as revealed later, wants Val to support her monetarily, nudging Val to buy her artwork, sensing that Val has fallen for her. Jenny is a writer who has her own distresses. With advancing age come ailments. Symptoms of different kinds emerge to compromise overall wellbeing in an individual. Naomi is waiting for BRCA1 and BRCA2 test results and is too afraid to call her doctor, assuming that the diagnosis is cancer. Catherine keeps herself busy with work, and at one point feels left out. She feels her work is driving her away from her friends and they are excluding her from the itinerary. A drunk and distressed Abby gives in to the temptation of young Devon.

The scene in which all the women run down the hill one after the other is metaphorical. Each of these women eventually decides against discarding their garb of miseries and rolls into a new hope. They appear much happier standing there holding hands and rejoicing, encouraging each other to join in fast. Catherine is the last one to join them after an emotional speech at the top of the hill where no one can hear her and listening to her speech holds no significance for anyone else but her. It is a kind of monologue in which she pronounces her resolve to transform herself for good. She rejects a lucrative job offer to spend more time with her friends. It is important that women at midlife find each other's company in order to continue to feel wanted and important in some way to someone. Loneliness aggravates psychological restiveness, which in turn may exert a negative impact on a woman's physical health. Women are emotional beings who need constant support and encouragement to confront challenges. Naomi's test results come back negative. The film ends with them all sitting and drinking.

The Lost Daughter (2021)

A psychologically intense drama portraying how reminiscence about a failed motherhood renders middle-aged Leda entangled in her own inadequacies. Watching the exhaustion and unhappiness of a younger woman, Nina, in handling her small daughter Elena stirs up Leda's own memories of herself when bringing up Bianca and Martha, her own two daughters, was a daunting task. Leda as a young mother could not cope with the stress of dealing with the two constantly demanding small children and walked out on them, never seeing them for three years. She admits that going away from them was rather "amazing" for her, contrary to how society would see it. She never went back to them until she genuinely missed them. The film is genuine in depicting overwhelmed young mothers torn between their own selves and nagging young children, to the extent that absconding from such weariness seems most natural. Leda also indulged in an extramarital affair with a fellow professor. Her selfish and unnatural conduct as a mother afflicts her now at the age of 49: "I'm an unnatural mother," admits Leda to Nina. She warns Nina that her depression would not go in the way, she is looking for distractions. Leda finds the missing Elena and brings her back to the anxious Nina. However, she keeps Elena's doll, which is rather enigmatic. Leda starts obsessing over the doll and treats it as her companion. She hides it away inside a kitchen cabinet, takes out and wipes it clean, presses mud and worms from its insides, buys it new clothes and hugs it tight in sleep. The doll becomes objective-correlative for Leda's emotions about her own motherhood which she now regretfully misses.

Midlife is that plateau where the life's stillness becomes visible and pressingly realisable. In that silence, the tunes of the past start echoing hauntingly. The acquired wisdom enforces a self-assessment which deepens wounds by excavating all those choices that appeared rational during younger days. Leda sees her own reflection in Nina. Nina's desperation to break herself free from an overbearing family is relatable to Leda. Leda now has absolutely no power to erase the consequences of her selfishness which detached her from Bianca and Martha and estranged her husband, who had then pleaded to her to stay. A surging wave wakes an exhausted Leda, who then makes a phone call to Bianca. Both her daughters are together and sound cheerful on the phone and apparently were not distressed about not hearing from their mother for a long time. They casually tell Leda that they had assumed she was "dead".

The film does not have a happy ending and may not fill one with optimism. However, it is crucial that one confronts one's fears and regrets to learn from them and work through mistakes in order to alleviate their impacts. Women who can relate with Leda may realise that regretting the past is normal and most common. Seeing someone repenting may help them relieve themselves of their own deep-seated guilt.

Happiness for Beginners (2023)

Helen is a divorcee. She signs up for a hiking trip through which her goal is to hit the "reset" button of her life. Her checklist of expected outcomes for herself from the trip is interesting to note:

1. Find a deeper connection to nature.
2. Rise up from my own ashes like a freaking Phoenix.
3. Earn a damned certificate.

The choice of phrase, "rise up from my own ashes" indicates her latent wish to find a renewed purpose to life. In her forties, Helen realises that she is the oldest among the hiking group members. A day before the start of the trip, Helen introduces herself to the fellow hikers. Her agitated mind refers to her past as "rash". She describes the conflicts she had with her partner that led to divorce a year ago. Her husband's infidelity had long distanced them, but divorce made it official. The psychological impact of this broken marriage has lingered like a "rash", as she calls it. She wants to fix it because for her, one may not realise it, but it surely takes a toll somewhere, somehow. She wants a change in perspective through a literal change in territory. She had dreams about a happy family that turned into "shit" as a miscarriage happened not long before she separated from her husband: "And so I am here because I want to stop breaking promises to myself, and I want to start keeping them." She has made several promises to herself, and intends to keep them. This trip is the first of such promises.

During the course of their hike, Helen is often heard reiterating her purpose in taking the trip to others, probably reassuring herself in this way. She repeats her resolve to push her boundaries; transform her identity and modify her stereotypical image. She wants to relieve herself of the past's baggage. She took the trip because she wanted a new challenge, to defy her own limitations and kind of revive herself, which she calls a "reset". She wants to earn a certificate that will elevate her from being that old, lame teacher who is stuck in the mundanity of a fixed routine. To quote her: "This is the new and improved Helen. And this Helen spits in the face of danger and pees in the woods," and "Why did I come here? Um … You know I think I just sort of got sick of being fed up with myself." While talking to Hugh, Helen agrees that life's mistakes cannot be corrected, and since there is no going back now, it would be wise to admit them out loud.

Hugh: I could've been a lot of things in my life, you know. Somewhere along the way, I just took a wrong turn and can't find my way back. Now I realise it's probably too late. It's okay. I've come to terms with it, and it feels good to say it loud.
Helen: Well, I know how that feels.

At the end of the trip, Helen emerges as a new person who knows herself better and feels different: "I knew! I knew! Something had changed." The anger and guilt which she has always carried since her childhood has now left her. She is willing to start over afresh.

In her middle years, Helen's realisation that she needs to reset her life is crucial. Her decision to experience hiking is her way of exploring new trails to look forward to. Tendencies to uplift themselves from mundanity and search for new purposes to cope with life's agonies are often found in midlifers, and the idea has been made into several films about midlife crisis in women. The key is that the women protagonists should find solace in travel and feel liberated from their pasts so that it kindles hope in the audience.

Faraway (2023)

The opening of the movie shows a middle-aged Zeynep looking far away with a smile. Thereafter, it is about how Zeynep found that happiness and embraces it. The movie thus promises yet another journey undertaken toward the discovery of a happy self. Zeynep seems irritated as she juggles a chaotic household and job. Neither her husband nor her daughter are of any help. She has just lost her mother and has to deal with the tantrums of an ageing father. All she expects from her family is to be together in mourning. Her husband is attracted toward his much younger female colleague. For her teenage daughter, Zeynep is embarrassing. Zeynep's efforts in managing a muddled household stay unnoticed and unappreciated. Overwhelmed, she suffers a mental breakdown. The husband blames Zeynep for his infidelity, and the daughter is disrespectful toward her.

It is from this tipping point where Zenep's narrative starts taking a rather eventful turn. Impulsively, she decides to drive away to Croatia. She does not think any further than that. She wants to get away from her demanding father, insensitive husband and insolent daughter. She longs for solitude. She seeks purpose in living life and hopes her mother's property will provide her with it.

The movie from this point onward takes a somewhat lighthearted, romantic-comedic turn. She meets a man who lives in her mother's property. This man, Josip, is unwilling to part with the property, being moored to the place since his childhood. Several events roll by, and eventually Zeynep is seen to have fallen deeply in love with Josip. She has finally found a partner who understands and respects her. She now has a purpose in life, too. When her daughter, husband and father come to Croatia to take her back, she emerges to them as a more composed and confident woman who is capable of surviving on her own. Zeynep has now found a right path which she feels has been paved for her by her mother. In her walk toward self-discovery, her mother's diary is her beacon. With the discovery of her true self comes emancipation from a past in disarray. The toxicity of her past is now behind her. She hugs her daughter and assures her that she understands her confusion and shock. She makes peace with her husband, too, who finding her transformed self, decides to part with her. The last scene of the film is a typical rom-com ending.

Faraway is another film which reiterates the importance of taking a journey toward self-discovery – a journey that not only helps Zeynep in getting away from her chaotic present, but also potentially lifts her from the abyss into which she is gradually descending. However, life is not always a romantic-comedy like Zeynep's story, and one may not find a new partner like Josip, or a new purpose as she had ultimately, yet one must strive hard to look for new paths to choose from because it is essential for a woman in midlife to deliberately uplift herself, lest the chaos may consume her completely.

Conclusion

The age range of 40 to 65 is the most challenging stage in women's lives. The plots of the films discussed here address almost all the major setbacks middle-aged women usually confront. However, the degrees of their suffering and consequent treatment vary across social groups. Crises in women owing to bodily changes, altered familial situations, professional stagnancy, stalled personal growth and, above all, fear of death give rise to a strong urge to escape. Journeying toward a new destination to overcome the past's woes, finding a new partner, discovering an unknown facet about oneself or identifying a new purpose to look forward to are some of the messages which these films promote. Watching characters grappling with similar circumstances, feeling overwhelmed or suffocated, and then embarking on a mission or act to rise above their depressive state imparts a perspective, a palpable solution. If films do not suggest a way, they certainly help women discern that what they are undergoing is a crisis and they are by no means alone in it.

Works Cited

Aldwin, C. (n.d.). Stress, coping, and health at mid-life: A developmental perspective. In M. E. Lachman (Ed.), *The handbook of midlife development* (pp. 2–38). Wiley.

Brie Turns, P. M. (2016, January 14). Cinema narrative therapy: Utilizing family films to externalize children's 'problems'. *Journal of Family Therapy, 37*(4), 590–606. https://doi.org/10.1111/1467-6427.12098

Clausen, J. (1990). My interesting condition. Journal of Sex Research, 27(3), 445-459.

Crow, M. L. (1987). Midlife crisis: A growth opportunity for women educators. *The Clearing House, 60*(9), 413–415. Retrieved December 31, 2023, from http://www.jstor.org/stable/30180988

Diah, N. M. (2018). *Physical changes as part of midlife crisis: The case of urban Malay women. Malaysian Journal of Social Sciences, 3*(1). https://unimel.edu.my/journal/index.php/JSS/issue/view/57

Kuriansky, J. (2009). Introduction to this Special Issue. Counselling Psychology Quarterly, 22(1), 1-2.

Lee, S.-Y. (2014, February 28). Effects of the degree of preparation for later life and mid-life crisis on the marital satisfaction of married, middle-aged women. *Journal of Family Resource Management and Policy Review, 18*(1), 29–46. Retrieved December 31, 2023, from https://koreascience.kr/article/JAKO201410438897197.page

Li Ping Wong, H. A. (2012). Midlife crisis perceptions, experiences, help-seeking, and needs among multi-ethnic Malaysian women. *Women & Health, 52*(8), 804–819. https://doi.org/10.1080/03630242.2012.729557

Lieblich, A. (1986). Successful career women at midlife: Crises and transitions. *The International Journal of Aging and Human Development, 23*(4), 301–312. https://doi.org/10.2190/P5T6-BHVP-GK6B-T69L

Linda Berg-Cross, P. J. (1990). Cinematherapy: Theory and āpplication. *Psychotherapy in Private Practice, 8*(1), 135–156. https://doi.org/10.1300/J294v08n01_15

McQuaide, S. (1998, January). Women at midlife. *Social Work, 43*(1), 21–31.
Mihailova Lilia, R. S. (2022, August 1). Factors determining the choice of the inertia-development alternative by women during the midlife crisis. In *The contemporary issues of the socio-humanistic sciences* (pp. 92–108). Retrieved December 31, 2023, from https://ibn.idsi.md/vizualizare_articol/162123
Moen, P., & Wethington, E. (1999). Midlife development in a life course context. In Life in the middle (pp. 3-23). Academic Press.
Niemiec, R. M. (2020, August). Character strengths cinematherapy: Using movies to inspire change, meaning, and cinematic elevation. *Journal of Clinical Psychology, 76*(8), 1447–1462. https://doi.org/10.1002/jclp.22997
Orchowski, L. M. (2006). Cinema and the valuing of psychotherapy: Implications for clinical practice. *Professional Psychology: Research and Practice, 37*(5), 506–514. https://doi.org/10.1037/0735-7028.37.5.506
Sacilotto, E. (2023). Convergence between Cinematherapy and neuropsychology: exploring the use of art as a cognitive and emotional therapeutic tool
Schmidt, S. (2018). The feminist origins of the midlife crisis. *The Historical Journal, 61*(2), 503–523. https://doi.org/10.1017/S0018246X17000309

Index

β-amyloid plaques 45–46

abuse 35, 51, 112, 124, *147*–148, 155, 158, 239
accommodative changes 101
active ageing 34, 36
adjustment 4, 9, 10, 72, 101, 112, 121, 156, 205
aging 20–21, 24, 26–27, 31, 33, 36, 47, 76
ageing parents 10, 39, 71, 99, 100, 106, 124, 125, 128, 142, 216
Ainsworth, M. 70, 84
alcoholism 59, 112, 155, 184
aliveness 111
altruism 86, 113
Alzheimer's disease 44–46, 53–54, 132
andropause 122–123
anthropomorphization 86
anxiety 14, 21, 38, 58, 69, 71–73, 79, 85, 104–105, 125, 129–131, 133, 144–146, 148–149, 153–156, 158, 159, 182, 199, 205, 238, 243–244
anxious 70–71, 85, 200, 205, 245
apolipoprotein E type 4 53, 59
assimilative changes 101
assisted reproduction 102
attachment 5, 10, 69–77, 80, 84–86, 91, 172, 217–218, 235
authenticity 110, 234
autonomy 14, 21, 76, 78, 85, 172, 217–218, 224, 227, 234–235
avoidant 70–72, 85

baby boomers 5, 98, 125
Baltes, M. M. 15, 182
Baltes, P. B. 4, 7, 15, 52, 121, 182, 183
Bartholomew, K. 72
beliefs 17, 23, 56, 72, 74, 79, 87, 110, 133, 169, 205, 207–209, 218, 229, 232
bereavement 69, 77, 105, 112
Bhagvad Gita 24
bilateral 47
biological clock 23, 59
body image 32, 35, 38–39, 216–217
bottom-up 182, 185
Bowlby, John 70, 73, 84
brain injury 60
Buhler, Charlotte 15
bulldozer parenting 102
burden 25, 100, 104, 112, 128–129, 134, 147, 157, 159, 175, 204, 206
burnout 85

Cameron, P. 9
career 3, 9, 12, 15, 26, 39, 48, 69, 84, 88–90, 111, 125–126, 130, 201–203, 205, 238, 241–243
caregiver 69–70, 76–77, 84, 97, 103, 106, 113, 124, 125, 128, 130, 185
challenges 3, 9–11, 40, 58, 69, 76–79, 89, 112, 121–134, 142, 149, 151, 154, 159, 187, 192, 201, 216–218, 232–234, 236–237, 244
childlessness 125–126
child with special health needs 103
cholesterol 55
chronic health conditions 123, 180
chronic physical ailments 184
cinematherapy 238–248
claustrophobic 224
cognitive decline 44–45, 47–48, 51, 53, 56, 60, 61, 79, 101, 132, 154
cognitive function 44, 46–48, 52, 55, 59–60, 114, 128, 130, 132
cohort-centrism 32
commitment 6, 12, 75, 77, 86–87, 91, 110, 123–124, 169, 181
community 26, 36, 83, 104, 115, 128, 132–134, 151, 153, 157, 159, 168–170, 172–174, 181, 184–186,

187–191, 192, 219, 221, 229–230; intervention 180–181, 184–185
community-based participatory research (CBPR) 184, **191**–193
compassion 75, 106, 113
connectedness 5, 104, 111, 114, 174
contract 87, 155, 242
co-residency 98
coronaphobia 144
cortex 45–47, 55
couple parenting 99, 104
COVID-19 131–132, 142–160, 173
covidence 186
crisis 6, 14, 20–22, 25, 28, 31–32, 70, 75–80, 99, 103, 112, 121, 125, 130, 142, 154, 156, 160, 170, 181, 183, 199–211, 214, 216, 223–227, 238–243, 246, 248
crystallized intelligence 51

death 21, 24, 26, 31, 78, 111, 132, 144–145, 150, 181, 183, 199–200, 202–205, 210, 238, 240–242, 248
defence 24, 72
dementia 44, 46, 52, 54, 59–60, 79, 100, 125, 132, 190, 225, 226
demography 99
depression 55, 59–60, 69, 77–80, 101, 112–114, 121, 123–124, 127, 129–133, 147–149, 154–156, 159, 182, 243, 245
despair 168, 183, 201, 210
de St. Aubin, E. 6, 12, 126, 181
diabetes mellitus 54
diet 57, 100, 129, 131, 152
discrimination 37, 105, 132, 146–*147*, 157, 159, 169–170, 173, 175, 220
disorganized 71
dissatisfaction 38, 71, 78–79, 200
divorces 124
domestic violence 158
downward spirals 183
Drevenstedt, J. 9

education 33, 39, 54, 56, 88, 98, 102, 114, 122, 127, 133, 152, 173, 182, 183, 192, 219, 221, 230, 231, 235
ego strength 235
embodiment 25, 214, 221
emotional intimacy 73–74
emotional processing 51
emotional regulation 48, 58, 84, 183
emotion regulation 101, 181
employment 17, 40, 83, 89, 90, 99, 114, 129–130, 143, 145, *147*, 156, 157, 167, 173, 182, 192; unemployment 69, 130, 159
empty-nest 6, 69, 76–77, 79, 121–122, 216
engagement 55–56, 71, 83, 89, 103, 111, 127–128, 131, 134, 174, 185, **188**, **190**, 201, 225–227
epidemiology 99
episodic memory 46, 50, 54–57, 133
Erikson, E. H. 5–6, 12, 24, 83, 99, 106, 125, 142, 181, 227, 229
established adulthood 3
executive functioning 49, 57
exercise 48, 57, 110, 120, 152, 170, **187**, **189**

family 3, 5, 10–11, 21, 38–39, 69–70, 74–76, 83, 88, 90, 98–100, 102–104, 106, 112, 113, 122, 124–125, 128–129, 131–134, 143, 145, 147, 150, 151, 154, 156–158, 168, 171–175, 183, 184, 202, 203, 205, 208, 219–222, 235, 238, 240, 243, 245–247
fears 200–201, 240, 242, 245
feminist 21, 36, 169, 218
financial minorities 100
Freud, S. 10, 25, 27, 84
friendship 74–75, 154, 221, 223, 224, 227, 233
Fromm, E. 110
frontline workers 144

Gandhi, M. K. 24–25, 27–29
gender 5, 20–21, 25, 32, 35–38, 54, 70, 78, 88–91, 103, 106, 132, 145, 158, 170, 171, 174–176, 182, 192, 215–222, 225, 230, 231; based violence 158; crossover 217; culture bias 106; fluidity 5
generation Alpha 5
generation X 5, 98
generation Z 5
generativity 5–6, 12, 21, 99, 113, 125–126, 133,.142, 181, 201, 211, 224, 229, 233, 235–237
genes 7, 53
Glass ceiling effect 89
glucose tolerance 54
grandparenting 127, 128, 133, 142
gray divorces 130
gray matter 48, 60, 64

Greatest Generation 4
guilt 14, 104, 201, 233, 245–246

happiness 69, 77, 181, 182, 204, 232–233, 235, 245, 247
Havighurst, R. J. 4, 14–15
Hazan, C. 84–85
healthcare providers 148, 159
hedonic set-point 69
helicopter 102, 127
helicopter parenting 102
herd behaviour 144
heteronormative 104, 175
Horowitz, L. M. 72
hypertension 54, 150, 183

identity 5, 12, 33, 35–36, 38, 83, 86, 91, 101, 105, 111, 132, 142, 153, 168–176, 201, 205, 216–217, 219, 222, 225, 231–233, 235, 236, 246
illness anxiety 155
implicit memory 50
industrialisation 33
inferior quality of life 106
information and communication technology 143
integrity 45, 111, 113
intellectual intimacy 74
intergenerational ambivalence 76, 78, 98, 102, 110
intergenerational solidarity 76
intergenerational ties 103
internal working models 73
interspecies family 104
intervention 44, 102, 121, 134, 160, 181, 183–185, *186*, **187–191**, 192, 214, 216, 239
intimacy 5, 12, 69–75, 80, 127, 154

James, William 110
job satisfaction 84–85, 91
Jung, C. G. 9, 11, 14, 111, 142, 181, 199, 217, 229

Kakar, S. 23, 26, 106, 217
Katz, D. 86
Kay Heath 24, 202
Keder 9

labour market volatility 130
Lachman, M. E. 3, 5, 11, 13, 31, 39, 51–52, 56, 83, 101, 121–122, 133, 181–183, 248
leader-follower relationships 84
Lefebvrean paradigm 215
Levinson, Daniel 13, 14, 99, 113, 207, 209
LGBTQ 99, 104, 132–134, 182, 184
LGBTQ+ couple parenting 104
life satisfaction 5, 58, 100, 106, 129, 131, 174, 182
lifestyle 21, 36, 53, 55, 61, 99–102, 121, 128–129, 131, *147*, 150–152, 183, 192, 199, 229, 233; factors 53, 55, 129
Linton, R. 34
lockdown 143–144, 146, 148–154, 157, 158
loneliness 59–61, 77, 79–80, 121, 124, 129–130, 154–155, 157, 168, 172, 203–204, 208, 244
loss 10–11, 15, 21, 26, 45, 48–52, 54, 60, 69–71, 76–78, 87, 112, 130, 143, 146–149, 153, 155, 157–159, 170, 173, 174, 181, 182, 184, **187**, 205, 209, 225, 227, 243
love 25, 69, 75, 77, 104, 124, 175, 202–207, 209–210, 221, 225–227, 231, 233, 236, 240–242, 247

Mahler, M. S. 10–11
marginalized 146–147, 159, 169–176
marital 5, 11, 39, 69, 75–79, 103, 113, 121, 123–125, 182, 192, 203, 210, 223, 224, 231, 235, 239, 245
masculine 11, 89, 181, 217, 238
maslow 142
maturation 15, 47, 71, 111, 236
McAdams, D.P. 6, 131, 132, 190
menopause 25, 36–37, 58, 106, 113–114, 123, 154, 216–217
mental health 48, 55, 58–59, 69, 73, 100–101, 103–105, 112–115, 123, 125, 129–132, 144, 146–149, 154, 156–160, 175, 182–183, 185, 192, 210
midlife crisis 20–22, 25, 31–32, 70, 75–80, 99, 121, 142, 181, 199–211, 216, 239, 242, 243, 246
midlife parenthood 97, 99, 103, 106
midlifer 4, 10, 13–17, 44, 48, 52, 55–60, 115, 175, 199–201, 204, 207, 209–210, 216, 224, 226, 234–237, 243, 246
MIDMAC 99
MIDUS 48
migrants 146–147, 169, 171, 173–175

mild cognitive impairment 44, 46, 54, 59
millennials 5, 98
minor children 100
modernisation 33
mood disorders 123, 154
multimorbidity 106
mystic writing pad 27–28

Neugarten, B. L. 4, 13, 39
neural activity 47, 54
neuroimaging 47
neuroplasticity 23, 44
new normal 144, 146, 152, 172
non-communicable diseases 159, 183
non-human children 104
non-human parenting 99
non-normative parenthood 102–105
normative parenthood 101–102
nutrition 129, *147,* 148–147, 149, 223

obesity 53–55, 58, 100, 123, 132, 150, 159, 183–184
obsessive compulsive disorder (OCD) 155
opportunities 3, 6, 36–37, 89–90, 111–112, 121–124, 127–128, 133, 145–146, 153–154, 160, 167–168, 192, 217–218, 229
optimism 80, 90, 201, 210, 221, 224, 238, 245
organizational citizenship 86

pain 10, 23, 36, 57, 79, 126, 143, 148, 155, 175, 192, 203, 205, 225–226, 239
pandemic 131–132, 142–143, 145–146, 148–156, 158–160
parental role perspective 97
parental roles 98, 105
parenthood 5, 39, 97–99, 101–106, 124–126
parenting practices 98
participatory action research (PAR) 185
partition of Bengal 230
patriarchal 21, 88, 176, 218, 222, 231
peace 9, 111, 206, 239, 241, 247
Peck, Robert 12
people living with HIV (PLWH) 147–148
personalised plasticity 7
phenomenological 25, 27–28
physical activity 57, 131, 150, 152, **188–189**
physical intimacy 74
physiological change 15, 122–123
positive plasticity 6–7, 115
post-modern 26–27, 98–99, 103, 105, 167–168
postponement of parenthood 102–103
post-traumatic stress disorder 154, 159
PRISMA *186*
problem solving 51–52, 220
processing speed 48–49, 52, 54, 57, 60
protective factor 48, 103, 184
proxy father-figures 84
psychiatric illness **147**, 154–157
psychobiograph 21, 25

quality of life 34, 36, 73, 103, 106, 113, 128, 154
quarantine 143, 146, 150, 155, 156, 159

reasoning 47, 51, 55–56, 58, 112, 220
religious orientation 110, 115
remarriage 103, 231
re-partnering 124
representation 3, 5, 32, 36, 73, 158, 168–169, 173, 199, 201, 207, 214–216, 219–223, 225–227
resilience 40, 78, 115, 126, 134, 152–154, 169–170, 172, 226–227, 233
Ribot's law 47
Riley, M. W. 31–32, 34
Rogers 142
roles 5, 9–10, 13–14, 21, 26, 32, 35, 39, 78, 84, 88, 90–91, 97–98, 100–101, 105–106, 112–113, 121, 125, 128–130, 151, 174, 181, 204, 211, 217–218, 220–222, 225, 230–232, 238
romantic 5, 73–74, 80, 84, 124, 154, 207–208, 221, 234, 240–241, 247

sandwich generation 6
sculpted creativity 216
secure 70–74, 84–85
Selective optimization 15, 181
self 4–6, 10, 12, 14–17, 22, 23, 28, 39, 78, 101, 103, 106, 111–115, 134, 167, 199, 207, 208, 211, 226, 239, 241, 242, 247
selfhood 101, 169, 226–227
serenity 111
sexism 222
sex-role orientation 217
Shanan, J. 9
Shaver, P. R. 84

shrinking safety net 99
silent generation 5, 98–99
single parenthood 103, 124
single parenting 99
sleep 57–59, 61, 100, 123, 125, 129, 151, 159, 184, 205–206, 245
sleep wake schedule 151
smoking 59
social clocks 4, 13
social engagement 56, 185
social isolation 59–60, 129, 132, 152, 155, 156, 172
socializing 75, 150, 153
social media 36–38, 40, 128–129, 131, 144, 157–159, 208
social safety net 145
social support 79, 103–104, 128–129, *147*, 152–155, 158, 160, 171, 174–175
socioeconomic status 40, 56, 130, 133, 153, 156, 173, 175
Socioemotional selectivity theory (SST) 105–106, 182
socio-relational evolution 97
spatial processing 50
spiritual intimacy 74
spirituality 110–115
STAC hypothesis 47
stagnation 12, 99, 142, 155, 181, 229
step-parenthood 99, 103
stereotypes in job 89
stigma 35–36, 78, 146, 148, 159, 160, 169, 174–176
Strengths and Vulnerability Integration Model 105
stress 14, 22, 26, 56–58, 61, 69, 71, 73, 76–77, 79, 80, 85, 97, 101–103, 123, 126–127, 130, 144, 147–149, 151–152, 154, 156, 159, 183, 185, **190**, **191**, 244
suicide 78, 146, 156–157, 175, 183
systematic review 185–186, **187**, 192

Tagore, R. N. 23, 25, 27, 28, 229–237
tau neurofibrillary tangles 46
tiger moms 127
tiger parenting 102
top-down 181, 185
trauma 24, 26–27, 70, 112, 132, 144, 151–152, 154, 159

urbanisation 33

Valliant, George 12
value 5, 7, 9, 12, 14, 17, 23–24, 26, 70, 74, 83, 86, 89–91, 101, 105–106, 111, 129, 133, 146, 168, 169, 185, 217, 221–223, 230–231, 234
vascular health 50, 53–54
violence 24, 29, 155, 157, 158, 176, 201

well-being 4–7, 12, 15, 33, 36, 72–79, 86, 89, 99–106, 115, 123, 125, 126, 128–134, 142, 151, 169, 171, 172, 174–176, 180–183, 185, 192, 217, 219, 229, 231, 236, 239, 244
white matter 45, 53
wholeness 110–111, 229
widowhood 124
wisdom 16, 26, 101, 183, 201, 236, 245
work centrality 86–87
work-family balance 128–129
work from home 150
working memory 47, 49–50, 52, 56

xenophobia 144

FSC
www.fsc.org
MIX
Papier | Fördert gute Waldnutzung
FSC® C083411

Kolibri 360 GmbH
Ferdinand-Jühlke-Straße 7
99095 Erfurt, Deutschland
produktsicherheit@kolibri360.de